Case Studies in Oral and Maxillofacial Surgery

Case Studies in Oral and Maxillofacial Surgery

Editor: Raphael Atkinson

AMERICAN
MEDICAL PUBLISHERS
www.americanmedicalpublishers.com

AMERICAN
MEDICAL PUBLISHERS
www.americanmedicalpublishers.com

Cataloging-in-Publication Data

Case studies in oral and maxillofacial surgery / edited by Raphael Atkinson.
p. cm.
Includes bibliographical references and index.
ISBN 979-8-88740-611-4
1. Face--Surgery. 2. Mouth--Surgery. 3. Maxilla--Surgery. I. Atkinson, Raphael.
RD523 .O73 2023
617.520 59--dc23

American Medical Publishers,
41 Flatbush Avenue,
1st Floor, New York,
NY 11217, USA

ISBN 979-8-88740-611-4 (Hardback)

Contents

Preface

Oral and maxillofacial surgery is a specialized branch of dentistry that focuses on the diagnosis and surgical treatment of various medical conditions which affect the face, jaws, mouth and associated structures. There are a wide variety of medical procedures which are undertaken within this field such as dental extractions, dental implant placement, corrective jaw surgery, facial trauma reconstruction, treatment of facial infections, removal of tumors or cysts in the jaw or facial area, management of temporomandibular joint (TMJ) disorders, and treatment of congenital facial deformities. Oral and maxillofacial surgery makes use of various diagnostic tools such as X-rays, CT scans, and 3D imaging to examine the condition and anatomy of the oral and facial structures. These help in planning and executing surgical procedures with precision and accuracy. This book provides comprehensive insights into the field of oral and maxillofacial surgery. It will serve as a valuable source of reference for graduate and postgraduate students.

The information contained in this book is the result of intensive hard work done by researchers in this field. All due efforts have been made to make this book serve as a complete guiding source for students and researchers. The topics in this book have been comprehensively explained to help readers understand the growing trends in the field.

I would like to thank the entire group of writers who made sincere efforts in this book and my family who supported me in my efforts of working on this book. I take this opportunity to thank all those who have been a guiding force throughout my life.

Editor

1

Long-Term Outcomes of Nonextraction Treatment in a Patient with Severe Mandibular Crowding

Vincenzo Grassia,[1] Ludovica Nucci,[1] Paola Martina Marra,[1] Gaetano Isola,[2] Angelo Itro,[3] and Letizia Perillo[1]

[1]Multidisciplinary Department of Medical-Surgical and Dental Specialties, University of Campania Luigi Vanvitelli, Naples, Italy
[2]Department of General Surgery and Surgical-Medical Specialties, School of Dentistry, University of Catania, Italy
[3]Complex Operative Unit of Stomatological Surgery in Developmental Age, University of Campania Luigi Vanvitelli, Naples, Italy

Correspondence should be addressed to Paola Martina Marra; pablati3@hotmail.it

Academic Editor: Khalid H. Zawawi

Objective. To describe a clinical case with a severe mandibular crowding treated without extraction and showing a long-term outcome. *Methods.* A 14-year-old boy in permanent dentition showed a class I molar and cuspid relationship, a severe deep bite of 8 mm, a constricted V-shaped upper arch with moderate crowding, and a severe crowding of about 12 mm in the lower arch. The panoramic X-ray showed an impacted upper right canine. The treatment started with the placement of a transpalatal bar and 0.022×0.028 in standard edgewise appliances in the upper arch and a lip bumper bonded on the second lower molars. Initial leveling of the teeth was accomplished with light Australian round wires. Finishing was then performed with rectangular wires. The phase with fixed appliances lasted 2 years and 9 months, and the patient was motivated and cooperative throughout the treatment, although with poor oral hygiene. The patient was treated without extractions. *Results.* The space was gained with the first and second upper molar derotations using the transpalatal bar and the gingival lip bumper in the lower arch. The upper right canine was well positioned, and the maxillary arch form was improved. The severe lower crowding was completely corrected, and a good overbite was achieved. *Conclusion.* A conservative, nonextraction treatment approach for this patient with class I malocclusion with severe mandibular crowding was effective, and the results have remained stable after a long-term follow-up (10 years).

1. Introduction

Mandibular anterior crowding represents one of the most frequent features of a malocclusion [1], and it is a critical issue due to its impact on treatment approach, prognosis, and long-term stability [2, 3].

Moreover, mandibular anterior crowding is the most common patient chief complaint.

It can be characterized by a discrepancy between the mesiodistal tooth widths of four permanent incisors and the available space in the alveolar process, although other variables such as the direction of mandibular growth, early loss of deciduous molars, incisor and molar inclinations, or perioral and oral musculature effect can occur [4].

The amount of crowding is the most important factor when deciding between extraction and nonextraction treatment [5], so the debate on which strategy can give better long-term results is still open [6]. Moreover, in the effort to identify an orthodontically ideal, long-lasting, and balanced position of the mandibular incisors, the anterior limit of the teeth [7] should always be considered.

For example, anatomic factors such as the mandibular symphysis and the labiolingual alveolar process thickness have to be evaluated [8].

Thus, in cases with narrow and high symphysis extensive orthodontic tooth movements with fixed appliances should be limited to avoid the risk of progressive bone loss of lingual and labial cortical plates [9].

Therefore, the choice of the treatment plan is greatly influenced by the morphology of the symphysis and the position of the mandibular incisors too [5–7].

Furthermore, other factors such as aesthetic features and the type of periodontium can affect the choice.

Thus, the resolution of crowding can require interproximal tooth reduction (IPR), extraction, or space gaining with increase of arch perimeter and widths and, if needed, incisor proclination [10].

One available appliance used to gain space in the mandibular arch is the lip bumper [5, 11].

The primary purpose of this appliance is to reduce dental arch crowding through an increase in arch width and length by modifying the equilibrium between the lips, cheeks, and tongue [5, 11–15, 21].

According to Buschang [14], lip bumper therapy, performed during the mixed dentition, produced useful treatment changes, with limited amounts of relapse and lasting long-term effects, which may be due to growth potential [16].

Several short-term papers confirmed this opinion along with only two long-term researches [16–18] and one clinical case [18].

However, the two systematic reviews, published later and reporting significant increase in intercanine, interpremolar, and intermolar widths, arch perimeter, and arch length concluded that the long-term effects of the lip bumper still need to be elucidated [19, 20].

Thus, it is useful for the clinician to know the long-term effects of the different treatment options offered to the patient in order to achieve the more stable result when retention is discontinued.

Many theories have been proposed although the cause of relapse is still uncertain.

According to some researches [21], final proclination and position of the mandibular incisors seem to be one of the important factors affecting stability.

On the other hand, other authors reported that the final mandibular incisor inclination and linear protrusion do not influence crowding relapse [22, 23].

In the recent years, instead, Raucci et al. showed both short- and long-term mandibular arch changes in patients treated with lip bumper followed by full fixed appliances [5]. After lip bumper treatment, they observed a significant increase in dental arch widths and perimeter along with a significant reduction in crowding and no change in arch length and incisor inclination. An average crowding of 5.39 mm was corrected with a small amount of relapse, 0.36 mm, at the follow-up lasting 6.3 years on average [5].

This clinical report shows a case with a severe mandibular crowding (12 mm) treated with a nonextraction treatment, using lip bumper followed by fixed appliance in a permanent dentition patient with a long-term outcome (10-year follow-up).

2. Materials and Methods

The patient was a 14-year-old boy in permanent dentition with a chief complaint of "crooked teeth." The extraoral examination showed a narrow smile with dark corners, a very flat and retrusive profile, with retruded upper and lower lips and an increased nasolabial angle. The occlusion showed a class I molar and cuspid relationship on the left side and a class I molar on the right one where the cuspid was impacted. A severe deep bite of 8 mm and an overjet of about 2 mm were observed.

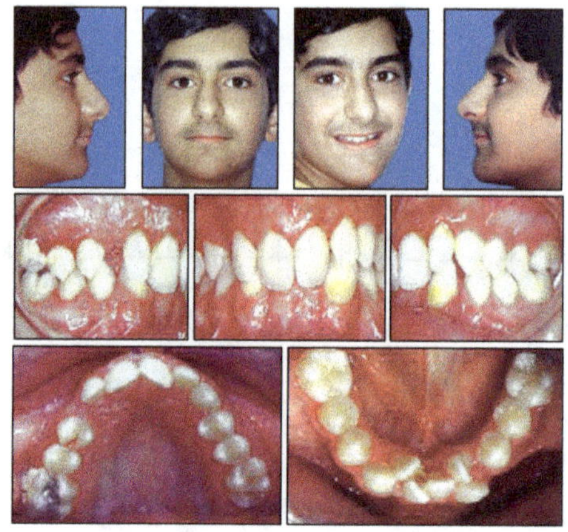

Figure 1: Pretreatment facial and intraoral photographs.

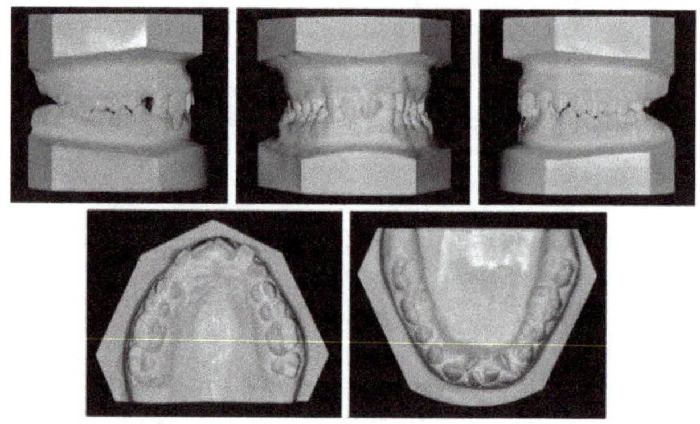

Figure 2: Pretreatment dental casts.

The upper arch was V-shaped with a moderate crowding, whereas a severe crowding of about 12 mm was present in the lower arch. A deep curve of Spee and lack of space for third molars were also noted (Figures 1 and 2).

The lateral cephalometric evaluation revealed a class I malocclusion (ANB, 2°) with a mesiofacial pattern (SnGoGn, 32°) and retroclined upper (1/SN, 83°) and lower incisors (IMPA, 85°) (Table 1).

Bolton analysis showed an overall ratio of 93% with lower anterior excess of 1.6 mm and an anterior ratio of 79% with a lower anterior excess of 1.2 mm.

The panoramic X-ray showed an impacted upper right canine and the presence of upper and lower third molar buds.

The impacted canine presented an angulation of 33° with respect to the midline; it was classified in the sector II according to Lindauer and sector IV according to Ericson and Kurol analysis [26, 27]. The distance between the canine cuspid and the occlusal plane was 12 mm.

All the measurements were hand traced under natural light, using 0.5 mm lead on 0.003 mm matte acetate tracing paper.

TABLE 1: Cephalometric measurement pre- and posttreatment.

	Pretreatment	Posttreatment	Mean SD
Sagittal skeletal relations			
Maxillary position S-N-A	76°	76.5°	82° ± 3.5°
Mandibular position S-N-B	74°	75.5°	80° ± 3.5°
Sagittal jaw relation A-N-Pg	2°	1°	2° ± 2.5°
Vertical skeletal relations			
Maxillary inclination S-N/ANS-PNS	11°	11°	8° ± 3.0°
Mandibular inclination S-N/Go-Gn	32°	32°	33° ± 2.5°
Vertical jaw relation ANS-PNS/Go-Gn	21°	21°	25° ± 6.0°
Dentobasal relations			
Maxillary incisor inclination 1-SN	83°	103°	110° ± 6.0°
Mandibular incisor inclination IMPA	85°	100°	94° ± 7.0°
Mandibular incisor compensation 1-A-Pg (mm)	-1.8 mm	1.0 mm	2 ± 2.0
Dental relations			
Overjet (mm)	2 mm	2.5 mm	3.5 ± 2.5
Overbite (mm)	8 mm	2.5 mm	2 ± 2.5
Interincisal angle 1/1	110.0°	127.0°	132° ± 6.0°

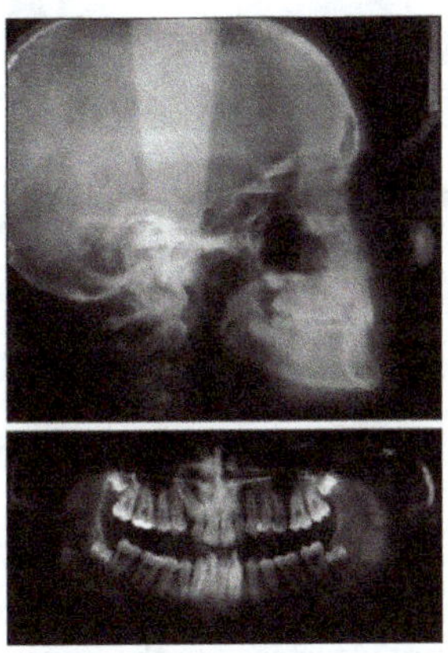

FIGURE 3: Pretreatment lateral cephalometric and panoramic X-rays.

No root resorption and bone loss were detected whereas the upper incisors showed slightly anomalous roots (Figure 3). The patient's medical and dental histories were unremarkable.

No previous orthodontic treatment was performed, and no signs or symptoms of temporomandibular joint disorder during mandibular movement were reported.

The oral hygiene was very poor with gingival inflammation in the upper and lower anterior and posterior areas. The patient's medical and dental histories were unremarkable.

The treatment objectives for this patient were to gain the space needed to guide the impacted upper right canine into the arch and to solve the crowding, to reduce the increased overbite correcting the incisor inclination, and to improve the arch forms, the smile, and the profile.

Before starting and after obtaining the informed consent from the patient's parents, we considered the following treatment options:

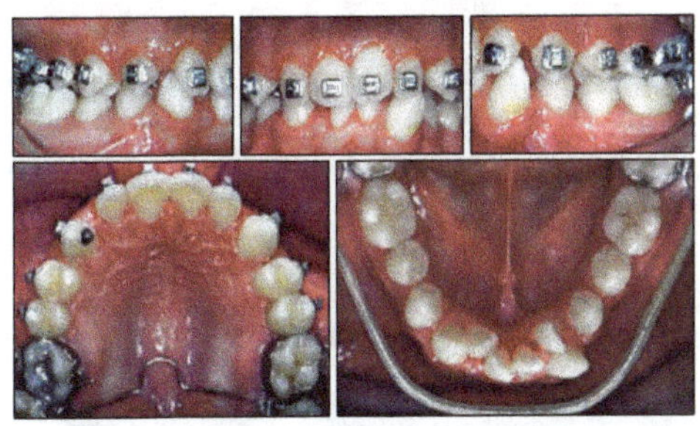

FIGURE 4: Transpalatal bar in the upper arch and lip bumper in the lower arch.

(1) Treatment with extractions of the upper and lower first premolars

(2) Treatment with extraction of a mandibular incisor, along with anterior stripping or incisor proclination, although this would create a tooth-size discrepancy of the anterior occlusion that would make correction of the overbite more difficult

(3) Treatment without extractions in which in this option the space can be gained with the first and second upper molar derotations using a transpalatal bar in the upper arch and a gingival lip bumper in the lower arch positioned on the second molars. In addition, space can be gathered through the correction of the upper and lower incisor inclination with a favorable effect on smile and profile. Correct biomechanics to achieve the right torque of the lower incisors was needed

(4) No treatment if not accepted by the patient's parents

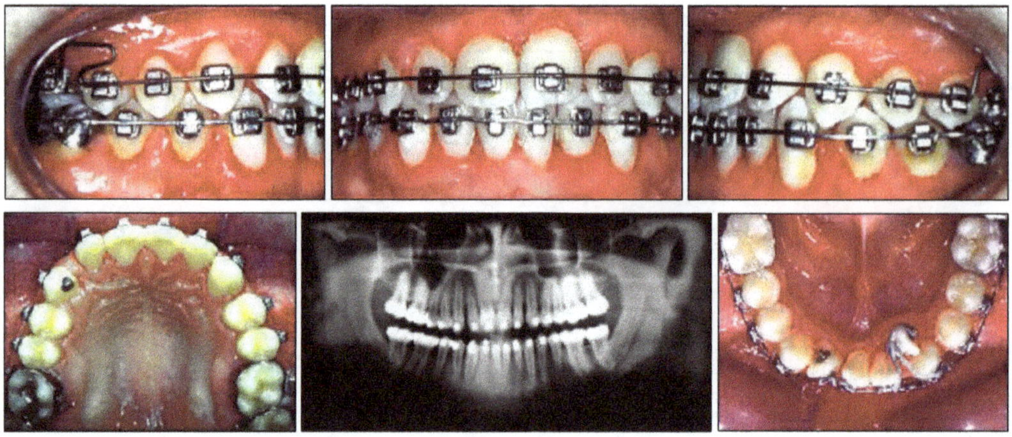

Figure 5: Leveling in both arches with space gaining with lateral incisor derotations in the lower arch along with panoramic X-ray before brace removal.

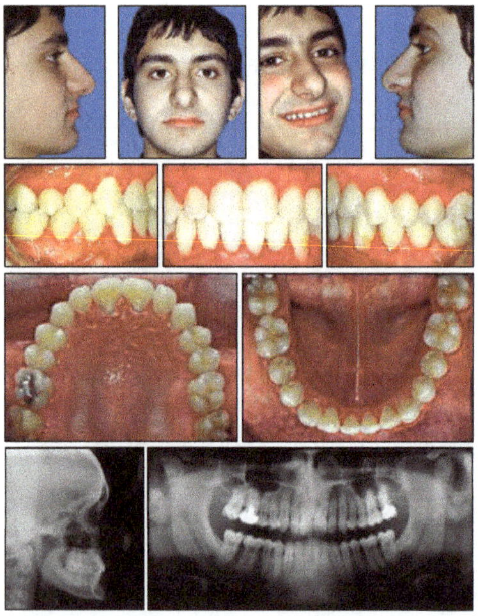

Figure 6: Posttreatment facial and intraoral photographs and X-rays.

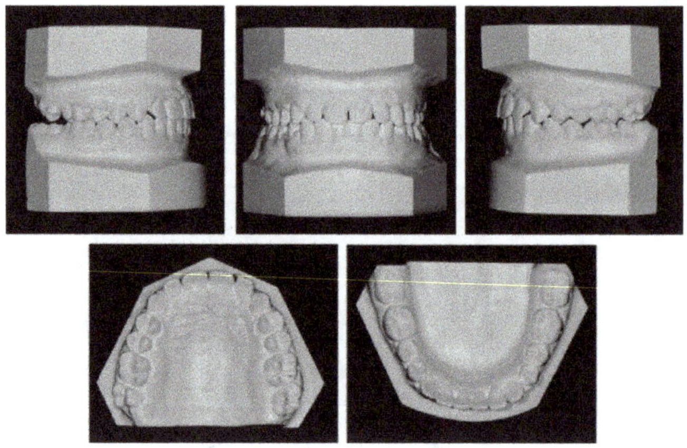

Figure 7: Posttreatment dental casts.

The third option seemed to be the easiest and more rational choice considering the occlusal and aesthetic features and the patient's expectations.

Treatment started with an interceptive first phase, including a double transpalatal bar in the maxillary arch and a lip bumper on the second lower molars (Figure 4).

After 1 year and 8 months of treatment, the upper and lower molars were derotated and an improvement of upper and lower crowding was detected; consequently, the shapes of both arches were changed.

The recovery of space in the upper arch resulted in the physiological eruption of the upper right canine.

The second phase of treatment began with the placement of 0.022 × 0.028 in standard edgewise appliances.

An intrusion arch with round Australian wire 0.016 in was used for bite opening.

The leveling of the teeth was accomplished with light Australian round wires, before 0.016 and then 0.018 in wires.

Open coil springs were used in the lower arch to gain space whereas lingual buttons along with elastomeric chains were applied to both lateral incisors to allow their derotation and correct placement in the arch. During the treatment, third molar bud extractions were performed. Considerable time and effort were required for the finishing procedures, including torquing, uprighting, and root paralleling (Figure 5).

After active orthodontic treatment, the brackets were removed. Maxillary and mandibular Hawley retainers were used for retention.

The fixed phase lasted 2 years and 9 months, and the patient was motivated and cooperative throughout the entire treatment.

3. Results

The overall treatment objectives were achieved. The patient appeared with a really improved smile and profile. The occlusion showed a well-aligned dentition with class I molar and canine relationships. The patient had a consonant smile arc, interdigitation of the teeth was good, the upper right canine

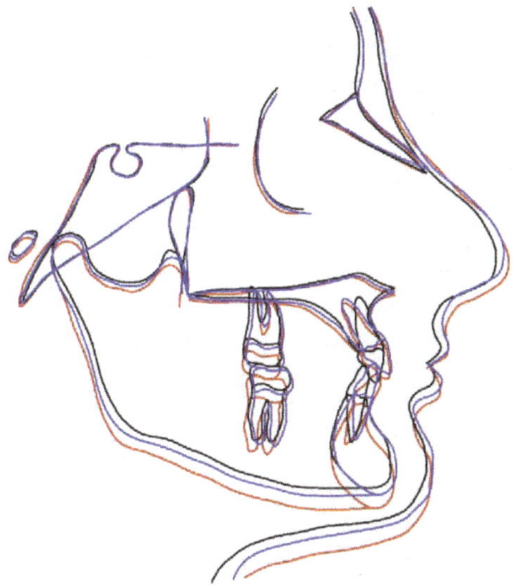

FIGURE 8: Superimposition tracings.

was well positioned, and the maxillary arch form was improved. The severe lower crowding was completely corrected, and a good overbite was achieved. The posttreatment panoramic radiograph showed nice root parallelism and the absence of the upper and lower wisdom teeth. Superimpositions revealed a proclination of upper and lower incisor inclination (1/SN, 103°; IMPA, 100°, respectively) (Figures 6–8; Table 1). The treatment lasted 4 years and 5 months and the retention period 2 years. Both the patient and his parents were pleased with the outcome. After 10 years of postretention, the occlusion was well maintained (Figures 9 and 10).

4. Discussion

In orthodontic diagnosis, mandibular incisor crowding is a critical and frequently a limiting factor when planning a treatment. Decisions regarding extractions in the mandible many times are greatly influenced not only by the extent of crowding but also by the relationship between basal bone and incisor position [3]. For over 6 mm of crowding, extractions seem to be the best choice whereas between 3 and 6 mm the decision is not so clear and affected by other factors such as the aesthetic and the type of periodontium.

A major goal of orthodontic treatment is to achieve a long-term stability of posttreatment occlusion [24, 25] although it is a challenge for the orthodontists; it is almost impossible to guarantee the absolute posttreatment stability, even in a case with borderline crowding [26].

For these reasons, the long-term stability after extraction or nonextraction treatment is still a controversial topic [22, 25].

According to many authors [27–32], avoiding completely the relapse is not possible in the extraction cases as well as in nonextraction cases treated in permanent dentition [32].

In particular, Cansunar and Uysal [31] pointed out that there were no significant differences among extraction and nonextraction treatments for several features such as alignment, marginal ridge height, buccolingual inclination, overjet, and interproximal contact measurements. However, nonextraction patients had both better sagittal dental relationship and root angulations [29, 33]. Moreover, in extraction treatments, the arch width reduction creates unaesthetic triangles at the corners of the mouth with negative spaces lateral to the buccal segments [32] and undesirable dental retraction; worsening facial aesthetics are possible [6]. Thus, the trend of nonextraction treatment has changed due to the new aesthetic concepts of facial soft-tissue profile in orthodontics [32–36]. The present case shows a patient with a severe mandibular crowding, treated without extractions and with a postretention long-term stability (10-year follow-up).

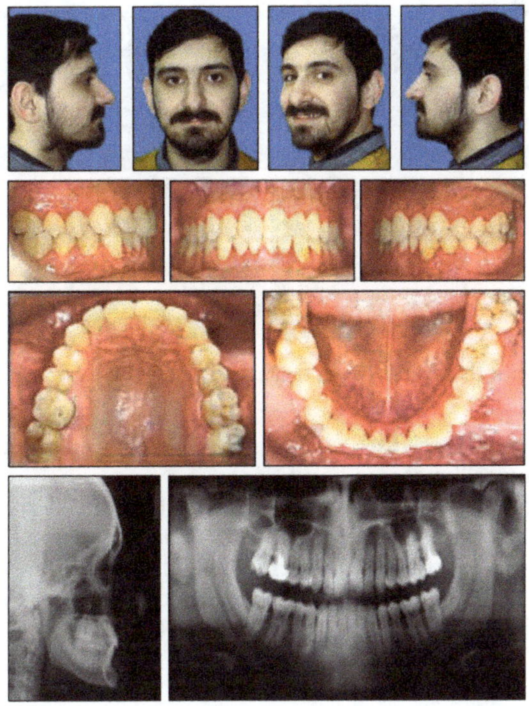

FIGURE 9: Facial and intraoral photographs, lateral and panoramic X-rays after 10-year retention.

The severe lower crowding was completely corrected, and the improvement of overbite was obtained. The overall treatment objectives were achieved. The patient showed a better smile and profile, although the superimpositions revealed a lower incisor proclination.

A possible limitation of this treatment could be the time to gain the outcomes showed. This is due to the choice of an early treatment and the need of two phases of treatment: one in mixed dentition and one in permanent. This therapeutic option can be slowed down by the patient's dental exfoliation times. Fortunately, this strategy allows to have an early treatment, to take advantage of growth, and to prevent dental extractions.

A possible explanation for such long-term stability was that the major changes in arch dimensions were primarily achieved during the lip bumper phase, whereas the final alignment was obtained with fixed appliances [5].

So, primarily, cheek and lip muscular pressures were involved, suggesting on the one hand that gaining of space before bracket placement may help to keep the correction stable and on the other hand that a new muscular balance was achieved to allow stability of the 12 mm crowding after

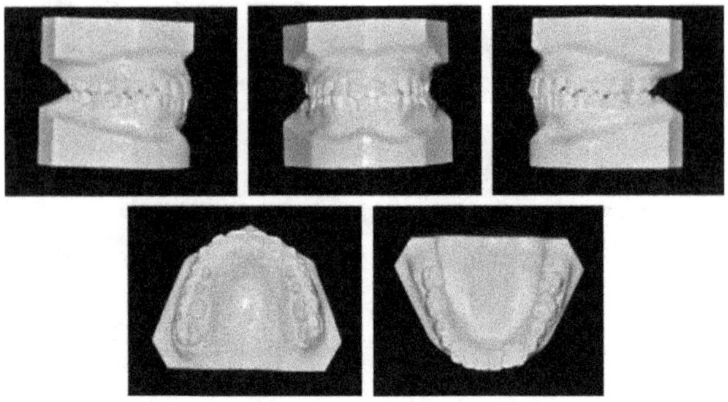

Figure 10: Posttreatment dental casts after 10-year retention.

10 years. The relapse of 0.5 mm in the upper and lower arch was clinically not significant.

This result can be more than satisfactory considering that the only other case report showed a mandibular crowding of 7 mm treated with lip bumper in late mixed dentition with 5 years and 3 months of follow-up including two-year retention [18].

5. Conclusions

An early treatment can be considered a valid choice to resolve the inclusion of a permanent canine reducing the risk of side effects and to gain space in the lower arch for the resolution of severe crowding avoiding dental extractions. The postretention stability results are remarkable because a very light relapse (0.5 mm) of the lower crowding was observed after 10 years along with an aesthetic and functional outcome.

Authors' Contributions

PMM, GI, and LN are responsible for the literary review and writing of the manuscript. LP, VG, and AI conceived the ideas of the manuscript and revised the drafts. All authors read and approved the final manuscript.

References

[1] L. Perillo, C. Masucci, F. Ferro, D. Apicella, and T. Baccetti, "Prevalence of orthodontic treatment need in southern Italian schoolchildren," *The European Journal of Orthodontics*, vol. 32, no. 1, pp. 49–53, 2010.

[2] M. O. Sayin and H. Türkkahraman, "Malocclusion and crowding in an orthodontically referred Turkish population," *The Angle Orthodontist*, vol. 74, no. 5, pp. 635–639, 2004.

[3] T. Uysal, A. Yagci, T. Ozer, I. Veli, and A. Ozturk, "Mandibular anterior bony support and incisor crowding: is there a relationship?," *American Journal of Orthodontics and Dentofacial Orthopedics*, vol. 142, no. 5, pp. 645–653, 2012.

[4] M. O. Sayin and H. Türkkahraman, "Factors contributing to mandibular anterior crowding in the early mixed dentition," *The Angle Orthodontist*, vol. 74, no. 6, pp. 754–758, 2004.

[5] G. Raucci, C. Pachêco-Pereira, M. Elyasi, F. d'Apuzzo, C. Flores-Mir, and L. Perillo, "Short- and long-term evaluation of mandibular dental arch dimensional changes in patients treated with a lip bumper during mixed dentition followed by fixed appliances," *The Angle Orthodontist*, vol. 86, no. 5, pp. 753–760, 2016.

[6] R. M. A. Lima Filho and A. L. Lima, "Long-term outcome in a patient with class I malocclusion with severe crowding treated without extractions," *American Journal of Orthodontics and Dentofacial Orthopedics*, vol. 126, no. 4, pp. 495–504, 2004.

[7] A. Gracco, L. Luca, M. C. Bongiorno, and G. Siciliani, "Computed tomography evaluation of mandibular incisor bony support in untreated patients," *American Journal of Orthodontics and Dentofacial Orthopedics*, vol. 138, no. 2, pp. 179–187, 2010.

[8] K. Nauert and R. Berg, "Evaluation of labio-lingual bony support of lower incisors in orthodontically untreated adults with the help of computed tomography," *Journal of Orofacial Orthopedics / Fortschritte der Kieferorthopädie*, vol. 60, no. 5, pp. 321–334, 1999.

[9] H. Wehrbein, W. Bauer, and P. Diedrich, "Mandibular incisors, alveolar bone, and symphysis afterorthodontic treatment. A retrospective study," *American Journal of Orthodontics and Dentofacial Orthopedics*, vol. 110, no. 3, pp. 239–246, 1996.

[10] L. O. Duncan, L. Piedade, M. Lekic, R. S. Cunha, and W. A. Wiltshire, "Changes in mandibular incisor position and arch form resulting from Invisalign correction of the crowded dentition treated nonextraction," *The Angle Orthodontist*, vol. 86, no. 4, pp. 577–583, 2016.

[11] G. Raucci, C. Pachêco-Pereira, M. Elyasi, F. d'Apuzzo, C. Flores-Mir, and L. Perillo, "Predictors of postretention stability of mandibular dental arch dimensions in patients treated with a lip bumper during mixed dentition followed by fixed appliances," *The Angle Orthodontist*, vol. 87, no. 2, pp. 209–214, 2017.

[12] W. R. Proffit, "Equilibrium theory revisited: factors influencing position of the teeth," *The Angle Orthodontist*, vol. 48, no. 3, pp. 175–186, 1978.

[13] S. O'Donnell, R. S. Nanda, and J. Ghosh, "Perioral forces and dental changes resulting from mandibular lip bumper treatment," *American Journal of Orthodontics and Dentofacial Orthopedics*, vol. 113, no. 3, pp. 247–255, 1998.

[14] P. H. Buschang, "Maxillomandibular expansion: short-term relapse potential and long-term stability," *American Journal of Orthodontics and Dentofacial Orthopedics*, vol. 129, no. 4, pp. S75–S79, 2006.

[15] H. N. Nance, "The limitations of orthodontic treatment. II. Diagnosis and treatment in the permanent dentition," *American Journal of Orthodontics*, vol. 33, no. 5, pp. 253–301, 1947.

[16] T. Ferris, R. G. Alexander, J. Boley, and P. H. Buschang, "Long-term stability of combined rapid palatal expansion-lip bumper therapy followed by full fixed appliances," *American Journal of Orthodontics and Dentofacial Orthopedics*, vol. 128, no. 3, pp. 310–325, 2005.

[17] M. J. Solomon, J. D. English, W. B. Magness, and C. J. McKee, "Long-term stability of lip bumper therapy followed by fixed appliances," *The Angle Orthodontist*, vol. 76, no. 1, pp. 36–42, 2006.

[18] R. Sabri, "Treatment of a severe arch-length deficiency with anteroposterior and transverse expansion: long-term stability," *American Journal of Orthodontics and Dentofacial Orthopedics*, vol. 137, no. 3, pp. 401–411, 2010.

[19] J. O'Neill, "Do lip bumpers work?," *Evidence-Based Dentistry*, vol. 10, no. 2, pp. 48-49, 2009.

[20] D. I. Hashish and Y. A. Mostafa, "Effect of lip bumpers on mandibular arch dimensions," *American Journal of Orthodontics and Dentofacial Orthopedics*, vol. 135, no. 1, pp. 106–109, 2009.

[21] M. Weinberg and C. Sadowsky, "Resolution of mandibular arch crowding in growing patients with class I malocclusions treated nonextraction," *American Journal of Orthodontics and Dentofacial Orthopedics*, vol. 110, no. 4, pp. 359–364, 1996.

[22] K. M. Freitas, M. R. de Freitas, J. F. Henriques, A. Pinzan, and G. Janson, "Postretention relapse of mandibular anterior crowding in patients treated without mandibular premolar extraction," *American Journal of Orthodontics and Dentofacial Orthopedics*, vol. 125, no. 4, pp. 480–487, 2004.

[23] R. J. Schulaf, R. W. Allen, R. D. Walters, and M. Dreskin, "The mandibular dental arch: part I, lower incisor position," *The Angle Orthodontist*, vol. 47, no. 4, pp. 280–287, 1977.

[24] S. Ericson and J. Kurol, "Radiographic examination of ectopically erupting maxillary canines," *American Journal of Orthodontics and Dentofacial Orthopedics*, vol. 91, no. 6, pp. 483–492, 1987.

[25] S. J. Lindauer, L. K. Rubenstein, W. M. Hang, W. C. Andersen, and R. J. Isaacson, "Canine impaction identified early with panoramic radiographs," *The Journal of the American Dental Association*, vol. 123, no. 3, pp. 91–97, 1992.

[26] M. F. Francisconi, G. Janson, K. M. S. Freitas et al., "Overjet, overbite, and anterior crowding relapses in extraction and nonextraction patients, and their correlations," *American Journal of Orthodontics and Dentofacial Orthopedics*, vol. 146, no. 1, pp. 67–72, 2014.

[27] R. M. Little, "Stability and relapse of dental arch alignment," *British Journal of Orthodontics*, vol. 17, no. 3, pp. 235–241, 2019.

[28] K. C. Dyer, J. L. Vaden, and E. F. Harris, "Relapse revisited–again," *American Journal of Orthodontics and Dentofacial Orthopedics*, vol. 142, no. 2, pp. 221–227, 2012.

[29] A. T. Kamal, A. Shaikh, and M. Fida, "Improvement in Peer Assessment Rating scores after nonextraction, premolar extraction, and mandibular incisor extraction treatments in patients with class I malocclusion," *American Journal of Orthodontics and Dentofacial Orthopedics*, vol. 151, no. 4, pp. 685–690, 2017.

[30] S. Ciger, M. Aksu, and D. Germeç, "Evaluation of posttreatment changes in class II division 1 patients after nonextraction orthodontic treatment: cephalometric and model analysis," *American Journal of Orthodontics and Dentofacial Orthopedics*, vol. 127, no. 2, pp. 219–223, 2005.

[31] H. A. Cansunar and T. Uysal, "Comparison of orthodontic treatment outcomes in nonextraction, 2 maxillary premolar extraction, and 4 premolar extraction protocols with the American Board of Orthodontics objective grading system," *American Journal of Orthodontics and Dentofacial Orthopedics*, vol. 145, no. 5, pp. 595–602, 2014.

[32] G. Janson, F. R. T. Maria, and R. Bombonatti, "Frequency evaluation of different extraction protocols in orthodontic treatment during 35 years," *Progress in Orthodontics*, vol. 15, no. 1, p. 51, 2014.

[33] V. Grassia, F. d'Apuzzo, D. DiStasio, A. Jamilian, A. Lucchese, and L. Perillo, "Upper and lower arch changes after mixed palatal expansion protocol," *European journal of paediatric dentistry: official journal of European Academy of Paediatric Dentistry*, vol. 15, no. 4, pp. 375–380, 2014.

[34] V. Grassia, A. Lombardi, H. Kawasaki et al., "Salivary microRNAs as new molecular markers in cleft lip and palate: a new frontier in molecular medicine," *Oncotarget*, vol. 9, no. 27, pp. 18929–18938, 2018.

[35] S. Eslami, J. Faber, A. Fateh, F. Sheikholaemmeh, V. Grassia, and A. Jamilian, "Treatment decision in adult patients with class III malocclusion: surgery versus orthodontics," *Progress in Orthodontics*, vol. 19, no. 1, p. 28, 2018.

[36] A. Scalzone, C. Flores-Mir, D. Carozza, F. d'Apuzzo, V. Grassia, and L. Perillo, "Secondary alveolar bone grafting using autologous versus alloplastic material in the treatment of cleft lip and palate patients: systematic review and meta-analysis," *Progress in Orthodontics*, vol. 20, no. 1, p. 6, 2019.

2

The "3D Versascrew": An Innovative Approach for Management of Bilateral Cleft Lip and Palate Case

M. V. Ashith[1] **NS Suma**[2] **K. Mithun**[3] **and Dhruv Ahuja**[1]

[1]*Department of Orthodontics and Dentofacial Orthopedics, Manipal College of Dental Sciences Mangalore(Manipal Academy of Higher Education Manipal), Mangalore, Karnataka, India*
[2]*Department of Orthodontics, SVS Institute of Dental Sciences, Mahabubnagar, India*
[3]*Department of Orthodontics, AJ Institute of Dental Sciences, Mangalore, Karnataka, India*

Correspondence should be addressed to M. V. Ashith; ashith.mv@manipal.edu

Academic Editor: Rui Amaral Mendes

The purpose behind the innovation of modified nasoalveolar moulding appliance was to achieve simultaneous anteroposterior and transverse correction in bilateral cleft cases with minimal vomeroid bending. This paper presents a 3D Versascrew appliance that has been used for presurgical nasoalveolar moulding in a 15-day-old neonate with bilateral cleft. Treatment was initiated at 30 days and continued for 90 days following which mild expansion of posterior maxilla with establishment of arch continuity and concomitant improvement in nasal morphology was achieved towards the end.

1. Background

The primary challenge in the management of bilateral cleft lip and palate disorder arises from the deficient columella and ectopic premaxilla [1]. The objective of nasoalveolar moulding in bilateral cleft cases is to reconstruct a symmetrically balanced lip and nose with good columellar length before surgery [2, 3]. Literature review shows different techniques by Grayson, Figueora, and Liou for presurgical management of the bilateral cleft palate [4]. Nevertheless, when rapid and large movements are performed in the patient, the vomer can be deformed, injured, and even fractured, especially at the prevomerine suture [1]. Another critical factor in presurgical nasoalveolar moulding is the timing of the treatment. This article presents the case report of a neonate with bilateral cleft treated by a 3D Versa appliance where presurgical nasoalveolar moulding was performed, the method of appliance fabrication and perusal of nasal outcome has been thoroughly explained. The innovative appliance used here is named 3D Versascrew as it consists of a 3D screw and after its versatility of correction in all 3 dimensions- transverse, vertical, and antero-posterior dimensions whereas, previous studies have shown correction with jack screw, which provides control in antero-posterior dimension [4].

2. Case Presentation

A 15-day-old male infant with bilateral cleft lip and palate was referred to our department. The parent's chief complaint was impaired facial appearance of the child and difficulty in feeding. The medical history of the child and parents was conventional.

Extraoral and intraoral examination of the child revealed protruding and rotated premaxilla with the lip segments wide apart (Figure 1).

Depressed alar domes with reduced columella were other clinical features. Bird's eye view showed premaxilla almost obscuring the left nostril. After thorough clinical examination, the treatment method was explained to the parents and informed consent was obtained. The core intention of PNAM is to bring about correction of premaxillary position with minimal vomeroid bending, reduction in the cleft defect by approximation of segments, columellar lengthening, and improvement of nasal morphology. Minimal

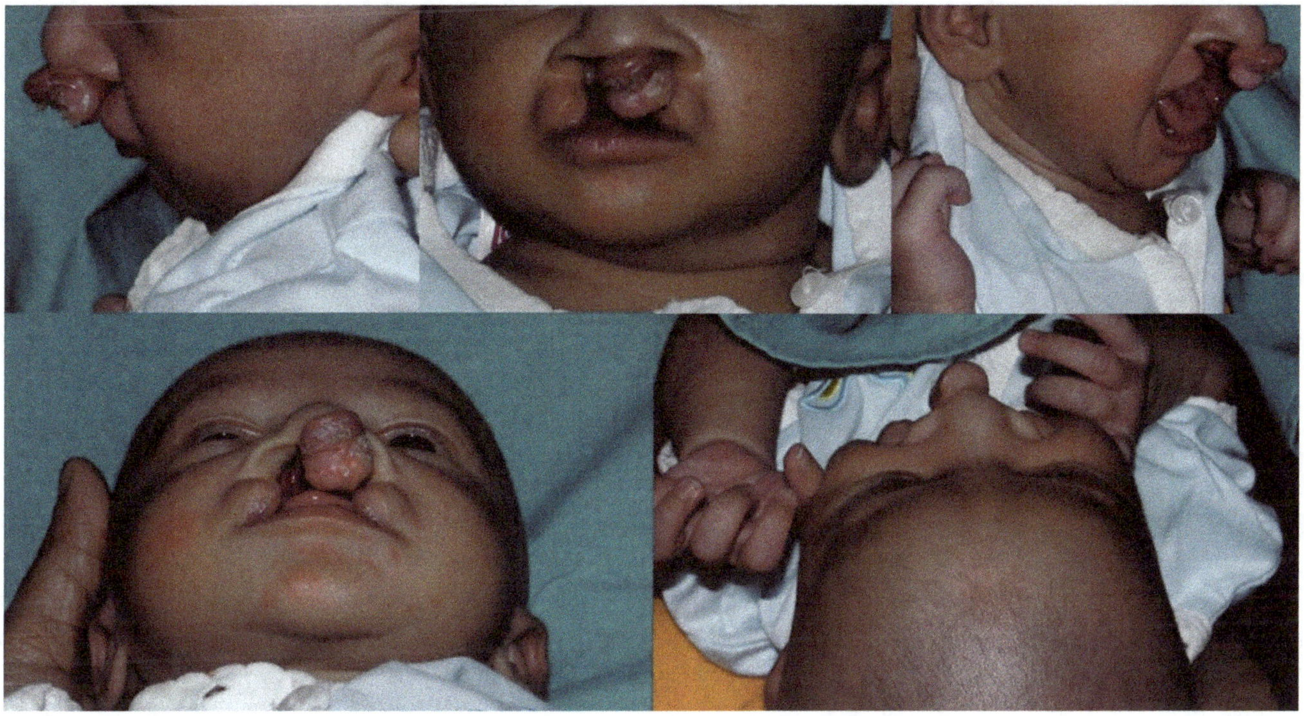

Figure 1: Pre-treatment: extraoral.

scarring is expected as the defect is minimized. The acrylic plate also functions as an obturator and aids in better feeding of the infant. As the patient reported difficulty in reporting for follow up appointments, we decided to treat the infant with a 3D Versascrew appliance, which is an active moulding plate incorporating a 3-way screw so that activations can be performed at home.

3. Treatment

Primary impression of the infant's maxillary gumpad was made with moulding wax (Figure 2(a)). A special tray fabricated from the primary cast was used to make a definitive impression (Figure 2(b) and 2(c)). Impression of the upper gumpad was made using polyvinyl siloxane (Figure 2(d)) (REPROSILR, DENTSPLY) with the infant's head at a lower level than the rest of the body. A study model and a working model were poured using dental stone. Wax block outs were given to relieve the undercuts and alginate separating medium was deliberately applied all over the surface of the working model. 3D screw (Leone Company) was positioned slightly off-centred for premaxillary rotational correction with the anterior screw completely open to facilitate premaxillary retraction on activation. The screw position corresponded to the centre of the rotated predictive normal palate in the midst of posterior gum pad region (Figure 2(e)). Cold cure acrylic resin in dough stage was adapted uniformly over the cast surface and curing under pressure was done to ensure appliance with minimal porosity.

Nasal stent wires were fabricated using TMA wire bent at almost right angle and further near the nasal bone the wire is bent at approximately at 80°. The ends of the wires were recurved to form a loop, which was covered with acrylic and coated with soft tissue liner to elevate the nasal dome. A thin layer of acrylic was then used to attach nasal stent wires to the appliance proper. These wires serve to initiate nasal correction from the very initial stages of treatment. Also, acrylic extensions to engage elastics were attached bilaterally to the appliance proper. The elastic was gently stretched and secured to cheek by means of a tape which served to prevent unseating of the appliance (Figure 2(f)). Finishing and polishing of the appliance were done to ensure a smooth surface and the appliance was placed in room temperature water overnight for leaching of excess monomer. Dynaplast (Johnson's) was used for active lip taping (Figure 3).

In order to prevent cheek irritation due to repeated active lip taping, Micropore tape (3 M) was placed on both the cheeks. This exerts a compressive force on the prolabium region, thus aiding in correction of premaxillary protrusion.

The appliance was activated by closing the anterior screw and opening the posterior screw. Nasal stent wires were incorporated in the first visit to reduce the need for alteration of the appliance and to reduce the frequency of the visit. Activations were carried out only when cleft defect was ≤5 mm. The key to successful activation is the appearance of tissue blanching clinically. Biweekly activations were planned for the anterior screw to actively retract and centre the premaxilla. Posterior expansion was only minimally required to ensure the arch continuity; therefore, the posterior screw was activated only once a week. Prior to appliance insertion, the activation which is produced is 1–1.5 mm, which will not displace the nasal stent remarkably, the nasal stent wires are incorporated to elevate the nasal dome

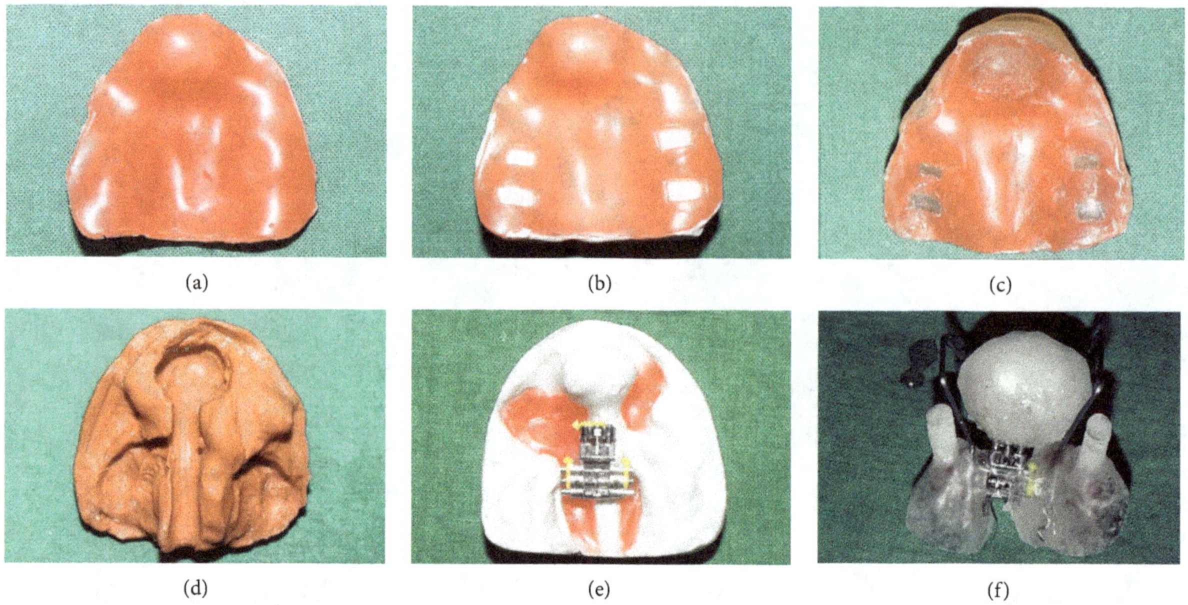

FIGURE 2: Steps in appliance fabrication (a) Primary wax impression. (b) Primary cast with wax spacer and tissue stops. (c) Special tray. (d) Polyvinylsiloxane impression. (e) Master cast with 3D screw in position. (f) 3D Versascrew appliance.

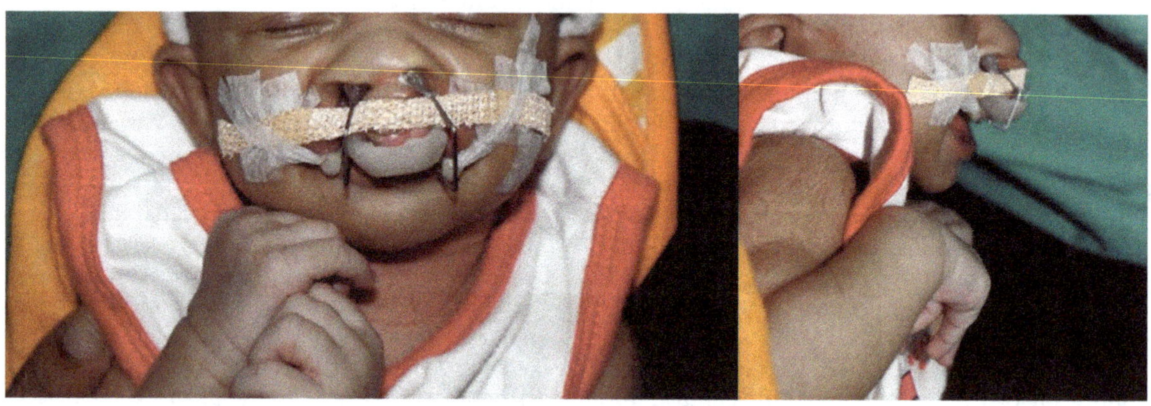

FIGURE 3: Insertion of a 3D Versascrew appliance.

simultaneously the anterio-posterior screw activation will retract the premaxilla thus increasing the columella length and off-centred screw position to correct the deviation and rotation of the premaxilla (Figure 4). The gum pads were gently wiped to clear off the debris, and active lip taping was done using elastic adhesive bandage (Dynaplast). Customized activation protocol chart was given to the patient's parents and the method of activation and lip taping was demonstrated.

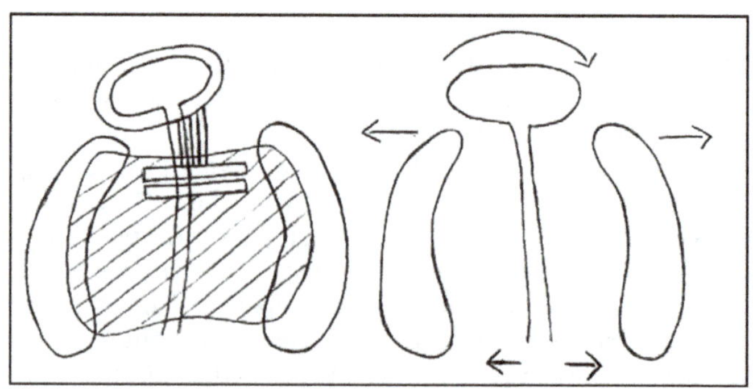

FIGURE 4: Off-centred screw position to correct the rotation of premaxilla.

4. Outcome and Follow-up

By the end of active treatment, which on an average lasted about 2.5 months, we could achieve our treatment objectives with minimal vomeroid bending. The chief reason for this result was the anteroposterior rotation of premaxilla unlike pure retraction in conventional techniques. This also aided in deepening of the maxillary labial vestibule. The acrylic hood encasing the premaxilla passively depressed the premaxilla, which aided in establishing a good arch continuity.

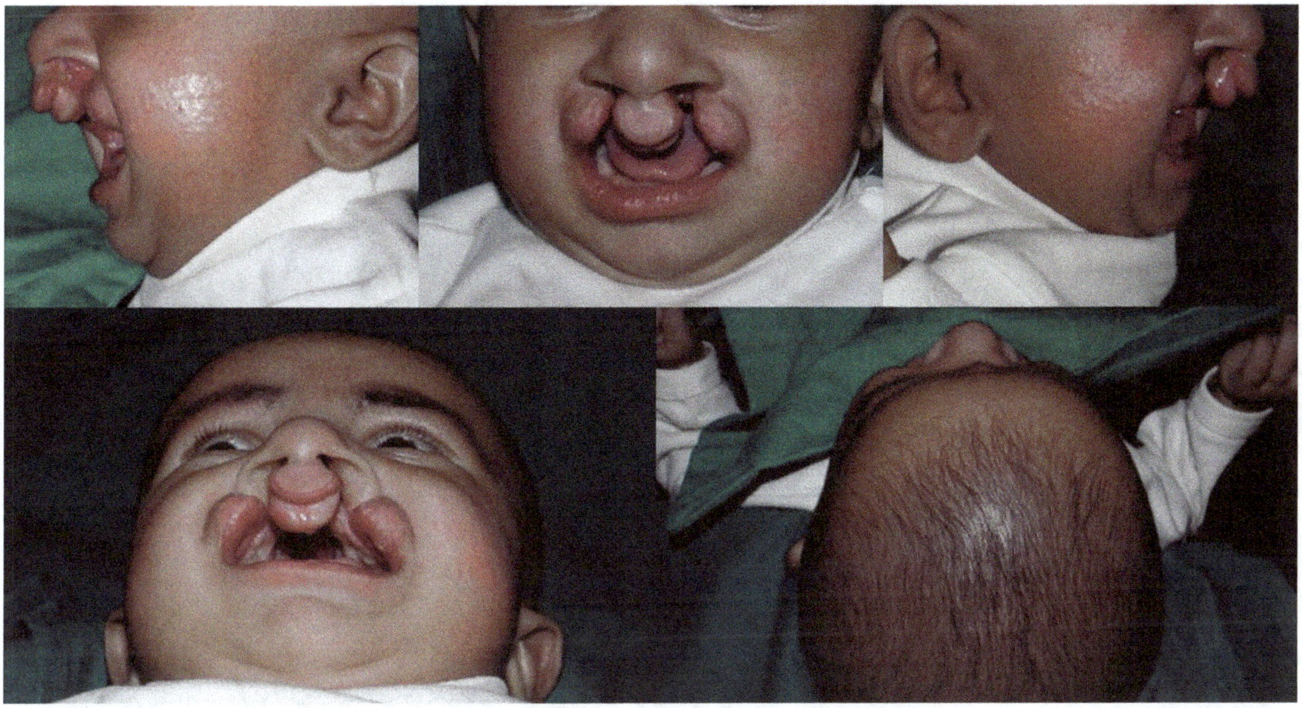

Figure 5: Post 3D Versascrew appliance: extraoral.

The treatment outcomes are listed herewith (Figure 5):

(1) Correction of premaxillary position

(2) Improved nasal contour with lengthening of columella

(3) Deepening of the maxillary labial vestibule

(4) Approximation of lip segments facilitating suturing without tissue tension

(5) Appreciable reduction in cleft defect

(6) Minimal vomeroid bending

The primary lip and palate repair was done at 6 months and 14 months, respectively. The approximation of the alveolar segments permits the surgeon to perform for better repair. A 4-year follow-up of the case shows the improvement in facial esthetics (Figure 6).

5. Discussion

Naso-alveolar moulding significantly improved the overall facial appearance of the infant by normalizing the premaxillary position, reduction of the alar base width, approximation of lip segments, columellar lengthening and increased nostril volume. The reduction in the cleft deformity and nasal correction prior to surgery makes lip closure less complicated and aids in better esthetics due to minimal scar tissue formation. Grayson stated that the plasticity of the cartilage faded over the first 6 months of age and a state of elasticity eventually set in [3]. In our case, as the patient presented at a very early age, we could make full advantage of plasticity of the cartilage and achieved good nasal moulding.

A study by Wojciech et al. [5] concluded that preoperative NAM in combination with primary gingivoperiosteoplasty reduces the need for secondary alveolar bone grafting by 60% in patients with unilateral cleft lip and palate. Similarly, in our study, naso-alveolar moulding achieved expansion of collapsed posterior segments which in turn, aided in accommodation of the retracted premaxilla and helped us achieve a good arch continuity. The permanent teeth were expected to erupt with a better periodontal support as the alveolar segments were aligned well and there were increased bony bridges across the cleft. In a study conducted by Severens et al. [6], it was found that the overall costs in cleft care were reduced by the lesser number of surgeries involved in the treatment. The same was achieved in our case with the decrease in the number of visits to the hospital and by achieving appreciable results in a short treatment duration.

A study by Neha et al. [4] advocated active retraction but posterior expansion was not performed whereas in our study, a 3D Versascrew appliance helped us achieve simultaneous premaxillary retraction and posterior maxillary expansion. Active retraction was preferred over passive in order to hasten the process of premaxillary retraction so that nasal moulding could be initiated at the earliest and also to facilitate at home activations. The activations were planned to keep the force levels gentle and to prevent any deleterious effects on the delicate vomer bone and maxillary segments. Furthermore, this is supported by a study done by the same authors, Neha et al., [7], where they have mentioned about the early correction of cleft with 3D expansion screw for simultaneously retraction and expansion using external nasal stents, whereas

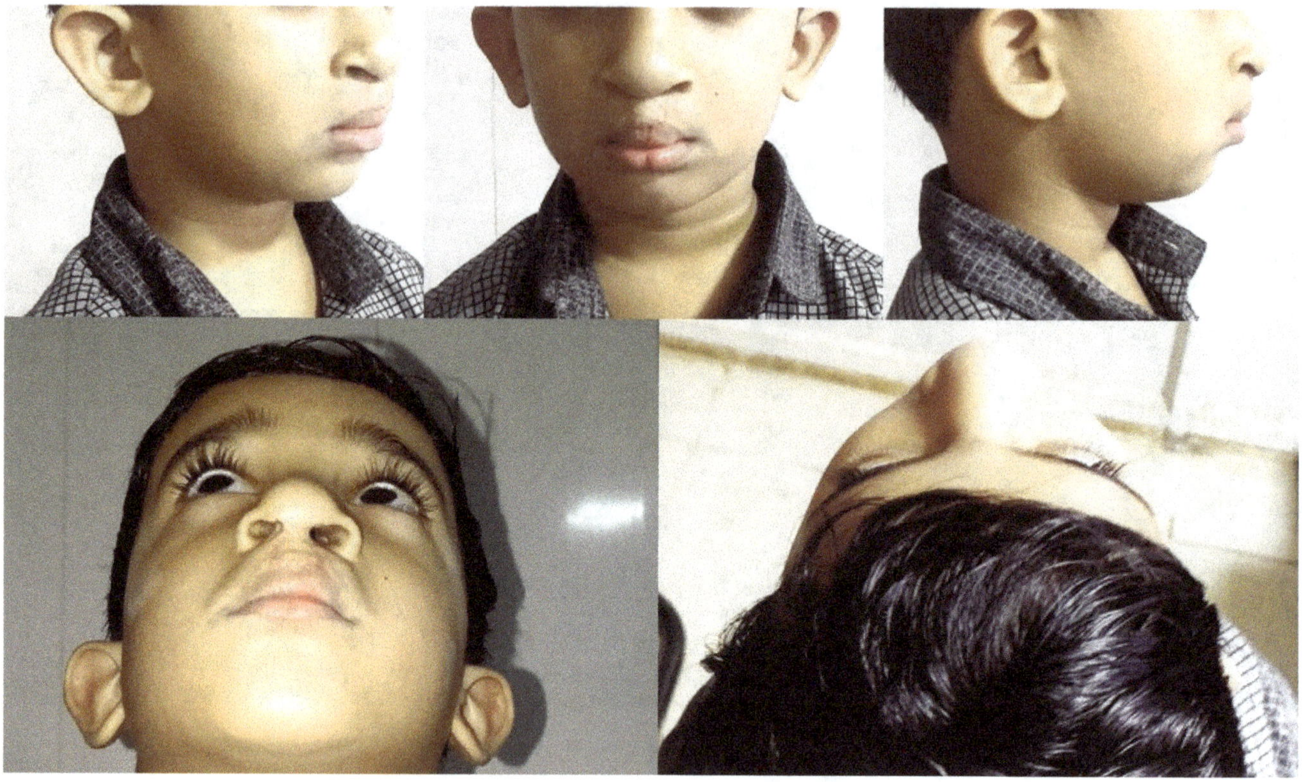

FIGURE 6: Four-year follow-up: extraoral.

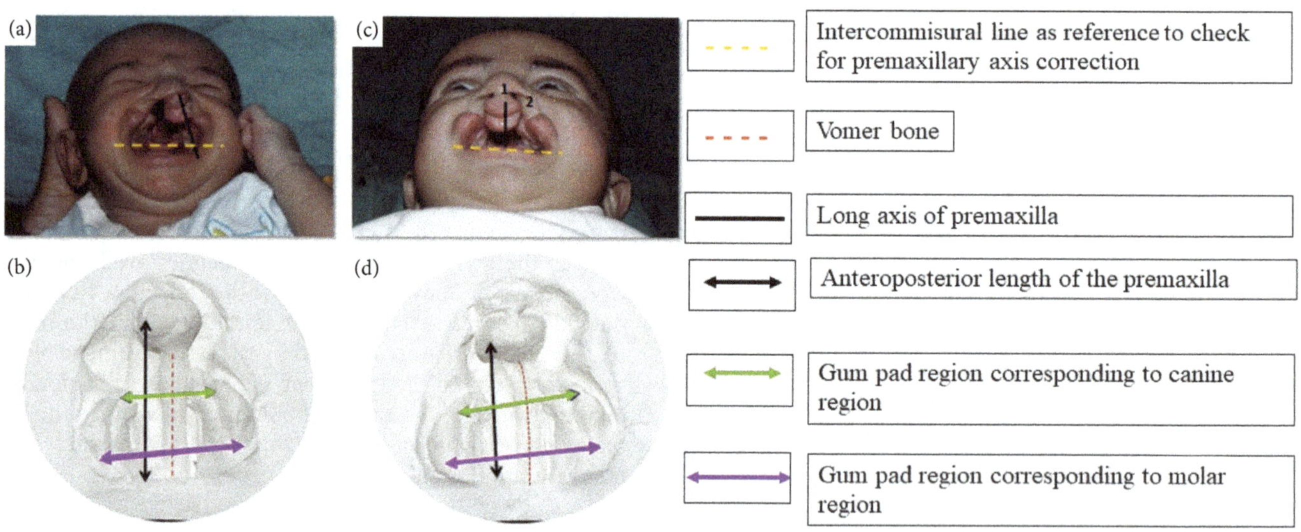

FIGURE 7: Comparison of pre- (a, b) and post-3D Versascrew appliance (c, d).

3D Versacrew is a single appliance in which nasal stents are incorporated within the appliance for ease of use by the baby.

Construction of imaginary lines was done to quantify the correction achieved with the therapy. Imaginary line drawn connecting the most distal points of the posterior segments to mark the posterior extent of palate was labelled as posterior reference line. Premaxillary retraction was quantified by measuring the distance between the most prominent point on the superior aspect of the premaxilla and midpoint of posterior reference line (Figure 7).

Retraction of 4.5 mm was achieved in a period of 2.5 months. As controlled retraction was performed, there were minimal effects on the delicate vomer bone. An imaginary line drawn connecting the most mesial points of the posterior segments was labelled as anterior reference line and served as a guide to quantify the expansion measured at future canine region. Expansion of 2.5 mm was achieved in the mentioned period (Table 1). Appreciable reduction in the cleft defect was seen bilaterally minimizing the need for bone grafting in the future.

Table 1: Comparative values of pre- and post-3D Versascrew appliance model analysis.

Parameter	Pre-treatment	Post-treatment
Antero-posterior length	38.5 mm	34 mm
Intercanine region of gumpad	21.5 mm	24 mm
Intermolar region of gumpad	33 mm	34.5 mm

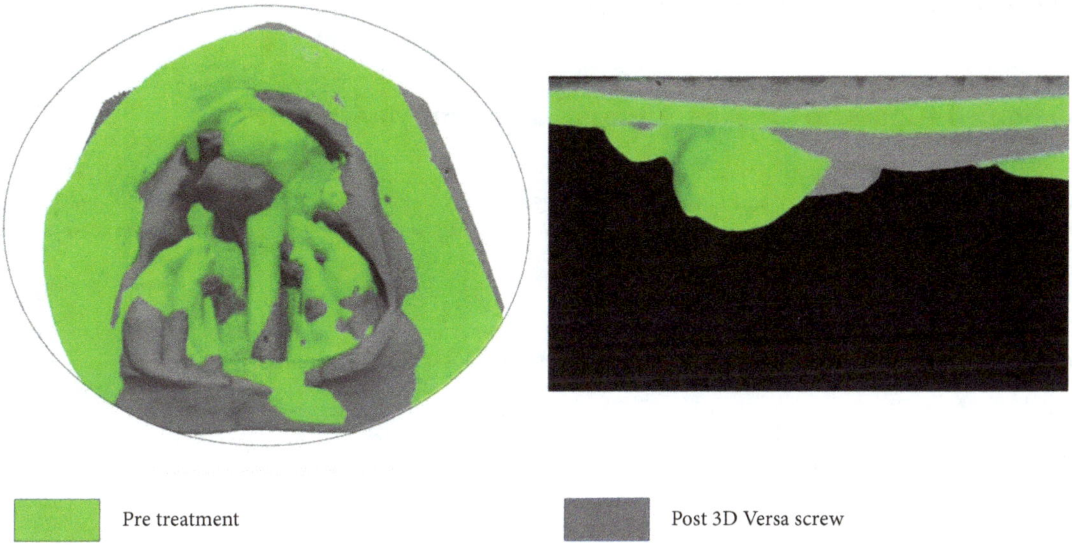

Figure 8: 3D Superimposition of models.

The acrylic hood enclosing the premaxilla resulted in downward descent of the premaxilla and overcame the effect of premaxillary extrusion, while retraction, which was a concern with the previous techniques, and these changes can be appreciated in superimposition of pre- and post-treatment casts (Figure 8).

Thus, the “3D Versascrew appliance” results favourably in centering, retraction and passive depression of premaxilla with minimal vomeroid bending, modest posterior maxillary expansion with initiation of arch continuity and collateral refinement in nasal morphology and is indeed a versatile appliance true to its name.

6. Learning Points/Take Home Messages

(1) Commencement of treatment of nasoalveolar moulding should be initiated at the earliest, preferably within 15 days of life

(2) Nasoalveolar moulding decreases the number and cost of review-surgical procedures required for nasal defect rectification

(3) 3D Versascrew appliance allows the growth of the alveolar processes in the right direction with minimal vomeroid bending, reshapes the flattened nose, and helps in minimizing the extent of complex surgeries

References

[1] A. T. Vachiramon, J. N. Groper, and S. Gamer, “A rapid solution to align the severely malpositioned premaxilla in bilateral cleft lip and palate patients,” *The Cleft Palate-Craniofacial Journal*, vol. 45, no. 3, pp. 229–231, 2008.

[2] B. H. Grayson and D. Maull, “Nasoalveolar molding for infants born with clefts of the lip, alveolus, and palate,” *Clinics in Plastic Surgery*, vol. 31, no. 2, pp. 149–158, 2004.

[3] B. H. Grayson and J. S. Garfinkle, “Early cleft management: the case for nasoalveolar molding,” *American Journal of Orthodontics and Dentofacial Orthopedics*, vol. 145, no. 2, pp. 134–142, 2014.

[4] T. T. Neha, P. Rai, and P. S. Bhandari, “Nasoalveolar molding: use of reverse expansion screw in retraction of cleft premaxilla in a case of bilateral cleft lip and palate,” *Journal of Cleft Lip Palate and Craniofacial Anomalies*, vol. 2, pp. 143–146, 2015.

[5] W. Dec, P. R. Shetye, E. H. Davidson et al., “Presurgical nasoalveolar molding and primary gingivoperiosteoplasty reduce the need for bone grafting in patients with bilateral clefts,” *The Journal of Craniofacial Surgery*, vol. 24, no. 1, pp. 186–190, 2013.

[6] J. L. Severens, C. Prahl, A. M. Kuijpers-Jagtman, and B. Prahl-Andersen, “Short-term cost-effectiveness analysis of presurgical orthopedic treatment in children with complete unilateral cleft lip and palate,” *The Cleft Palate-Craniofacial Journal*, vol. 35, no. 3, pp. 222–226, 1998.

[7] B. Neha, T. Tripathi, and P. Rai, “Active nasoalveolar molding using 3-directional expansion screw for arch alignment in bilateral cleft lip and palate,” *American Journal of Orthodontics and Dentofacial Orthopedics*, vol. 2, no. 1, pp. 20–25, 2022.

3

Nonsyndromic Generalized Radiculomegaly of Permanent Dentition: A Rare Case Report

Mohammed Alhussain,[1] **Naif Almosa**,[2] **and Hourya Alnofaie**[3]

[1]*Ministry of Health, Riyadh, Saudi Arabia*
[2]*Department of Pediatric Dentistry and Orthodontics, College of Dentistry, King Saud University, Riyadh, Saudi Arabia*
[3]*Division of Oral and Maxillofacial Surgery, Basic Dental Sciences Department, College of Dentistry, Princess Nourah Bint Abdulrahman University, Riyadh, Saudi Arabia*

Correspondence should be addressed to Mohammed Alhussain; mosaalhussain@moh.gov.sa

Academic Editor: Giovanni Mergoni

Introduction. Radiculomegaly (marked elongation of dental roots) is a distinct dental abnormality with a major clinical significance that is closely related to oculofaciocardiodental syndrome (OFCD). Since OFCD syndrome was first identified in 1996, only a few cases of nonsyndromic/nonfamilial radiculomegaly have been reported. We report a new nonsyndromic/nonfamilial radiculomegaly case and the association of OFCD syndrome with the dental challenges. *Case Presentation.* 18-year-old medically free male presented to the screening dental clinics complaining of teeth malposition. Panoramic radiograph incidentally revealed extremely long and wide roots of almost all dentition. Apical radiographs and cone-beam computed tomography (CBCT) were taken to confirm this anomaly and to rule out any artifact. The images confirmed the excessive length of the roots. A cephalometric X-ray was performed on the patient to rule out any dentofacial deformity. History and physical examinations were negative for ocular or cardiac anomalies. Due to lack of evidence of physical signs and symptoms consistent with OFCD syndrome, genetic testing was not performed. *Conclusion.* Dentists need to be informed of the clinical and radiographic features of different dental anomalies, especially radiculomegaly, as it is considered one of the significant features of OFCD syndrome. Challenges related to radiculomegaly face dentists while the current literature has not yet provided a solid baseline for managing such patients. The challenges include repairing the root canals, extracting and/or moving the teeth orthodontically. Early diagnosis of the syndrome is crucial to prevent dental challenges and provide the best dental care services.

1. Introduction

The normal mechanism of crown and root development is a complex process, where three stages are included in the process: bud, cap, and bell stages. Hertwig's epithelial root sheath, a double layer of the epithelial sheath, provides guidance for root development when the crown is about to be completed [1]. The most common root malformations in humans arise from either developmental disorders of the root alone or disorders of radicular development as part of general tooth dysplasia [2]. Despite that, little is known about the mechanisms of root morphogenesis and elongation [3]. Hyperdontia, hypodontia, oligodontia, multiple roots, and taurodontia are all examples of abnormal tooth morphology and number [4].

Radiculomegaly, dental root gigantism, or extremely long dental roots is a rare dental anomaly affecting the roots of teeth, and canines are mostly affected. This condition has rarely been reported in the literature. The first reports of radiculomegaly [5–7] related it as a characteristic feature of the X-linked rare congenital syndrome, oculofaciocardiodental syndrome (OFCD). OFCD syndrome is an X-linked dominant trait with potential male lethality [4, 8, 9], which affects the ocular, facial, cardiac, and dental aspects, with

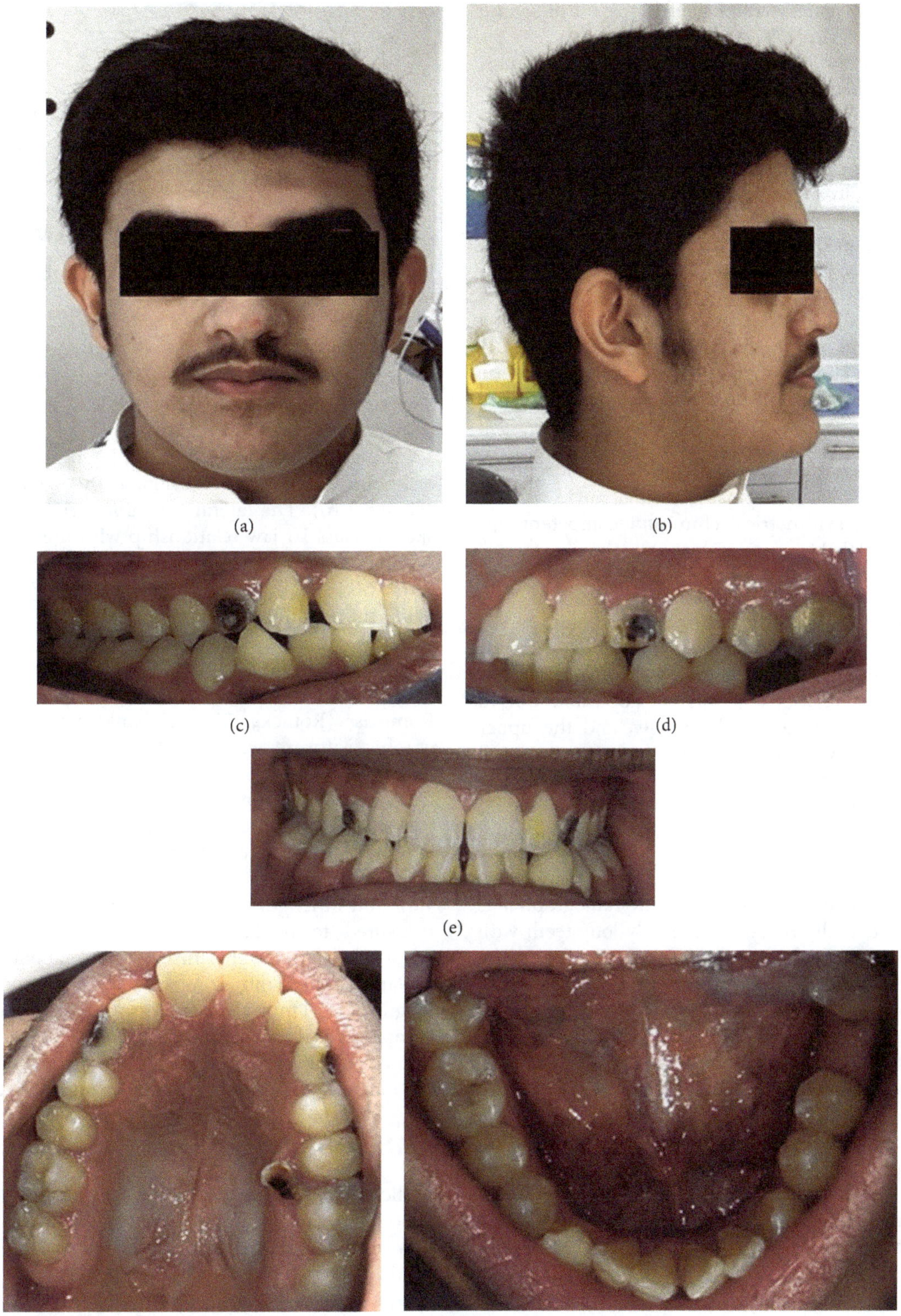

(a) (b) (c) (d) (e) (f) (g)

Figure 1: A clinical frontal view of the patient's face and neck (a), lateral profile view (b), intraoral lateral view of the patient's left side (c), IO right side (d), IO frontal view (e), IO upper occlusal view (f), and IO lower occlusal view (g).

an incidence of less than 1 in 1 million people [4, 8–11]. Among different dental anomalies that can be found with OFCD syndrome, radiculomegaly of the canines is highly related to this syndrome [4, 8, 12–14]. OFCD syndrome is characterized by heterogeneous clinical features such as dental radiculomegaly, congenital cataracts, facial dysmorphism, and congenital heart disease, which only affects females [10, 11, 15]. On the other hand, it was later identified as a defining feature of males with Klinefelter syndrome and Cockayne syndrome [16, 17].

To date, only a few nonsyndromic/nonfamilial radiculomegaly cases have been reported in the literature [8, 12, 18]. This case report aims to report a rare case of a nonsyndromic/nonfamilial generalized radiculomegaly case of an 18-year-old Saudi male patient and to investigate the association of OFCD syndrome with dental challenges.

2. Case Presentation

2.1. Patient History. An 18-year-old Saudi male patient with no relevant medical history is presented to the screening clinic at the College of Dentistry, King Saud University, Saudi Arabia. The chief complaint of the patient that he has "crooked teeth," with an unremarkable family history of any disease.

2.2. Extraoral Examination. The patient has a mesocephalic face with a concave profile, normal nasolabial angle, normal labiomental sulcus, symmetrical chin, and competent lips (Figures 1(a) and 1(b)).

2.3. Intraoral Examination. The examination showed poor oral hygiene with plaque and calculus accumulation on the lingual surface of the lower anterior teeth and multiple dental caries. The patient has a dental class III molar relationship, while canines' relationship was not applicable due to the missing permanent canines bilaterally, and the upper and lower midlines were centered. He has average vertical proportions, with 3 mm overjet and normal overbite. Moreover, the patient has retained maxillary primary canines, missing lower right first molar, upper mild spacing, and lower mild crowding (Figures 1(c)–1(g)).

2.4. Radiographic Assessment. A panoramic radiograph was taken which incidentally revealed extremely long teeth with relatively wide roots in almost all dentition (Figure 2). The permanent maxillary canines were impacted with notably long roots.

The roots of the maxillary teeth appear superimposed on the maxillary sinus and extend to about the level of the middle meatus. Maxillary second molars showed very long root trunks.

All mandibular teeth were long, especially the left second molar, which appears to be close to the inferior border of the mandible. The roots of mandibular third molars were developing in the inferior alveolar canals. The coronal portions of all teeth did not show any abnormalities in the aspect of shape or size. Further investigation to confirm the roots gigantism and to rule out any artifact was performed by taking periapical radiographs (Figure 3(a)). Due to the abnormal appearance of the roots, oculofaciocardiodental (OFCD) syndrome was included as a differential diagnosis. Thus, ophthalmology and cardiology teams were consulted for baseline assessment to rule out any association with OFCD syndrome. The ophthalmologic examination and investigation have included external eye examinations, visual acuity, extraocular muscles, visual fields, and intraocular pressure, while cardiology investigations have included

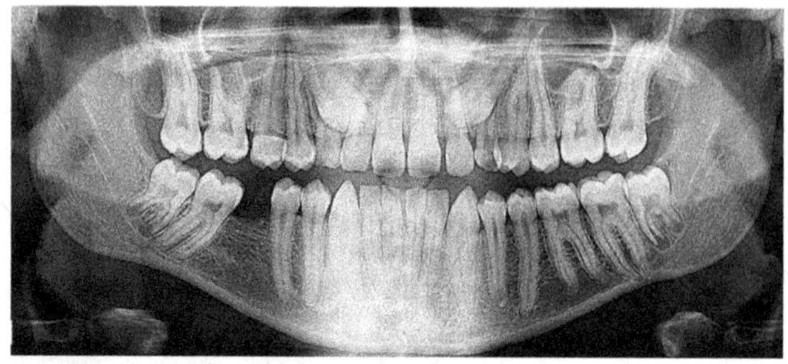

FIGURE 2: A panoramic radiograph showing the elongated roots of the teeth.

CVS auscultation, ECG, and echocardiogram. Both investigations did not show any ophthalmological or cardiac abnormalities. Furthermore, there was no family history of ocular or cardiac abnormalities.

A lateral cephalometric radiograph was taken for orthodontic purposes to evaluate the skeletal relationship (Figure 3(b)). The lateral cephalometric analysis showed a skeletal class III jaw relationship with mild maxillary retrusion and normal mandibular position (ANB, -2.1°; SNA, 77.6°; SNB, 79.8°). The maxillary incisors were proclined while the mandibular incisors exhibited lingual inclination (U1-PP, 121.4°; L1-GoGn, 79.3°). All measurements were done compared to the normative values (Figure 3(b)).

Cone beam computed tomography (CBCT) Planmeca Romexis® (Romexis 5.2.0., Helsinki, Finland) dental radiographic software was used to measure the length of the patient's entire set of teeth. Measurements were made from the apex to the tip of the cusps in a slice orientation manner (Figure 4). It has generally been reported that the vertical lengths of teeth share similar averages [19]. In this case, periapical radiographs (PAs) and CBCT revealed a significant variation in length. Permanent upper second premolar was measured to be 32.06 mm compared to the maximum reported length of 26.4 mm, the permanent upper second molar was 30.73 mm compared to the maximum reported length of 26.4 mm, permanent lower canine was 36.65 mm compared to the maximum reported length of 27.4 mm, and permanent lower second molar was 29.73 mm compared to the maximum reported length of 25.8 mm (Figure 4) [19].

3. Discussion

Radiculomegaly, or the marked elongation of the dental roots, is a rare congenital anomaly that has seldom been reported in the literature. The canine is the most affected tooth. The mandibular canine's length in a typical adult ranges from 24.6 to 27.4 mm with an average of 26 mm; therefore, a tooth is considered elongated when it is more than that [19]. Moreover, the apices of the canines do not close until adulthood, and mandibular roots with radiculomegaly often closely approach the lower border of the mandible [13]. Hayward was the first to describe radiculomegaly in 1980 [5]. Then, two more cases of radiculomegaly were described in the literature after Hayward's report [6, 7]. Only a few cases of nonsyndromic/nonfamilial radiculomegaly have been reported in the literature since the description of

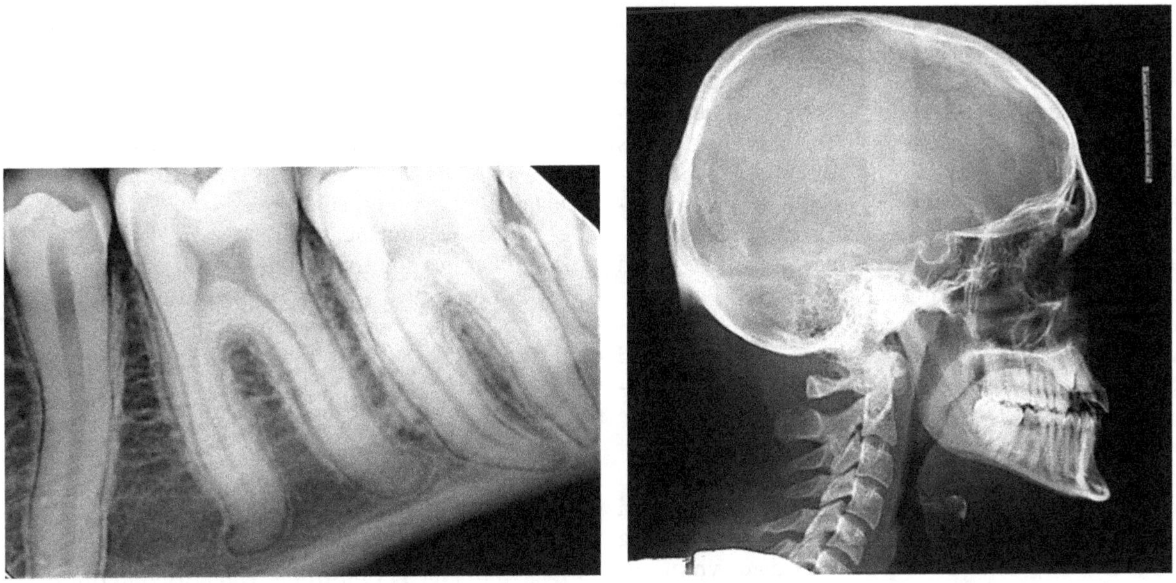

(a) (b)

FIGURE 3: Periapical radiograph shows long roots of teeth #35, 36, 37 (a) and lateral cephalometric radiograph of the patient (b).

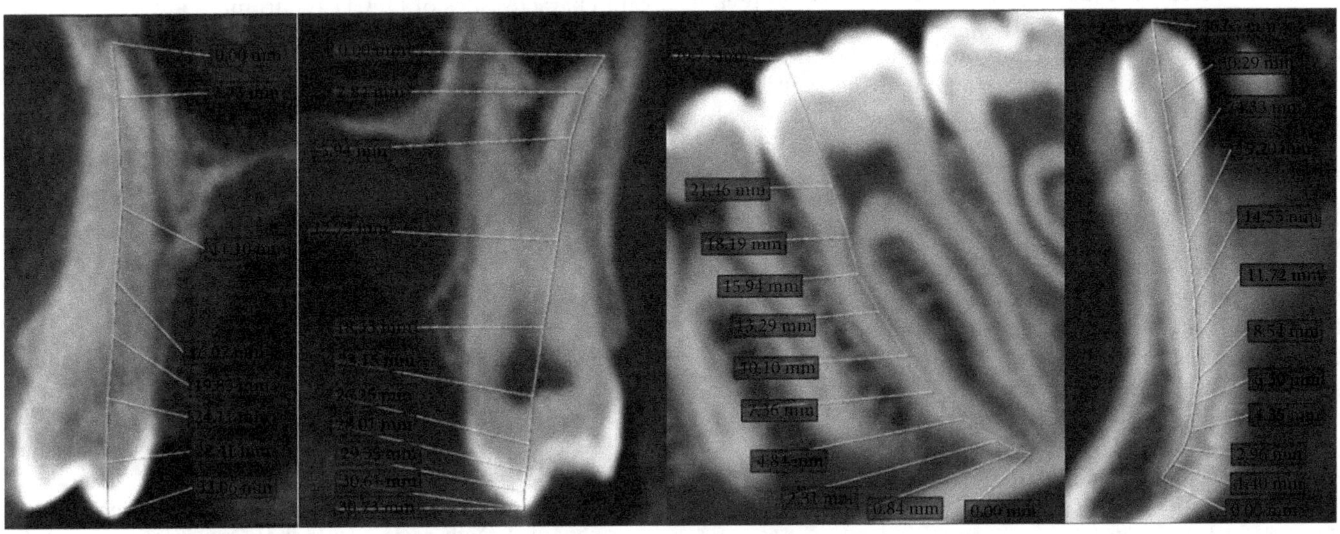

FIGURE 4: Sagittal section from cone beam computed tomography (CBCT) showing tooth sizes with radiculomegaly.

OFCD in 1996, and all of them are not related to OFCD syndrome [8, 12, 18]. Similar to our case, the patient reported by Kemoli and Junior presented with a dental class III molar relationship [12]. Likewise, Al-Obaida noted that the patient in his case has a protruded mandible [18]. However, both cases reported a V-shaped maxilla in their patients. Unlike our patient, who presented with a U-shaped maxillary arch [12, 18]. It is worth mentioning that crowding in the upper anterior segment was noted in the comparable cases. While our patient presented with an upper mild spacing [12, 18]. Interestingly, radiculomegaly was found rarely in males prior to our report [6, 11, 16–18]. OFCD syndrome is an inherited disorder with a dominant X-linked pattern with potential lethality of male hemizygotes that may happen in the early stages of embryonic development even before pregnancy is observed [11, 20]. The cause of the disorder is believed to be a truncated mutation in the BCOR (BCL-6 interacting corepressor) gene [21–24]. All published reports about OFCD syndrome patients have been females and rarely found in males, and none of them were having OFCD according to the literature [6, 11, 16–18]. Among the male cases, one case was an OFCD syndrome patient's brother [11], one was born with Cockayne syndrome [17], the third case was a report showing root elongation of an extracted tooth without related primary clinical data [6], the fourth case was diagnosed with Klinefelter syndrome [16], and the last case was a nonsyndromic generalized radiculomegaly in a Saudi individual [18]. Wilkie and Chambers, in a case of a mother and her daughter, reported that before the syndromic daughter was born, 2 miscarriages happened to the mother [7]. The authors suggested that the dominance of the mutated X chromosome may have caused the abortion, which is considered fatal in males [4, 8, 9]. Hedera and Gorski reported that having a skewed pattern of X chromosome methylation and a nonrandom inactivation pattern are found in patients with OFCD syndrome after they were confirmed by a thorough genetic investigation [25]. The authors indicated that in other X-linked conditions such as incontinentia pigmenti and focal dermal hypoplasia, a similar incident of male lethality was reported [25]. Although, in the investigated family and in other reported cases, they noted no indication of spontaneous male abortion [25]. Radiculomegaly of a tooth is mostly observed with other dental, ocular, facial, and cardiac anomalies, and the condition is called oculofaciocardiodental syndrome (OFCD) [11]. The phenotypic spectrum of OFCD includes mostly microphthalmia, microcornea, secondary glaucoma, and congenital cataract of the eyes [26–28]. The facial dysmorphic features are often elongation of a narrow face with a high nasal bridge and broadening of the nasal tip with separated cartilages, long philtrum, and cleft palate [26–28]. The cardiac symptoms are mainly atrial septal defect, ventricular septal defect, and mitral valve prolapse [26–28]. Syndactyly of toes 2-3, septate vagina, and sensorineural hearing loss are less frequently related manifestations [26–28]. In the present case, although the patient reported a dental history of overretained primary maxillary canines and impaction of the permanent ones in addition to the extraction of the permanent mandibular right first molar, he did not report any other medical problems. No personal or family history of ocular or cardiac abnormalities was observed after examining the patient. The absence of typical characteristics found in OFCD syndrome patients makes the diagnosis unlikely for the present patient. So far, root gigantism of all teeth from incisors to molars was documented in a few reports [11, 18, 27, 29]. Here, we report a new instance of generalized radiculomegaly of permanent teeth and the association of OFCD syndrome with dental challenges [19]. In endodontic treatment, poor prognosis is usually in teeth with extraordinary long roots and open apices [14, 30]. Besides, accessing the root canal system surgically should be avoided in treating lower teeth due to the flap size required to reach the apex that can damage critical anatomic structures such as the inferior alveolar nerve [30]. Although root canal therapy is difficult in teeth with unusual lengths, special endodontic methods can be used in treating such cases [14, 30]. In cases with very deep caries, the immediate treatment of them and the use of vital pulp therapy make it possible to preserve the function of the tooth and to avoid complicated endodontic procedures [30]. Maden et al., 2010, and Barthelemy et al., 2001, suggested that devitalization and early endodontic intervention to induce apical closure can be effective as preventive procedures for gigantic roots [14, 31]. Careful periodical dental examination and oral hygiene instructions in patients with radiculomegaly are essential to prevent dental caries and subsequent root canal treatment [30]. Moreover, root gigantism may complicate orthodontic treatment and would extend the treatment time. However, alignment of the dental arches can be achieved using light forces to minimize the risk of ankylosis or shortening of the roots [32]. Uribe et al., 2011, showed that teeth with radiculomegaly can be repositioned with traction on skeletal anchorage without causing ankylosis [33]. Sakaguchi et al., 2012, proved that teeth with long roots in patients with skeletal problems can be treated effectively with surgical orthodontic treatment with a light force so as not to cause ankylosis [34]. Likewise, the large size of the roots entails difficulties that make the extraction challenging because of the great amount of resistance during the removal [5]. Finally, this report demonstrates the important role of dental professionals in screening clinics to recognize unusual incidental findings which can be essential in providing information for the diagnosis of OFCD syndrome.

4. Conclusion

Radiculomegaly is rarely found as a nonsyndromic/nonfamilial generalized abnormality in male gender that is not related to OFCD syndrome, as reported in this patient. Dental professionals need to be informed of the clinical and radiographic features of different dental anomalies, especially radiculomegaly, as it is considered one of the significant characteristics of OFCD syndrome.

Consent

Written informed consent was taken from the patient to write the case report.

References

[1] X.-F. Huang and Y. Chai, "Molecular regulatory mechanism of tooth root development," *International Journal of Oral Science*, vol. 4, no. 4, pp. 177–181, 2012.

[2] H. U. Luder, "Malformations of the tooth root in humans," *Frontiers in Physiology*, vol. 6, p. 307, 2015.

[3] N. Suda and K. Moriyama, "Human diseases associated with abnormal tooth roots," *Journal of Oral Biosciences*, vol. 51, no. 4, pp. 199–204, 2009.

[4] J. Kato, K. Kushima, and F. Kushima, "New radiological findings and radiculomegaly in oculofaciocardiodental syndrome with a novel BCOR mutation: a case report," *Medicine (Baltimore)*, vol. 97, no. 49, article e13444, 2018.

[5] J. R. Hayward, "Cuspid gigantism," *Oral Surgery, Oral Medicine, and Oral Pathology*, vol. 49, no. 6, pp. 500-501, 1980.

[6] F. S. Weine, "A very long cuspid!," *Journal of Endodontia*, vol. 12, no. 2, pp. 80-81, 1986.

[7] G. J. Wilkie and I. G. Chambers, "A very large maxillary cuspid," *Oral Surgery, Oral Medicine, and Oral Pathology*, vol. 70, no. 2, pp. 159-160, 1990.

[8] M. H. Smith, D. M. Cohen, I. Bhattacharyya, N. M. Islam, and D. Kashtwari, "Radiculomegaly: a case report of this rare dental finding with review of the associated oculo-facio-cardio-dental syndrome," *Oral Surgery, Oral Medicine, Oral Pathology, Oral Radiology*, vol. 126, no. 4, pp. e220–e227, 2018.

[9] A. Davoody, I.-P. Chen, R. Nanda, F. Uribe, and E. J. Reichenberger, "Oculofaciocardiodental syndrome: a rare

case and review of the literature," *The Cleft Palate-Craniofacial Journal*, vol. 49, no. 5, pp. 55–60, 2012.

[10] A. O. Wilkie, D. Taylor, P. J. Scambler, and M. Baraitser, "Congenital cataract, microphthalmia and septal heart defect in two generations: a new syndrome?," *Clinical Dysmorphology*, vol. 2, no. 2, pp. 114–119, 1993.

[11] R. J. Gorlin, A. H. Marashi, and H. L. Obwegeser, "Oculo-facio-cardio-dental (OFCD) syndrome," *American Journal of Medical Genetics*, vol. 63, no. 1, pp. 290–292, 1996.

[12] A. M. Kemoli and T. M. Junior, "Bilateral second premolars agenesia together with a unilateral canine radiculomegaly," *Contemporary Clinical Dentistry*, vol. 8, no. 1, pp. 151–154, 2017.

[13] M. Iwase, H. Nishijima, G. Kondo, and M. Ito, "Radiculomegaly of permanent canines and first premolars: report of two cases in conjunction with oculo-facio-cardio-dental syndrome," *International Journal of Case Reports and Images*, vol. 6, no. 3, p. 189, 2015.

[14] M. Maden, A. Savgat, and G. Görgül, "Radiculomegaly of permanent canines: report of endodontic treatment in OFCD syndrome," *International Endodontic Journal*, vol. 43, no. 12, pp. 1152–1161, 2010.

[15] A. H. Marashi and R. J. Gorlin, "Radiculomegaly of canines and congenital cataracts–a syndrome?," *Oral Surgery, Oral Medicine, and Oral Pathology*, vol. 70, no. 6, pp. 802-803, 1990.

[16] R. Lähdesmäki and L. Alvesalo, "Root lengths in the permanent teeth of Klinefelter (47,XXY) men," *Archives of Oral Biology*, vol. 52, no. 9, pp. 822–827, 2007.

[17] A. Bloch-Zupan, M. Rousseaux, V. Laugel et al., "A possible cranio-oro-facial phenotype in Cockayne syndrome," *Orphanet Journal of Rare Diseases*, vol. 8, no. 1, p. 9, 2013.

[18] M. Al-Obaida, "A rare case of nonsyndromic generalized radiculomegaly with a literature review," *Case Reports in Dentistry*, vol. 2020, Article ID 3974829, 7 pages, 2020.

[19] A. M. Bjorndal, W. G. Henderson, A. E. Skidmore, and F. H. Kellner, "Anatomic measurements of human teeth extracted from males between the ages of 17 and 21 years," *Oral Surgery, Oral Medicine, and Oral Pathology*, vol. 38, no. 5, pp. 791–803, 1974.

[20] Z. Fan, T. Yamaza, J. S. Lee et al., "BCOR regulates mesenchymal stem cell function by epigenetic mechanisms," *Nature Cell Biology*, vol. 11, no. 8, pp. 1002–1009, 2009.

[21] H. E. Feberwee, I. Feenstra, S. Oberoi et al., "Novel BCOR mutations in patients with oculofaciocardiodental (OFCD) syndrome," *Clinical Genetics*, vol. 85, no. 2, pp. 194–197, 2014.

[22] D. Horn, M. Chyrek, S. Kleier et al., "Novel mutations in BCOR in three patients with oculo-facio-cardio-dental syndrome, but none in Lenz microphthalmia syndrome," *European Journal of Human Genetics*, vol. 13, no. 5, pp. 563–569, 2005.

[23] E. Hilton, J. Johnston, S. Whalen et al., "BCOR analysis in patients with OFCD and Lenz microphthalmia syndromes, mental retardation with ocular anomalies, and cardiac laterality defects," *European Journal of Human Genetics*, vol. 17, no. 10, pp. 1325–1335, 2009.

[24] D. Ng, N. Thakker, C. M. Corcoran et al., "Oculofaciocardiodental and Lenz microphthalmia syndromes result from distinct classes of mutations in _BCOR_," *Nature Genetics*, vol. 36, no. 4, pp. 411–416, 2004.

[25] P. Hedera and J. L. Gorski, "Oculo-facio-cardio-dental syndrome: skewed X chromosome inactivation in mother and daughter suggest X-linked dominant inheritance," *American Journal of Medical Genetics. Part A*, vol. 123A, no. 3, pp. 261–266, 2003.

[26] A. H. Marashi and R. J. Gorlin, "Radiculomegaly of canine teeth and congenital cataracts: confirmation of a syndrome," *American Journal of Medical Genetics*, vol. 42, no. 1, p. 143, 1992.

[27] B. R. Schulze, D. Horn, A. Kobelt, G. Tariverdian, and A. Stellzig, "Rare dental abnormalities seen in oculo-facio-cardio-dental (OFCD) syndrome: three new cases and review of nine patients," *American Journal of Medical Genetics*, vol. 82, no. 5, pp. 429–435, 1999.

[28] E. McGovern, M. Al-Mudaffer, C. McMahon, D. Brosnahan, P. Fleming, and W. Reardon, "Oculo-facio-cardio-dental syndrome in a mother and daughter," *International Journal of Oral and Maxillofacial Surgery*, vol. 35, no. 11, pp. 1060–1062, 2006.

[29] H. Tsukawaki, M. Tsuji, T. Kawamoto, and K. Ohyama, "Three cases of oculo-facio-cardio-dental (OFCD) syndrome," *The Cleft Palate-Craniofacial Journal*, vol. 42, no. 5, pp. 467–476, 2005.

[30] R. Pace, V. Giuliani, and G. Pagavino, "Endodontic management in oculo-facio-cardio-dental syndrome: a case report," *Journal of Endodontia*, vol. 37, no. 4, pp. 558–561, 2011.

[31] I. Barthelemy, L. Samuels, D. M. Kahn, and S. A. Schendel, "Oculo-facio-cardio-dental syndrome: two new cases," *Journal of Oral and Maxillofacial Surgery*, vol. 59, no. 8, pp. 921–925, 2001.

[32] A. T. Altug-Atac, "Oculofaciocardiodental syndrome and orthodontics," *American Journal of Orthodontics and Dentofacial Orthopedics*, vol. 131, no. 1, pp. 83–88, 2007.

[33] F. Uribe, A. Davoody, and R. Nanda, "Orthodontic treatment of a transposed gigantic canine –a case report," *Journal of Orthodontics*, vol. 38, no. 4, pp. 282–289, 2011.

[34] K. Sakaguchi, T. Yagi, J. Nagata, T. Kubota, K. Sugihara, and S. Miyawaki, "Patient with oculo-facio-cardio-dental syndrome treated with surgical orthodontics," *American Journal of Orthodontics and Dentofacial Orthopedics*, vol. 141, no. 4, pp. S159–S170, 2012.

4

Postsurgical Prosthetic Rehabilitation after Mandibular Ameloblastoma Resection: A 7-Year Follow-Up Case Report

C. Moreno-Soriano,[1] A. Estrugo-Devesa,[1,2] P. Castañeda-Vega,[1] E. Jané-Salas,[1,2] and J. López-López[1,2,3]

[1]Department of Odontostomatology, Faculty of Medicine and Health Sciences (Dentistry), University of Barcelona, L'Hospitalet de Llobregat, Barcelona, Spain
[2]Oral Health and Masticatory System Group, Institut d'Investigació Biomédica de Bellvitge (IDIBELL, Bellvitge Institute of Biomedical Research), L'Hospitalet de Llobregat, Barcelona, Spain
[3]Medical-Surgical Area of Dentistry Hospital University of Barcelona-University of Barcelona, L'Hospitalet de Llobregat, Barcelona, Spain

Correspondence should be addressed to J. López-López; jl.lopez@ub.edu

Academic Editor: Kenji Yamagata

Ameloblastomas are benign but locally invasive odontogenic tumors most frequently located in the mandible. The gold standard of treatment is the surgical resection of the tumor with safety margins. Postsurgical defects generate a significant morbidity that needs reconstruction and oral rehabilitation to restore the oral functions. This case report describes the prosthetic rehabilitation of a 42-year-old male after resection of a mandibular ameloblastoma. Excision of the lesion by segmental mandibulectomy and mandibular reconstruction by microvascularized fibula flap was performed. After placement of 6 dental implants, the patient was rehabilitated with a lower hybrid prosthesis fabricated using computer-aided design-computer-aided manufacturing. During a 7-year and 5-month follow-up, some clinical complications were observed.

1. Introduction

Ameloblastomas are benign but locally invasive odontogenic tumors derived from odontogenic epithelium. Their most frequent location is the mandible. No predilection for gender is described and a higher prevalence is shown between the 3rd and 4th decades of life [1]. These lesions represent 1% of oral tumors and 9-11% of all odontogenic tumors [2].

The recurrence rate is 90% if a conservative surgery such as curettage is performed. Otherwise, 15-20% recurrence rates can be achieved with marginal or segmental surgical resection [3].

Ameloblastomas can infiltrate up to 8 mm beyond the apparently healthy margin. Consequently, the gold standard of treatment is surgical resection with ≥1 cm safety margins [3].

Postsurgical defects may generate a significant morbidity that needs reconstruction and rehabilitation techniques to restore the oral functions of patients, increasing their quality of life [4]. Bone reconstruction can be achieved by flaps or bone regeneration materials [5]. Dental implants are the main option for prosthetic rehabilitation. An individualized treatment plan is necessary, which requires multidisciplinary teams: maxillofacial surgeons, implantologists, and prosthodontists.

The aim of the present paper is to present a complex case report of an oral rehabilitation after mandibular ameloblastoma resection, mandibular reconstruction, and placement of six dental implants, with some clinical complications of the peri-implant tissue during the follow-up.

2. Case Presentation

A 42-year-old man was referred for prosthetic rehabilitation to the Department of Dentistry for Cancer and Immunocompromised Patients at the Dentistry Hospital of the University of Barcelona.

The patient reported a medical history of controlled arterial hypertension (AHT) and did not have any significant allergies. As toxic habits, he consumed 20 cigarettes daily for 20 years and 1-2 units of alcohol daily.

Initially, the patient was referred from his Primary Health Center with an inflammatory process in the right mandible, which was being treated as a dental abscess (Figure 1). Due to nonremission of signs and symptoms, he was referred to the Department of Maxillofacial Surgery of the Head and Neck Unit at Bellvitge Hospital (L'Hospitalet de Llobregat). The following complementary tests were performed: orthopantomography (OPG) (Figure 2), computed tomography (CT) (Figure 3), and biopsy. The final diagnosis was a follicular ameloblastoma.

A stereolithographic surgical template from CT scan was created prior to the surgery to design the reconstruction plate and plan the surgery (Figure 4). Excision of the lesion by segmental mandibulectomy of the body and mandibular symphysis of the right side and mandibular reconstruction by microvascularized flap of the right fibula with cutaneous island were performed (Figure 5). A temporary percutaneous tracheostomy was also required. After the first surgery, a 6-month period was allowed to achieve an adequate osseointegration of the flap and soft tissue metaplasia (Figure 6).

Six dental implants (Tapered Screw-Vent; Zimmer Biomet Dental, Warsaw, IN, USA) were placed in the fibula (Figure 7). After the osseointegration of the implants, the patient was referred to the Department of Dentistry for Cancer and Immunocompromised Patients again. After prosthetic planning, the decision was taken to rehabilitate the patient with a lower hybrid prosthesis fabricated by CAD-CAM (Figures 8–10).

Periodic follow-ups were done over a period of 7 years and 5 months. As maintenance program, the hybrid prosthesis was unscrewed and cleaned every six months. Curettage with a plastic curette around the peri-implant tissue and irrigation with chlorhexidine were performed in order to avoid peri-implant disease. In every appointment, oral hygiene instructions were reinforced.

As medical and surgical history, he suffered two myocardial infarctions (MI) and underwent coronary angioplasty with the placement of two stents during the follow-up.

Four years and 7 months after the prosthesis placement, explantation of the most distal implant on the right side had to be done due to a lack of osseointegration (associated with peri-implant disease). Nonetheless, this fact did not affect the stability of the prosthesis.

One year and 5 months later, a biopsy of the peri-implant tissues on the left side was performed to rule out recurrence of ameloblastoma. The histopathological diagnosis was granulation tissue with epithelial hyperplasia without atypical changes.

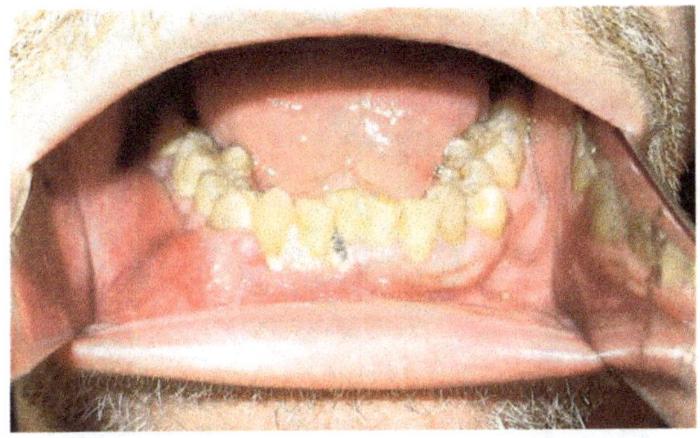

FIGURE 1: Intraoral image of the lesion. Note the swelling on the right mandibular premolar region.

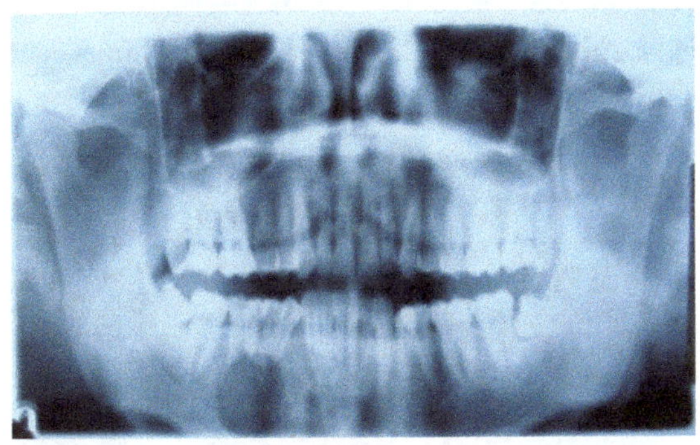

FIGURE 2: Preoperative orthopantomography.

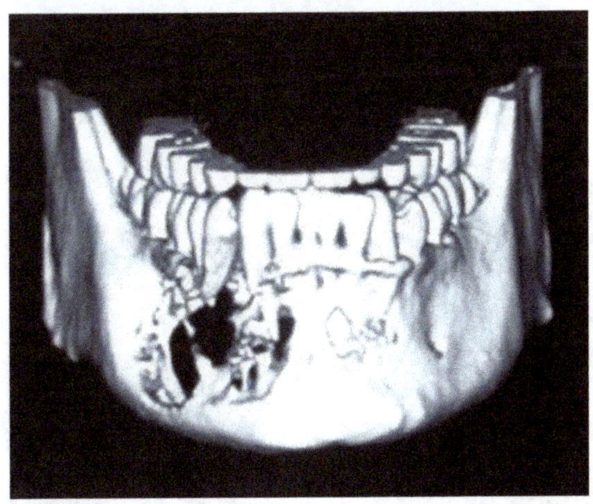

FIGURE 3: Preoperative computed tomography.

Six months later, the granulation tissue formation was observed on the right side. As a result, the prosthesis had to be removed. After a month, the tissues showed a clear improvement due to prosthesis removal.

Ten months later, as a solution to avoid the recurrence of granulation tissue due to the suspicion of a possible hypersensitivity reaction, the patient underwent partial removal of the metal reconstruction plate. After the healing process, the hybrid prosthesis was placed again and an improvement of the peri-implant tissue was observed after a 7-year and 5-month follow-up (Figure 11).

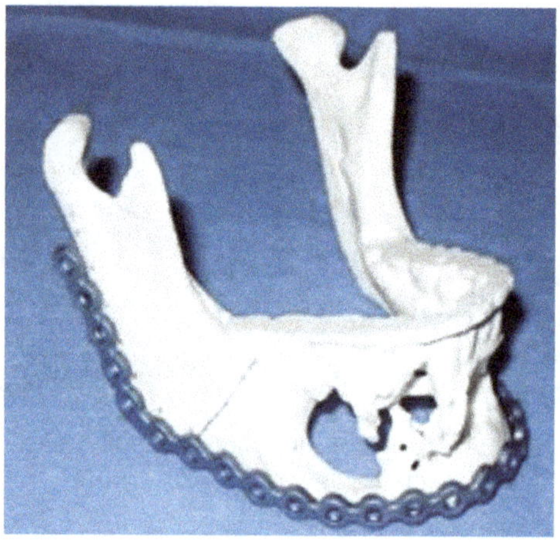

Figure 4: Stereolithographic surgical template from CT and reconstruction plate.

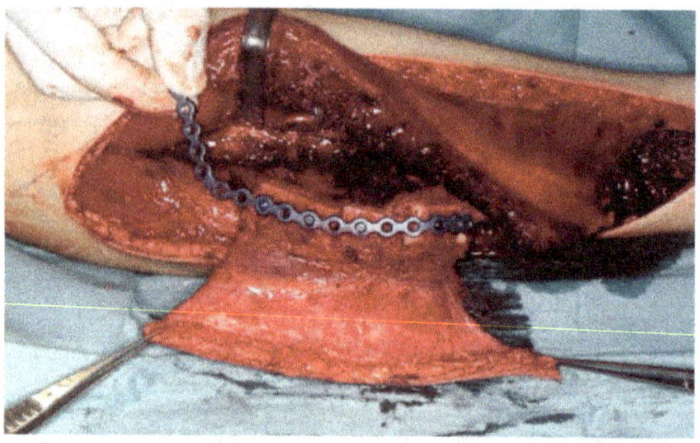

Figure 5: Microvascularized graft of the right fibula and reconstruction plate.

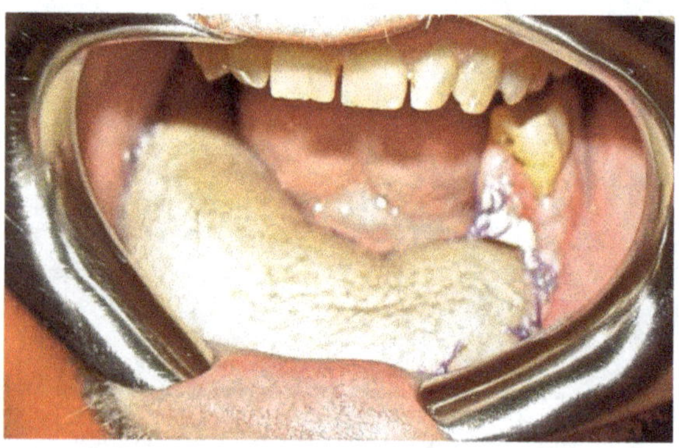

Figure 6: Postoperative intraoral image.

3. Discussion and Conclusion

Because of the high rate of recurrence of ameloblastomas when a conservative surgery is performed, the gold standard of treatment in extensive lesions is tumor resection with ≥1 cm safety margins [5]. Extensive curettages can compromise bone stability. This results in inadequate residual bone for implant placement, which can generate unpredictable results and long periods of oral rehabilitation. On the other hand, a surgery with safety margins ensures complete resec-

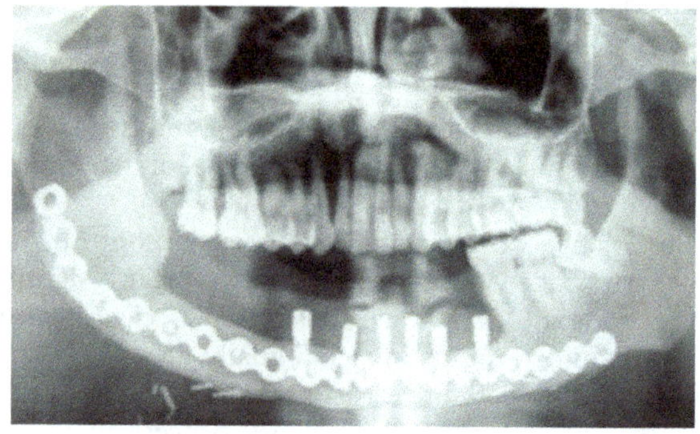

Figure 7: Orthopantomography after 6-implant placement on the fibula.

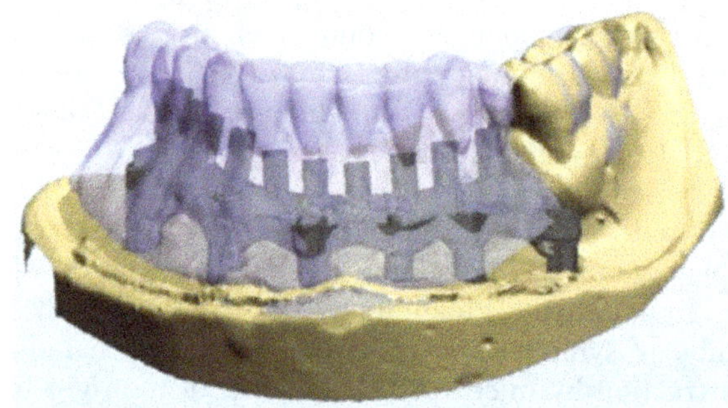

Figure 8: Design of the hybrid prosthesis by CAD-CAM.

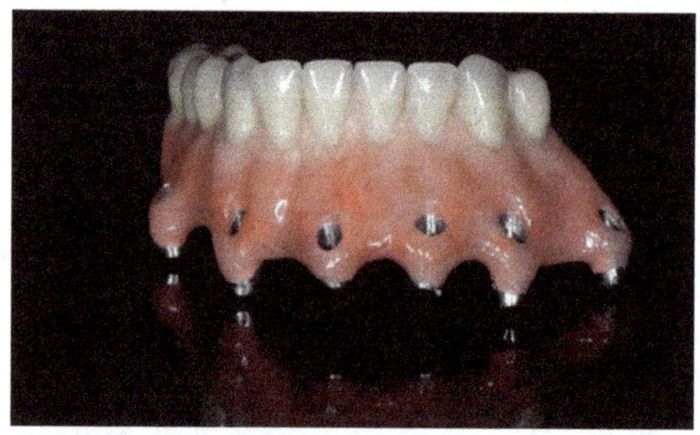

Figure 9: Frontal view of the finished lower hybrid prosthesis.

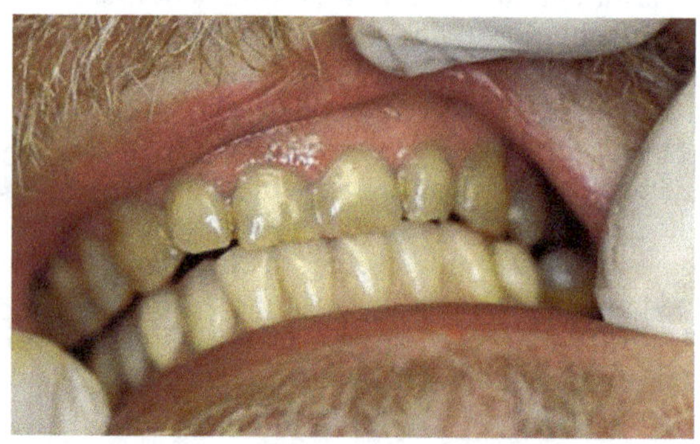

Figure 10: Intraoral image of the hybrid prosthesis placed into the mouth.

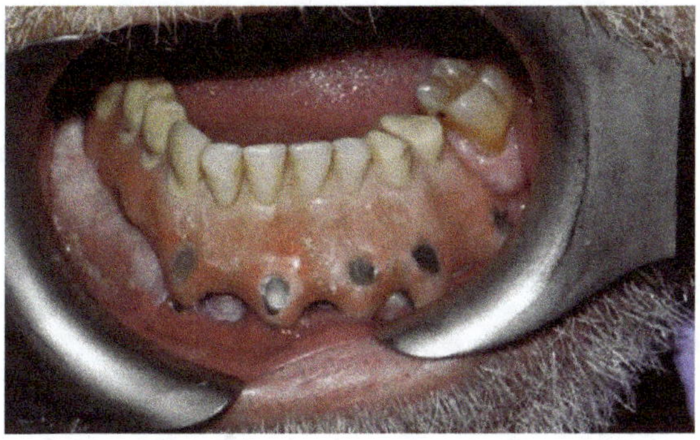

FIGURE 11: Intraoral image of the patient at the end of the treatment after a 7-year and 5-month follow-up.

tion of the tumor, prevents recurrence, and leads to a treatment with a faster and safer rehabilitation [6].

An immediate reconstruction of the postoperative defect is essential to avoid aesthetic problems and functional sequelae such as malocclusions, pathological fractures, or facial asymmetry, leading to concomitant psychosocial problems [5]. The functional reconstruction of large mandibular segments with microvascularized flaps and dental implants is considered the best option. This technique has been widely discussed during the last three decades [7].

Regarding the microvascularized flap, the fibula bone may not provide an adequate height, creating a considerable discrepancy between the reconstructed segment and the occlusal plane [8]. Consequently, implants need longer prosthetic structures in order to approach the occlusal plane, generating excessive leverage forces, overload in the prosthesis, and compromising its long-term success. Moreover, together with a poor oral hygiene, the aforementioned discrepancy between the implants and the occlusal plane creates an ideal space for bacteria growth around peri-implant tissues, which results in granulation tissue growth. To solve this problem, a double-bar fibular flap was proposed [9].

The most remarkable aesthetic and functional benefits are related to implant placement at the same time as the surgical resection of the lesion and mandibular reconstruction. This method allows for placement of implants in the fibula bone structure at a suitable height for a correct and restores occlusion in a single step. Furthermore, this speeds up the oral rehabilitation process and decreases the number of surgeries for the patient [10]. In this case report, implants were placed 6 months after the segmental mandibulectomy, so the patient underwent two different surgeries. As a matter of fact, dental implants were not in a prosthetically driven position because of the anatomy and the bone availability of the fibula, apart from proximity to the reconstruction plate, which compromises the choice of the prosthetic treatment plan.

In reference to oral rehabilitation, a screw-retained hybrid prosthesis was selected as prosthetic treatment due to implants' position with regard to the upper teeth. The possibility of an overdenture was considered, but the corresponding bar or abutments would be too buccally positioned compared to the occlusal plane, which would compromise long-term stability. Moreover, there was a lack of sufficient labial and buccal sulcus to create space for an overdenture flange.

Another important factor is the follow-up period. As a result of the high rate of recurrence of ameloblastoma, it is important to have an exhaustive control of patients. Nevertheless, there is no consensus in the follow-up time related to this type of lesions. Also, the complementary tests play an essential role in these patients. Oral hygiene measures and patient collaboration are vitally important, because clinical complications with the prosthesis may occur, especially food retention, peri-implant disease, and stimulation of the metaplastic tissue of the reconstruction flap. In this case, follow-up was performed over a period of 7 years and 5 months. As maintenance program, the hybrid prosthesis was unscrewed and cleaned every six months. Curettage with a plastic curette around the peri-implant tissue and irrigation with chlorhexidine were performed in order to avoid peri-implant disease. In every appointment, oral hygiene instructions were reinforced.

Consent

Written consent for publication was obtained from the patient.

References

[1] M. A. Oomens and I. van der Waal, "Epidemiology of ameloblastomas of the jaws; a report from the Netherlands," *Medicina Oral, Patología Oral y Cirugía Bucal*, vol. 19, pp. 581–583, 2014.

[2] R. Netto, W. Cortezzi, T. Nassif, M. Calasans-Maia, and R. S. Louro, "Rehabilitation with dental implants in microvascular iliac graft after solid ameloblastoma resection: a case report," *Implant Dentistry*, vol. 22, no. 6, pp. 561–565, 2013.

[3] S. Anil Kumar, N. K. Sahoo, and H. S. Sandhu, "Vascularised fibula osteocutaneous flap for mandibular reconstruction and multiple implant retained fixed prosthetic rehabilitation of a patient with mandibular ameloblastoma," *Medical Journal, Armed Forces India*, vol. 71, pp. 534–537, 2015.

[4] R. M. Lustosa, D. de Vasconcelos Macedo, L. C. V. Iwaki et al., "Continuity resection of the mandible after ameloblastoma - feasibility of oral rehabilitation with rhBMP-2 associated to bovine xenograft followed by implant installation," *Journal of Cranio-Maxillo-Facial Surgery*, vol. 43, no. 8, pp. 1553–1560, 2015.

[5] T. Bucci and P. F. Nocini, "Functional reconstruction of non-segmental mandibular defect with fresh frozen bone graft and delayed implants placement," *The Journal of Craniofacial Surgery*, vol. 28, no. 3, pp. 810–812, 2017.

[6] B. Bianchi, A. Ferri, S. Ferrari et al., "Mandibular resection and reconstruction in the management of extensive ameloblastoma," *Journal of Oral and Maxillofacial Surgery*, vol. 71, no. 3, pp. 528–537, 2013.

[7] M. C. Gil, T. Bucci, B. D. Ruiz, C. N. Vila, G. Marenzi, and G. Sammartino, "Implant mandibular rehabilitation postoncologic segmental resection: a clinical report," *Implant Dentistry*, vol. 21, no. 2, pp. 104–107, 2012.

[8] A. Kim, K. Kar, H. Nowzari, H. S. Cha, and K. M. Ahn, "Immediate free iliac bone graft after nonsegmental mandibular resection and delayed implant placement: a case series," *Implant Dentistry*, vol. 22, no. 5, pp. 438–443, 2013.

[9] Y. M. Chang, C. Y. Tsai, and F. C. Wei, "One-stage, double-barrel fibula osteoseptocutaneous flap and immediate dental implants for functional and aesthetic reconstruction of segmental mandibular defects," *Plastic and Reconstructive Surgery*, vol. 122, no. 1, pp. 143–145, 2008.

[10] Y. F. Shen, E. D. Rodriguez, F. C. Wei, C. Y. Tsai, and Y. M. Chang, "Aesthetic and functional mandibular reconstruction with immediate dental implants in a free fibular flap and a low-profile reconstruction plate: five-year follow-up," *Annals of Plastic Surgery*, vol. 74, no. 4, pp. 442–446, 2015.

5

Diode Laser Surgery as a Conservative Management of Hairy Tongue Lesion Resistance to Treatment

Nazanin Samiei[1] **Hadi Kaseb Ghane**[2] **and Reza Fekrazad**[3,4]

[1]*Periodontics Department, School of Dentistry, Tehran University of Medical Sciences, Tehran, Iran*
[2]*Department of Prosthodontics, Dental Branch, Islamic Azad University of Medical Sciences, Tehran, Iran*
[3]*Radiation Sciences Research Center, Laser Research Center in Medical Sciences, AJA University of Medical Sciences, Tehran, Iran*
[4]*International Network for Photo Medicine and Photo Dynamic Therapy (INPMPDT), Universal Scientific Education and Research Network (USERN), Tehran, Iran*

Correspondence should be addressed to Reza Fekrazad; rezafekrazad@gmail.com

Academic Editor: Gianluigi Caccianiga

Hairy tongue is a furry appearance on the dorsum surface of the tongue with variable colors. This lesion is due to defective shedding of filiform papillae. Various treatments are proposed for this condition like keratolytic agents, surgical procedure with a scalpel, or laser application. In this case study, we reported successful treatment of hairy tongue with a diode laser. The diode laser with wavelength 810 nm, power of 4 watts, a pulse width of 20 milliseconds, and an interval of 20 milliseconds by a 400-micron optical fiber was selected for treatment of this lesion. There was no bleeding during this minimally invasive surgery, and the patient experienced a low level of pain. Loss of taste function was completely resolved. Based on the result of this study, a diode laser can be a good alternative for minimally invasive surgical treatment of hairy tongue.

1. Introduction

Hairy tongue (HT), known as furred tongue, is referred to as an acquired benign tongue pathology. From the clinical view, HT is diagnosed through "hair-like" projections, developed when elongated, and hypertrophied filiform papillae are present on anterior 2/3 of dorsum aspect of the tongue. This pathology is the consequence of decreasing in cell desquamation and accumulation of keratinized layers [1].

HT may occur in various colors ranging from unpigmented, whitish, yellowish, bluish, tan, brown to black. Accordingly, what determines the color is an extrinsic factor that adheres to the lingual surface [2].

It may be prevalent within a wide range of 8.3 to 57% percent. Although there is no age limit for HT, its incidence and prevalence are positively correlated with age. It is reported to be more prevalent among men, yet females are also prone to this pathology [3]. According to a large cross-sectional study, an overall prevalence of HT was 11.3% with increased rates in men (18%) compared to women (6%) [4].

HT is associated with the following:1—poor oral hygiene; 2—smoking; 3—drugs (antibiotics such as penicillin, tetracycline, doxycycline, and erythromycin and medications inducing xerostomia including antidepressant, anticholinergics, and other drugs like olanzapine, aureomycin, and neomycin); 4—low fiber diets; 5—Candida albicans; 6—anemia; 7—alcohol; 8—dentures; 9—therapeutic radiation of head and neck. Scarcely has HT been found in human immunodeficiency virus (HIV) infection, graft versus host disease (GVHD), and internal malignancies [3].

It is asymptomatic and self-resolving in general, but patients may occasionally complain about halitosis, abnormal taste, gagging and tickling sensation, nausea, dysgeusia, and burning mouth sensation [5]. As the first-line treatment, it is necessary to identify and eliminate/modify predisposing factors; then, it comes to regularly brushing the tongue (gentle debridement with a toothbrush or tongue scraper) to promote desquamation and ultimately improve the oral hygiene [6].

Literature has also outlined the second-line therapy in different measures like topical retinoid, keratolytic agents (podophyllin), antimicrobial therapies, topical triamcinolone acetonide, gentian violet, salicylic acid, vitamin B complex, thymol, topical urea solution, and keratolytic agents like trichloroacetic acid. What merits attention is that the above-mentioned therapeutic measures are endowed with potential side effects from local irritation and possible systemic absorption. Surgical treatment of several oral lesions (namely, hemangioma, pyogenic granuloma, fibroma, and HT) can be addressed by laser application with different modalities like CO_2, Erbium family, Nd: YAG, and diode lasers [7, 8]. Less invasive nature along with excellent hemostasis, wound disinfection, and great patient comfort make it more popular than a conventional scalpel in the surgical treatment of oral lesions [9]. Meserendio and Pick in 1995 [10] first introduced diode laser in oral surgery. Since then, diode laser has become popular due to its small size, low cost, and user-friendly features. In this case study, we are reporting the treatment of hairy tongue by diode laser and explain different aspects of this treatment modality.

2. Case Presentation

A 22-year-old nonsmoker woman presented with whitish-yellowish discoloration on the dorsum of the tongue and was referred to a private dental office (Figure 1). The patient mentioned that with about 1.5 year of evolution, she had experienced ageusia. She denied any other symptoms, namely, tongue pain and halitosis. She had been prescribed different medications and treatments, but no perceived improvement was noticed. This issue affected her quality of life and made her frustrated.

Medical history was unremarkable. She did not take any medication. She mentioned that she had high-stress lifestyle due to her job. Intraoral examination showed good oral hygiene according to Silness and Löe [11] plaque index. On soft tissue examination, no abnormalities were detected on the buccal and labial mucosa and palate. The whitish-yellowish discoloration appeared as an elongation of the filiform papillae on the dorsum of the tongue. As it could not be wiped by gauze, the case was clinically diagnosed with HT.

After obtaining informed consent, a surgery was performed under local anesthesia (lidocaine HCL 2% with epinephrine 1:100,000). A diode laser (Twilight, Biolase Technologies, USA) was used by an expert surgeon. The laser enjoyed a wavelength of 810 nm, a power of 4 watts, a pulse width 20 milliseconds, and an interval of 20 milliseconds by a 400-micron optical fiber. The half of the lesion was removed by the laser in a slowly sweeping motion 4 mm above the surface and with a 30-degree angle relative to the tongue (to decrease penetration depth and reduce tissue damage) for 3-4 minutes, accompanied by high vacuum suction removal (Figure 2(a)). Special care was taken to remove only elongated filiform papillae and not to damage fungiform, circumvallate, and foliate papillae. Then, the surgical site was swept off with wet gauze. Chlorhexidine mouthwash (0.2%) was prescribed without any antibiotic therapies. No bleeding was reported after surgery. The patient experienced a low level of postoperative pain and just took few analgesics.

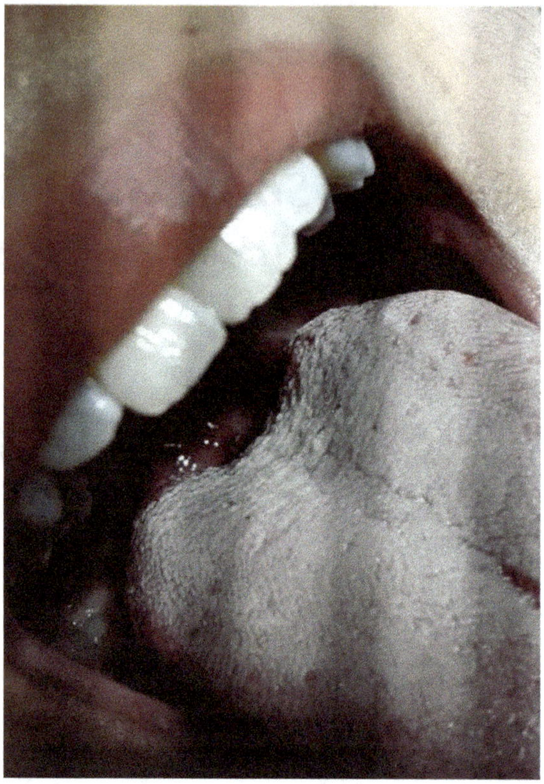

Figure 1: Dorsum of the tongue before treatment.

In the follow-up session after 1 and 2 weeks, partial healing was observed (Figures 2(b) and 2(c)). The other half of the lesion was removed by the same diode laser mode (Figures 3(a) and 3(b)). This procedure was done conservatively in two sessions in order to check the results in the follow-up sessions. After 1 month, complete healing was achieved with the resolution of ageusia. The patient was also examined 3 months later for assessing any sign of recurrence (Figure 4).

3. Discussion

HT is a relatively common abnormal coating on the dorsal surface of the tongue. This condition stems from elongation and lack of desquamation of filiform papillae, so they grow longer rather than falling off [12].

Various techniques have been employed to treat this lesion. We started with the second-line treatment (surgical procedure) as the patient's oral hygiene was good, and she did not have any risk factors (the requirements of the first-line treatment). Applying a knife to carry out the surgical excision of the papillae may be followed by some bleeding, where suturing is difficult and needs special skill. Also, it causes the removal of massive amount of tissue (with no control), which in turn increases the healing period and

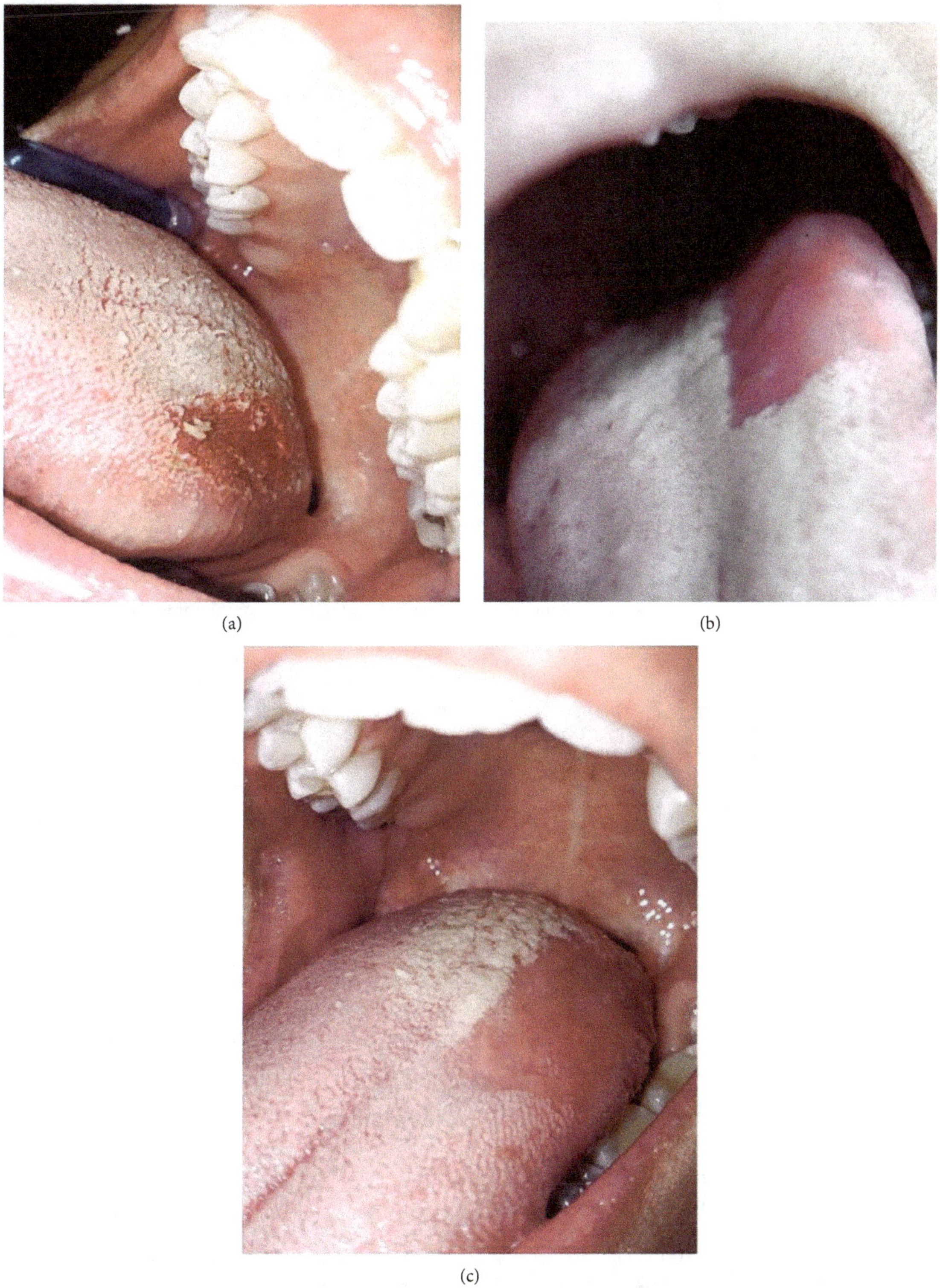

FIGURE 2: Clinical view of the tongue: (a) immediately after removing half of the lesion by the application of a diode laser; (b) one week after surgery; (c) two weeks after surgery.

levels of pain [13]. Laser technology could provide an escape from these complications. In this case, we could use different laser modalities. Due to low penetration depth and high absorption, CO_2 and Erbium family lasers are good options [14], but they are relatively high cost and not easily available [15]. The diode laser (450-1100) has become very popular in general dentistry as it is small in size and less costly, it enjoys fiber optic delivery, and it is user-friendly for minor oral soft tissues surgeries [16]. Regarding diode laser, research has shown that the wavelength around 810 nm is one of the most

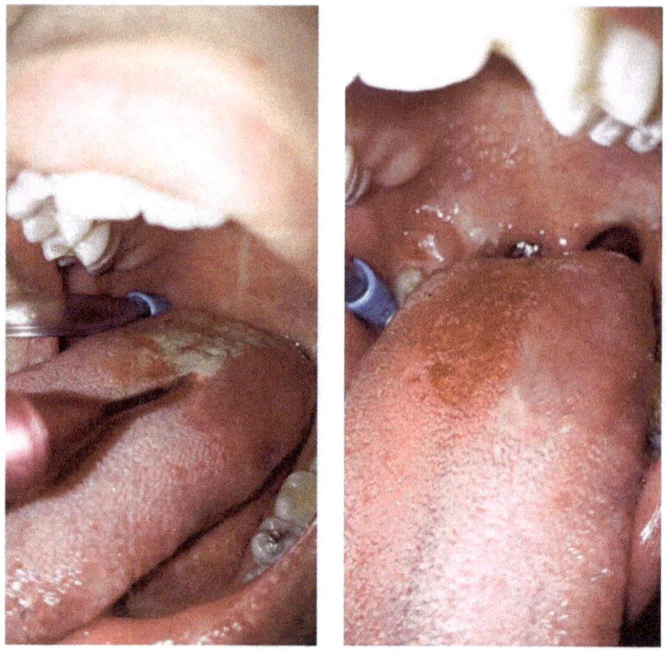

(a) (b)

FIGURE 3: Clinical view of the tongue: (a, b) removing the other half of the lesion by the same diode laser mode.

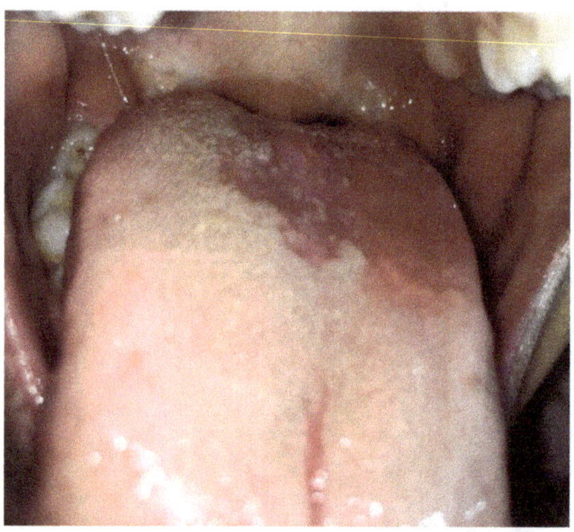

FIGURE 4: Three months after surgical procedure with a diode laser.

versatile wavelength ranges with regard to the number of different treatments it can be used for (soft tissue surgery, periodontal therapy, implantology, endodontics, photobiomodulation therapy, and teeth whitening) [17].

Thanks to the hemostasis and coagulation effect of the laser, the operator had an outstanding field visibility during the procedure and there was no need for suturing. Patients undergoing a diode laser surgery in the oral cavity seem to have less pain. In addition, it was proven that the diode laser can eliminate bacteria and disinfect the wound [18–20]; in this regard, there is no need for postsurgical antibiotics. Despite electrocutter and scalpel, the penetration depth of diode lasers can be adjusted; accordingly, it reduces tissue injury and improves wound healing.

In this study, the patient was satisfied with the result of the surgery and her ageusia was completely resolved. Consequently, her quality of life was significantly improved. To evaluate the lesion recurrence, she was examined 3 months later and there was no sign of recurrence. For further evaluation, long-term follow-ups were recommended.

4. Conclusion

Within the context of this study, application of the diode laser in the treatment of hairy tongue can be beneficial for both patients and clinicians. This modality provides minimal postoperative complications and a simple surgical procedure with the least possible side effects.

References

[1] M. Manabe, H. W. Lim, M. Winzer, and C. A. Loomis, "Architectural organization of filiform papillae in normal and black hairy tongue epithelium: dissection of differentiation pathways in a complex human epithelium according to their patterns of keratin expression," *Archives of Dermatology*, vol. 135, no. 2, pp. 177–181, 1999.

[2] D. M. Laskin, J. A. Giglio, and E. T. Rippert, "Differential diagnosis of tongue lesions," *Quintessence International*, vol. 34, no. 5, pp. 331–342, 2003.

[3] M. Z. Handler, D. F. Butler, D. Eisen, J. Burgess, D. P. Lynch, and G. L. Stafford, *Hairy tongue*, 2017.

[4] N. Avcu and A. Kanli, "The prevalence of tongue lesions in 5150 Turkish dental outpatients," *Oral Diseases*, vol. 9, no. 4, pp. 188–195, 2003.

[5] G. E. Gurvits and A. Tan, "Black hairy tongue syndrome," *World Journal of Gastroenterology: WJG*, vol. 20, no. 31, pp. 10845–10850, 2014.

[6] J. A. Byrd, A. J. Bruce, and R. S. Rogers III, "Glossitis and other tongue disorders," *Dermatologic Clinics*, vol. 21, no. 1, pp. 123–134, 2003.

[7] R. Fekrazad, F. Fazilat, K. A. M. Kalhori, N. Hakimiha, M. Amirmoini, and M. Nikhalat Jahromi, "Juvenile hyaline fibromatosis management with a diode laser: a rare case report," *Journal of Lasers in Medical Sciences*, vol. 11, no. 1, pp. 104–107, 2020.

[8] R. Fekrazad, H. Nokhbatolfoghahaei, F. Khoei, and K. A. Kalhori, "Pyogenic granuloma: surgical treatment with Er: YAG laser," *Journal of Lasers in Medical Sciences*, vol. 5, no. 4, pp. 199–205, 2014.

[9] R. M. Pick and B. C. Pecaro, "Use of the CO_2 laser in soft tissue dental surgery," *Lasers in Surgery and Medicine*, vol. 7, no. 2, pp. 207–213, 1987.

[10] L. J. Meserendio and M. Pick Robert, "Lasers in dentistry: quintessence," *Journal of the American Dental Association (1939)*, vol. 126, no. 10, pp. 1354–1356, 1995.

[11] J. Silness and H. Löe, "Periodontal disease in pregnancy II. Correlation between oral hygiene and periodontal condition," *Acta Odontologica Scandinavica*, vol. 22, no. 1, pp. 121–135, 1964.

[12] D. F. Thompson and T. L. Kessler, "Drug-induced black hairy Tongue," *The Journal of Human Pharmacology and Drug Therapy*, vol. 30, no. 6, pp. 585–593, 2010.

[13] P. Lopez-Jornet and F. Camacho-Alonso, "Comparison of pain and swelling after removal of oral leukoplakia with CO_2 laser and cold knife: a randomized clinical trial," *Medicina oral, Patologia oral y Cirugia Bucal*, vol. 18, no. 1, article e38, e44 pages, 2013.

[14] S. K. Verma, P. K. Chaudhari, S. Maheshwari, and R. K. Singh, "Laser in dentistry: an innovative tool in modern dental practice," *National Journal of Maxillofacial Surgery*, vol. 3, no. 2, pp. 124–132, 2012.

[15] R. Pick and L. Miserendino, Eds., *Quintessence. Lasers in dentistry*, Chicago, 1995.

[16] M. Asnaashari and S. Zadsirjan, "Application of laser in oral surgery," *Journal of Lasers in Medical Sciences*, vol. 5, no. 3, pp. 97–107, 2014.

[17] S. Pirnat, "Versatility of an 810 nm diode laser in dentistry: an overview," *Journal | Laser & Health Academy*, vol. 4, no. 2, pp. 1–9, 2007.

[18] A. Eliades, C. Stavrianos, A. Kokkas, P. Kafas, and I. Nazaroglou, "808 nm diode laser in oral surgery: a case report of laser removal of fibroma," *Research Journal of Medical Sciences*, vol. 4, no. 3, pp. 175–178, 2010.

[19] G. Caccianiga, G. Rey, M. Baldoni, P. Caccianiga, A. Baldoni, and S. Ceraulo, "Periodontal decontamination induced by light and not by heat: comparison between oxygen high level laser therapy (OHLLT) and LANAP," *Applied Sciences*, vol. 11, no. 10, p. 4629, 2021.

[20] G. Caccianiga, E. Urso, R. Monguzzi, K. Gallo, and G. Rey, "Efecto bactericida del láser de diodo en periodoncia," *Avances en Periodoncia e Implantologia Oral*, vol. 19, no. 3, pp. 131–140, 2007.

6

Management of Inflammatory Root Resorption of Maxillary Central Incisors following Traumatic Avulsion

Seyed Mohsen Sadeghi[1] **Samaneh Moradi**[2] **and Samaneh Soltani**[3]

[1]*School of Dentistry, Department of Endodontics, Qom University of Medical Sciences, Qom, Iran*
[2]*School of Dentistry, Department of Endodontics, Isfahan University of Medical Sciences, Isfahan, Iran*
[3]*School of Dentistry, Department of Periodontology, Qom University of Medical Sciences, Qom, Iran*

Correspondence should be addressed to Samaneh Soltani; sas_851050@yahoo.com

Academic Editor: Andrea Scribante

Background. Avulsion is among the most severe types of dental trauma, which often occurs at young ages and can compromise the long-term prognosis of the traumatized tooth. *Case Report.* Herein, we report replantation of two avulsed teeth. Our patient was an 11-year-old boy with two avulsed maxillary central incisors due to a bicycle fall 2 months earlier. The patient was referred to us after rigid splinting of his teeth by a surgeon. Long-term calcium hydroxide (CH) therapy was performed for the patient, and after healing of periodontal ligament (PDL), apexification was performed for both teeth followed by root canal therapy. During the 2-year follow-up, both teeth were functional and had no radiographic or clinical evidence of resorption or ankylosis. *Conclusion.* The reported case highlights the favorably high tissue healing potential following severe dental trauma, given that appropriate treatment is performed. Correct endodontic management can guarantee the long-term prognosis of teeth following severe dental trauma.

1. Introduction

Severe dental traumas often cause complex dental fractures or injuries and can simultaneously involve the dental hard tissue, periodontium, and dental pulp. The currently used classification for dental traumas differentiates between the fracture injuries and tooth displacement/luxation. Concussion and subluxation are the most common displacement traumas while avulsion has a lower prevalence and accounts for 7% to 23% of dislocation traumas. Horizontal root fracture of permanent teeth is an uncommon incidence, with a prevalence rate of 0.5% to 0.7% [1]. The prevalence of avulsion is higher in children between 7 and 9 years, and often involves a maxillary incisor. Falls, fights, and sport injuries are often the main etiology [1]. The long-term consequences of dental trauma can adversely affect the long-term prognosis of the traumatized teeth and can even lead to tooth loss and its consequent adverse functional and esthetic sequelae. Thus, early management and regular follow-ups are imperative to prevent these consequences [2]. The level of injury to the periodontium of the avulsed tooth determines its prognosis. Thus, timely endodontic intervention of avulsed teeth is imperative to improve their long-term prognosis. The chance of pulpal regeneration in avulsed teeth is low (around 10%) even under ideal conditions. Therefore, there is high risk of complications if endodontic interventions are postponed or not performed [3].

The time interval between the avulsion and replantation of the tooth, as well as the storage medium in which the tooth is stored during this time period, are critical factors determining the periodontal prognosis of the avulsed tooth. Periodontal injuries due to dehydration or immersion in a nonphysiological solution would cause inflammatory or replacement/substitutive root resorption, which would highly jeopardize the success of subsequent treatments. If endodontic treatment is not performed or is performed after a delay, the root canal system becomes infected. The infection can reach the injured cementum through the dentinal tubules and cause infection-related root resorption [2]. In case of occurrence of inflammatory root resorption, endodontic treatment and induced formation of a root-end barrier (apical plug) by the application of calcium hydroxide (CH), mineral trioxide aggregate (MTA), or other biomaterials should be considered [4].

Treatment of horizontal root fracture is often limited to repositioning of the coronal segment and semirigid splinting for 2 to 4 weeks to provide function and comfort for the patient. Dental pulp often remains viable in 80% of the cases. In case of occurrence of the signs and symptoms of pulpitis, root canal treatment of the coronal segment is performed. In most cases, the apical segment remains vital and apical closure occurs in some cases [5].

This case report describes the management and 2-year follow-up of an 11-year-old boy with external root resorption of his avulsed maxillary left central incisor and horizontal root fracture and inflammatory root resorption of his avulsed maxillary right central incisor.

2. Case Report

2.1. Dental History. Our patient was an 11-year-old boy with a history of bicycle fall 2 months earlier, with the resultant dental trauma. He was taken to a hospital immediately after the accident, and his avulsed maxillary central incisors were replanted with a rigid splint (arch bar) by a surgeon after storage in milk for about an hour. The splints were removed by the surgeon after 1 month and the patient was referred to the Endodontics Department of the School of Dentistry.

2.2. First Treatment Session (2 Months after Trauma). Two months after the accident, the patient was referred to us for the first time. The patient was systemically healthy, and his facial soft tissue and gingiva were normal. Clinical and periapical radiographic examinations revealed horizontal root fracture in tooth #8 and external root resorption in teeth #8 and #9 (Figure 1). CBCT was needed, but the patient's parents did not accept due to radiation. The pulp vitality tests were performed. The traumatized teeth did not respond to the cold, heat, or electric pulp tests but were both sensitive to percussion and palpation and showed grade II mobility. Since 2 months had passed since the avulsion, long-term CH therapy was considered to stop the progression of inflammatory root resorption. Written informed consent was obtained from the patient and his parents. In the first treatment session, after local infiltration injection and access cavity preparation, canals were disinfected with 5.25% sodium hypochlorite, and filled with CH (Golchai, Iran) with creamy consistency. The teeth were then temporarily restored with Cavisol (Golchai, Iran) (Figure 2).

2.3. Second Treatment Session (1 Week Later). The temporary restoration was removed; the root canals were rinsed with sodium hypochlorite, and filled with CH with powdery consistency. The teeth were followed-up monthly to accomplish the root canal treatment in case of observing a sound and intact periodontal ligament (PDL) and complete resolution of inflammatory root resorption (Figure 3).

2.4. Third Treatment Session (3 Months Later). The process of root resorption had been stopped, and a sound PDL was

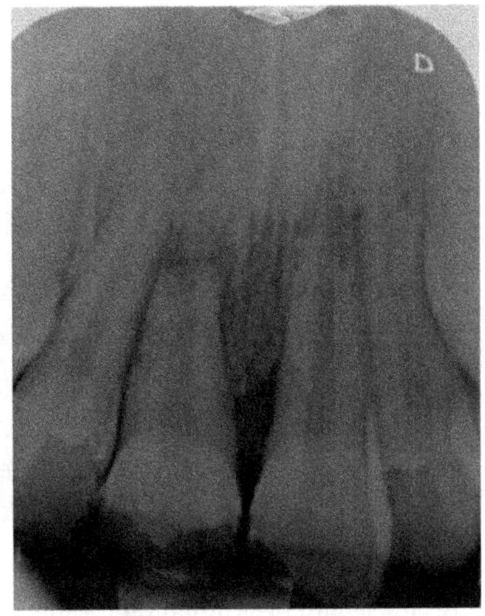

Figure 1: Periapical radiographs of the maxillary central incisors.

observed on the radiographs. Considering the poor patient cooperation, we decided to accomplish the endodontic treatment of the teeth within two sessions. Since the apices were open (larger than a #60 K-file), a 4 mm MTA plug was applied at the root end, and then the coronal part of the canal was filled by a warm vertical condensation technique. Fast-setting MTA Angelus (Angelus, Brazil) was used for filling the apical part of the root canal. In tooth #9, the apical 4 mm of the apex was instrumented with hand K-files after elimination of CH, rinsed with sodium hypochlorite and saline, dried with paper points, and filled with MTA Angelus. Next, the coronal part of the canal was filled with gutta-percha and AH-26 sealer using a warm vertical condensation technique (Figure 4).

2.5. Fourth Treatment Session. In tooth #8, the apical 4 mm of the canal was instrumented with hand K-files after elimination of CH, rinsed with sodium hypochlorite and saline, dried with paper points, and filled with MTA Angelus. The coronal part of the canal was then filled with gutta-percha and AH-26 sealer using a warm vertical condensation technique. The patient was then referred to the Operative Dentistry Department for restoration of both teeth (Figure 5).

2.6. Fifth Treatment Session (1 Year after Trauma). At the 1-year follow-up, tooth #9 showed discoloration (due to the bismuth oxide present in MTA Angelus) [6]. Thus, we decided to perform internal bleaching for correction of discoloration. The composite restoration of tooth #9 was removed, and gutta-percha was eliminated to 2 mm below the cementoenamel junction. A light-cured glass ionomer (GC, USA) was applied as a barrier, and sodium perborate was placed in the root canal as the bleaching agent. The tooth was then temporarily restored with the light-cured glass ionomer (Figure 6).

2.7. Sixth Treatment Session. One week later, the patient presented for continuation of bleaching treatment. Since the tooth color had been corrected, temporary restoration and sodium perborate were removed and the patient was

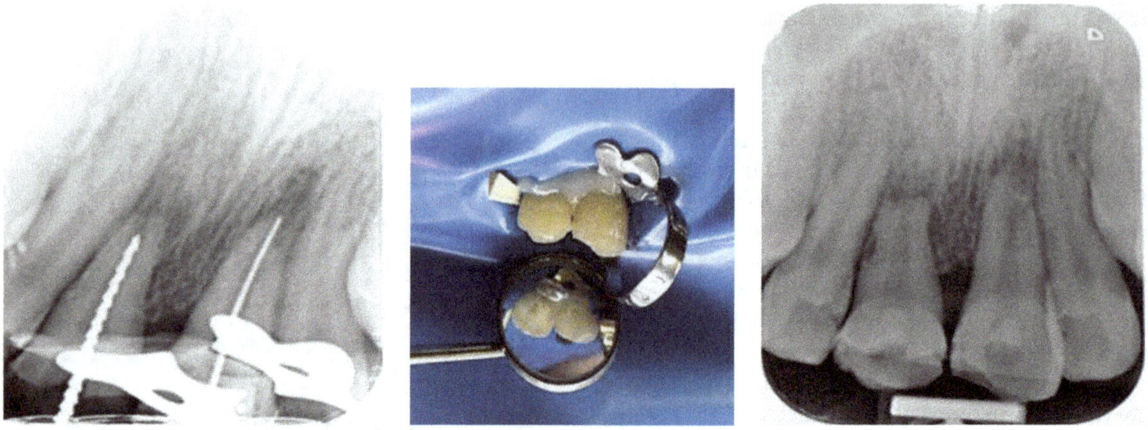

(a) (b) (c)

FIGURE 2: (a) Working length determination for the maxillary central incisors; (b) isolation with clamp, flowable composite, and wedge; (c) apexification with calcium hydroxide and temporary restoration of the access cavity.

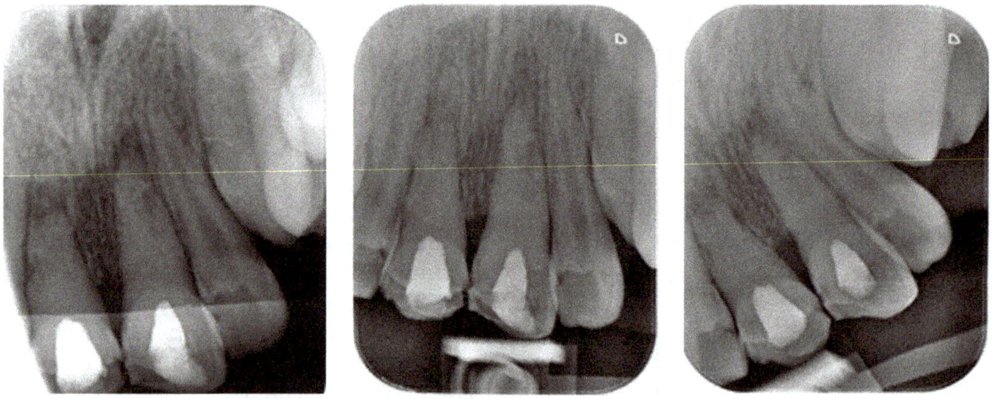

(a) (b) (c)

FIGURE 3: (a) Periapical radiograph taken at 1 month after the application of powdery calcium hydroxide; (b) periapical radiograph taken after 2 months; (c) periapical radiograph taken after 3 months, showing sound periodontal ligament.

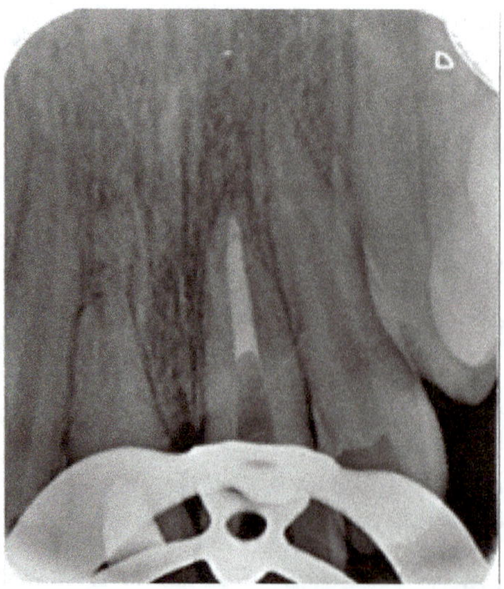

FIGURE 4: Periapical radiograph taken after one-session apexification of tooth #9 with MTA plug.

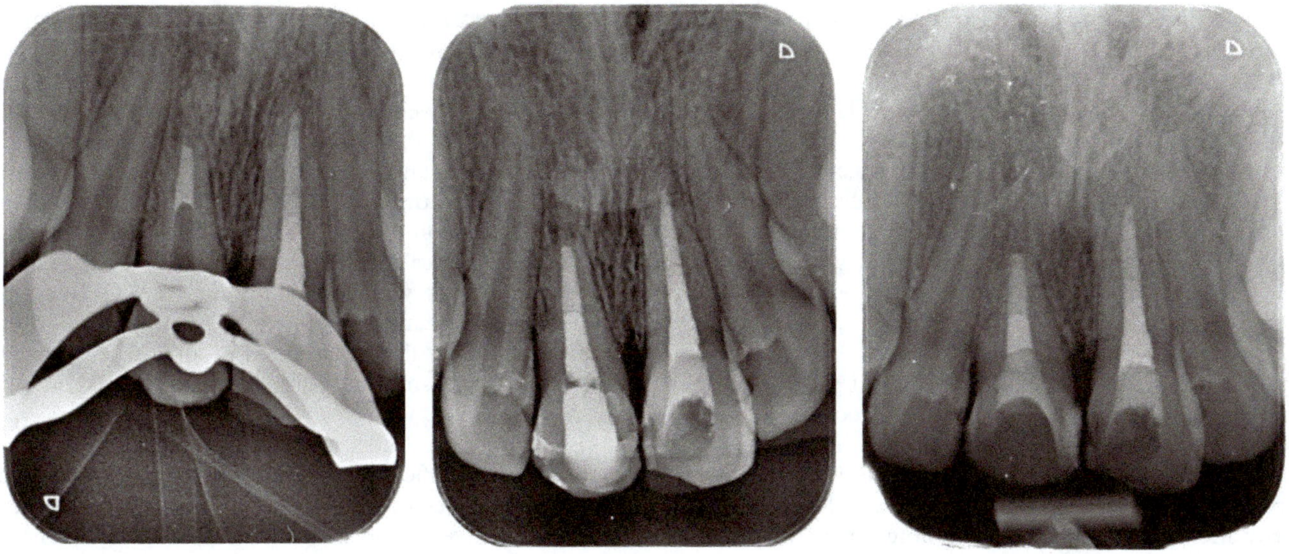

(a) (b) (c)

FIGURE 5: (a) Apexification of tooth #8 with MTA plug; (b) warm vertical root filling of teeth #8 and #9; (c) composite restoration of both teeth.

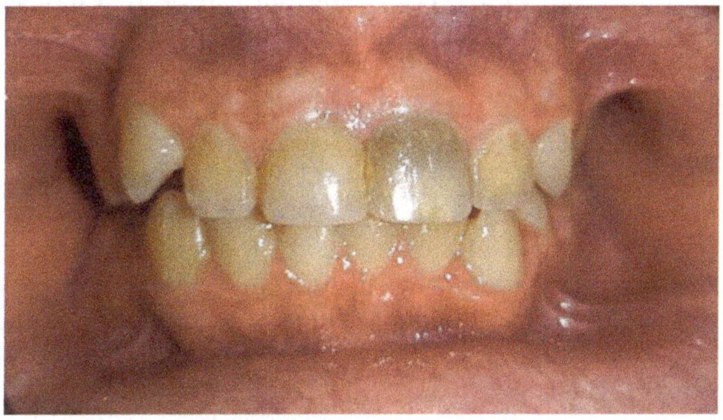

FIGURE 6: Discoloration of tooth #9 at the 1-year follow-up.

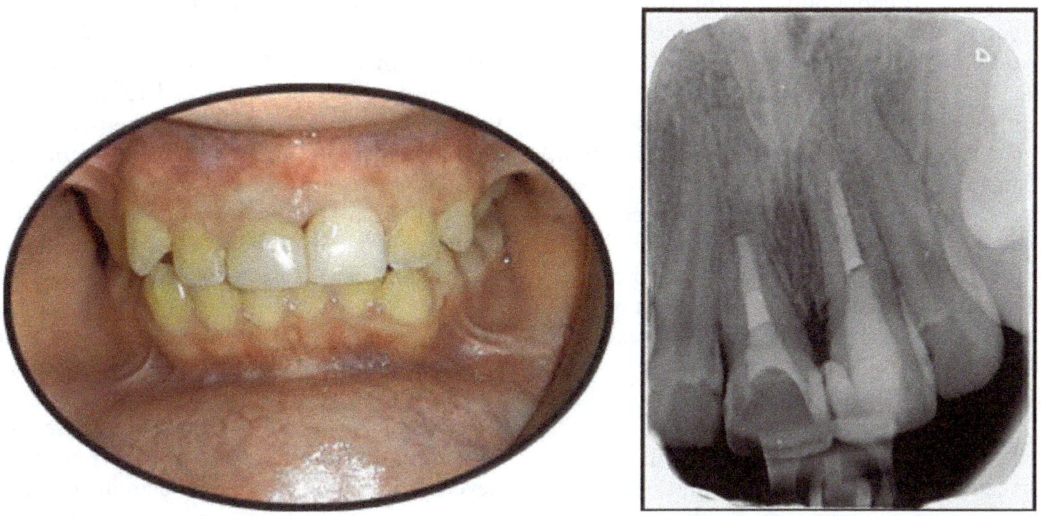

(a) (b)

FIGURE 7: Teeth showed optimal function and esthetics at the 2-year follow-up.

referred to the Operative Dentistry Department for permanent restoration of the tooth.

2.8. Follow-Up (2 Years after Trauma). The patient was completely satisfied with the function and esthetic appearance of his teeth. Both teeth were completely functional and had normal mobility. Radiographically, no periapical lesion was seen, and the inflammatory root resorption of both teeth had been completely resolved (Figure 7).

3. Discussion

Avulsion is a serious trauma to the dental pulp and PDL. Following avulsion and replantation, the tooth is at risk of infection and root resorption, which may compromise the prognosis of treatment and decrease the survival rate. Radiographic detection of root resorption and ankylosis is difficult shortly after replantation. Also, it is noteworthy that the risk of root resorption increases with time [7, 8]. Moreover, some cases with late complications following PDL healing can be falsely considered as healed if a follow-up session less than 1 year is scheduled [9].

The prevalence of dental trauma to permanent teeth is 25% to 33% [10], and crown fracture without pulp exposure is the most common type of dental trauma [11]. However, complex dental trauma as in our case rarely occurs. The study of complex and unusual cases of dental traumas can provide an insight into more efficient treatment of trauma cases.

In our patient, avulsed maxillary central incisors underwent rigid splinting by a surgeon after 1 h of storage in milk. Milk is a good storage medium considering its osmolarity and adequate pH and can preserve the PDL cells viable for up to 6 h [12]. Replanted teeth were clinically and radiographically followed-up for 2 years on a regular basis.

Current recommended clinical management of avulsed teeth includes intracanal CH placement initiated within 7–10 days after avulsion for a tooth with a closed apex to help prevent resorption. If endodontic treatment is started after this time period or after a resorptive root lesion is detected on a radiograph, CH is placed for an extended amount of time [13].

In our patient, since more than 2 weeks had passed since the avulsion, and the teeth showed external root resorption, long-term CH therapy was considered to stop the root resorption and then accomplish the root canal treatment. Radiographs were obtained on a monthly basis to assess the hard tissue formation and washout of CH, and also to accomplish endodontic treatment as soon as the root resorption stopped. Long-term treatment with CH may weaken the roots and make them susceptible to fracture. However, this effect was minimal in our case since CH was only used for 3 months [14].

Damage to the external root surface along with intracanal infection can cause inflammatory root resorption. Bacterial toxins originating from the root canal can reach the PDL through dentinal tubules and aggravate the external root resorption. Appropriate endodontic treatment can prevent the progression of resorption [15, 16].

The prognosis of horizontal root fracture depends on the site of fracture; the apical segment often survives while the coronal segment is necrotized in 25% of the cases. Also, fractures below the alveolar crest, as in our case (which was in the apical third of the root), often have good prognosis [5].

Apexification and revascularization have been considered effective treatment procedures for nonvital immature teeth. Apexification involves disinfection of the root canal, promoting an apical hard tissue barrier and obturating the empty canal space with root filling material. On the other hand, revascularization is aimed at promoting continued root development, the replacement of lost tissue, and function with stem cell-mediated growth of reparative tissue [17].

Endodontic treatment of immature teeth with horizontal root fracture is difficult due to the absence of an apical stop. In such teeth, one-session apexification with MTA can serve as an alternative to the traditional apexification with CH, and has shown promising results [18]. MTA can cause discoloration, and this property limits its application particularly in the anterior teeth [19]. According to recent studies, iron, manganese, and bismuth oxide are responsible for tooth discoloration. In fact, exposure of dentin collagen to bismuth oxide is responsible for tooth discoloration. Blood contamination is another cause of tooth discoloration. New bioceramic materials have the advantages of MTA without causing discoloration [20]. However, due to the unavailability of newer biomaterials in Iran and the need for fast-set MTA, MTA Angelus was used for our patient.

A rigid splint does not permit any physiological mobility of the tooth and thereby creates the conditions for complications in the sense of ankylosis or external resorption.

In the case of a semirigid splint, the physiological functional mobility of the traumatized tooth is possible, which is more favorable for the healing of PDL [21]. Semirigid splinting for 1 to 2 weeks is often recommended to prevent ankylosis. As most cases of avulsion occur in juvenile patients, it is of clinical importance to preserve the tooth and surrounding bone tissue to provide optimal, definitive, and prosthodontic rehabilitation under the possibility of later treatment with dental implants [22].

Splinting can be performed to immobilize the traumatized teeth whenever required. The prevalence of ankylosis after replantation of an avulsed tooth and rigid splinting is 57%-80%. Ankylosis in adults can be well managed by prosthetic and dental implant treatments. Rigid splinting is often contraindicated except for some certain cases of bone fracture, which can cause the death of PDL cells due to their compression, and can lead to subsequent root resorption. In our present case, due to the use of a rigid splint for 1 month, signs of inflammatory root resorption were noted at different parts of the root [23].

The follow-up radiographs of our case indicated healing of the PDL, and no further root resorption was noted. Several international surveys demonstrated the inadequate knowledge of dentists about emergency management of TDIs. As TDIs include other injuries and both GDPs and specialists in various dental disciplines can encounter such injuries in their practice, they must have sufficient knowledge on the emergency management of TDIs in general [24]. The current case report described successful management of maxillary central incisors following severe complex dental trauma.

References

[1] J. O. Andreasen and F. M. Andreasen, *tbook and Color Atlas of Traumatic Injuries to the TeethJohn*, Wiley & Sons, 2018.

[2] I. I. Hauert, F. Eggmann, and R. Weiger, "Horizontal root fracture with avulsion of the coronal segment: a case report with a 5-year follow-up," *Endo-Endodontic Practice Today*, pp. 112275–112283, 2018.

[3] M. T. Flores and M. L. Hicks, "International Association of Dental Traumatology guidelines for the management of traumatic dental injuries: 2. Avulsion of permanent teeth," *Pediatric dentistry*, vol. 37, no. 6, 2015.

[4] L. W. Lee, S. H. Hsiao, Y. H. Lin, P. Y. Chen, Y. L. Lee, and W. C. Hung, "Outcomes of necrotic immature open-apex central incisors treated by MTA apexification using poly(ε-caprolactone) fiber mesh as an apical barrier," *Journal of the Formosan Medical Association*, vol. 118, no. 1, pp. 362–370, 2019.

[5] M. Cvek, G. Tsilingaridis, and J. O. Andreasen, "Survival of 534 incisors after intra-alveolar root fracture in patients aged 7–17 years," *Dental Traumatology*, vol. 24, no. 4, pp. 379–387, 2008.

[6] M. A. Marciano, J. Camilleri, R. M. Costa, M. A. Matsumoto, B. M. Guimarães, and M. A. Duarte, "Zinc oxide inhibits dental discoloration caused by white mineral trioxide aggregate angelus," *Journal of Endodontics*, vol. 43, no. 6, pp. 1001–1007, 2017.

[7] L. Andersson, I. Bodin, and S. Sörensen, "Progression of root resorption following replantation of human teeth after extended extraoral storage," *Dental Traumatology*, vol. 5, no. 1, pp. 38–47, 1989.

[8] L. Andersson, L. Blomlöf, S. Lindskog, B. Feiglin, and L. Hammarström, "Tooth ankylosis: clinical, radiographic and histological assessments," *International Journal of Oral Surgery*, vol. 13, no. 5, pp. 423–431, 1984.

[9] J. O. Andreasen, M. K. Borum, H. L. Jacobsen, and F. M. Andreasen, "Replantation of 400 avulsed permanent incisors. 4. Factors related to periodontal ligament healing," *Dental traumatology*, vol. 11, no. 2, pp. 76–89, 1995.

[10] U. Glendor, "Epidemiology of traumatic dental injuries—a 12 year review of the," *literatureDental traumatology*, vol. 24, no. 6, pp. 603–611, 2008.

[11] E. Lauridsen, N. V. Hermann, T. A. Gerds, S. Kreiborg, and J. O. Andreasen, "Pattern of traumatic dental injuries in the permanent dentition among children, adolescents, and adults," *Dental Traumatology*, vol. 28, no. 5, pp. 358–363, 2012.

[12] M. Trope, "Clinical management of the avulsed tooth: present strategies and future directions," *Dental Traumatology*, vol. 18, no. 1, 2002.

[13] S. Heward and C. M. Sedgley, "Effects of Intracanal Mineral Trioxide Aggregate and Calcium Hydroxide During Four Weeks on pH Changes in Simulated Root Surface Resorption Defects: An In Vitro Study Using Matched Pairs of Human Teeth," *Journal of Endodontics*, vol. 37, no. 1, pp. 40–44, 2011.

[14] J. O. Andreasen, B. Farik, and E. C. Munksgaard, "Long-term calcium hydroxide as a root canal dressing may increase risk of root fracture," *Dental Traumatology*, vol. 18, no. 3, pp. 134–137, 2002.

[15] P. V. Abbott, "Prevention and management of external inflammatory resorption following trauma to teeth," *Australian dental journal*, vol. 61, pp. 82–94, 2016.

[16] J. V. Bastos, I. de Souza Côrtes, M. A. G. EM, E. A. Colosimo, R. S. Gomez, and W. O. Dutra, "Age and timing of pulp extirpation as major factors associated with inflammatory root resorption in replanted permanent teeth," *Journal of Endodontics*, vol. 40, no. 3, pp. 366–371, 2014.

[17] J. Silujjai and P. Linsuwanont, "Treatment outcomes of apexification or revascularization in nonvital immature permanent teeth: a retrospective study," *Journal of Endodontics*, vol. 43, no. 2, pp. 238–245, 2017.

[18] K. Ramnani, R. Shetty, and S. Shetty, "Evaluation of outcomes of recent materials used for single visit apexification," *Journal of Advanced Medical and Dental Sciences Research*, vol. 6, no. 6, pp. 76–80, 2018.

[19] J. Możyńska, M. Metlerski, M. Lipski, and A. Nowicka, "Tooth Discoloration Induced by Different Calcium Silicate-based Cements: A Systematic Review of In Vitro Studies," *Journal of Endodontics*, vol. 43, no. 10, pp. 1593–1601, 2017.

[20] M. Torabinejad, M. Parirokh, and P. M. Dummer, "Mineral trioxide aggregate and other bioactive endodontic cements: an updated overview—part II: other clinical applications and complications," *International endodontic journal*, vol. 51, no. 3, pp. 284–317, 2018.

[21] N. Hadziabdic, *The basics of splinting in dentoalveolar traumatology. In Oral and Maxillofacial Surgery—Practices and Updates*, IntechOpen, 2020.

[22] D. D. Müller, R. Bissinger, M. Reymus, K. Bücher, R. Hickel, and J. Kühnisch, "Survival and complication analyses of avulsed and replanted permanent teeth," *Scientific Reports*, vol. 10, no. 1, pp. 1–9, 2021.

[23] E. Bendoraitiene, S. Zemgulyte, and M. Borisovaite, "Reasonable outcome of avulsed permanent upper incisor after seven years follow-up period: a case report," *Journal of oral & maxillofacial research.*, vol. 8, no. 4, article e6, 2017.

[24] S. N. Al-Haj Ali, S. A. Algarawi, A. M. Alrubaian, and A. I. Alasqah, "Knowledge of general dental practitioners and specialists about emergency management of traumatic dental injuries in Qassim, Saudi Arabia," *International journal of pediatrics*, vol. 2020, Article ID 6059346, 7 pages, 2020.

7

Active Peripheral Osteoma in the Mandibular Notch: A Longitudinal Clinical Report

Jun Sasaki,[1,2] Shogo Hasegawa,[1] Hitoshi Miyachi,[1] and Toru Nagao[1]

[1]*Department of Maxillofacial Surgery, School of Dentistry, Aichi-Gakuin University, 2-11 Suemori-Dori, Chikusa, Nagoya, Aichi 464-8651, Japan*
[2]*Department of Maxillofacial Surgery, Okazaki City Hospital, 3-1 Goshoai, Koryujicho, Okazaki, Aichi 444-8553, Japan*

Correspondence should be addressed to Shogo Hasegawa; shogo@dpc.aichi-gakuin.ac.jp

Academic Editor: Yasuhiro Morimoto

Osteomas are benign osteogenic tumors composed of mature compact or cancellous bone and are characterized by slow, painless growth. A peripheral osteoma located in the mandibular notch is extremely rare. Here, we describe the case of a 38-year-old woman with an active peripheral osteoma in the mandibular notch for long-term follow up. Surgical resection of the lesion was performed, which resulted in the improvement of the mandibular function and temporomandibular dysfunction. This is the first report of resection surgery after confirming the activity of peripheral osteoma by bone scintigraphy. Creating a three-dimensional model of the mandible promises an accurate surgical plan.

1. Introduction

Osteomas are benign tumors composed of mature compact or cancellous bone and are characterized by slow, painless growth [1–3]. They can be peripheral, central, or extraskeletal [4, 5]. Most peripheral osteomas are known to occur in the mandibular body, angle, condyle, or coronoid process [2, 4, 5]. The occurrence of a peripheral osteoma in the mandibular notch is extremely rare, with an incidence of 1.6% among mandibular peripheral osteoma cases [4, 5]. Although several studies have described peripheral osteomas of the jawbone, only eight cases of peripheral osteomas in the Sigmoid notch of the mandible have been reported.

We report the case of an active peripheral osteoma in the mandibular notch of a 38-year-old woman in whom we were able to clarify the temporal course of the disease.

2. Case Presentation

A 38-year-old woman with complaints of pain during mandibular movement was referred to our department by a dental clinic. She had no significant medical history, and she was not taking any medication. The patient was evaluated based on preoperative clinical manifestations, panoramic radiography, computed tomography (CT), magnetic resonance imaging (MRI), and radioisotope imaging (RI). Panoramic radiography revealed a circular radiopacity between the right mandibular condyle and the muscle process (Figure 1(d)). On reviewing the patient's panoramic radiograph taken at the age of 18 and 21 years, no osteoma was found in the mandibular notch (Figures 1(a) and 1(b)). At the age of 26, a bone bulge was found in the right mandibular notch (Figure 1(c)). CT showed a 13.3×12.8×10.0mm lesion showing Hounsfield units (HU) equivalent to that of the mandible, arising from the right mandibular notch (Figures 2(a) and 2(b)). MRI showed uniform hypointense trabecular bone, and there was no continuity of fat signals in the bone marrow, suggesting the exclusion of the lateral pterygoid muscle due to bone lesions (Figure 2(c)). RI showed significant uptake of Tc-99m (Figure 2(d)). Bone scintigraphy showed circular area of strong radioisotope accumulation with indistinct boundaries, consistent with lesion in right mandibular notch. No neurological symptoms of the

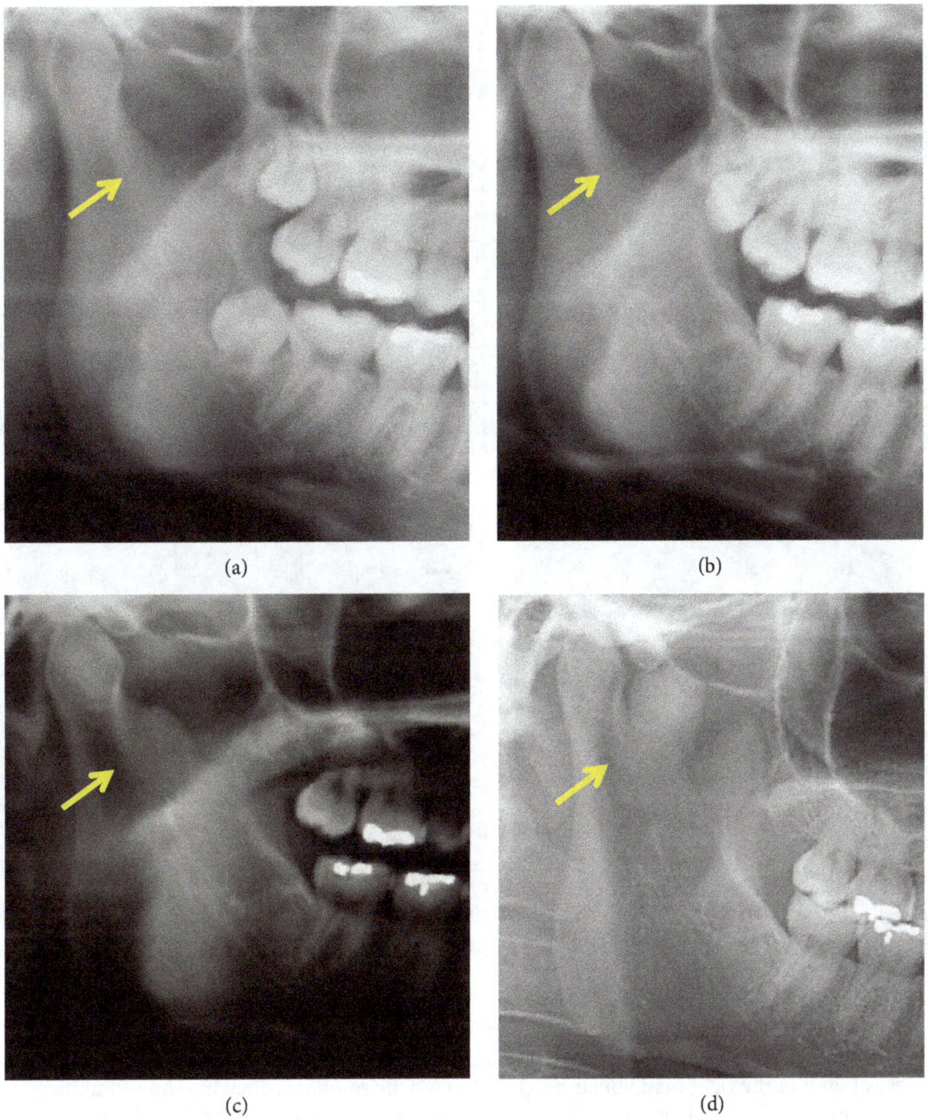

Figure 1: Time course of osteoma in the right mandibular notch by panoramic radiography. (a) At the age of 18, no osteoma was found in the right mandibular notch. (b) At the age of 21, no osteoma was found in the right mandibular notch. (c) At the age of 26, a bony bulge was found in the right mandibular notch. (d) At the age of 38, an oval radiodense mass was observed in the right mandibular notch.

mandible were observed, and there was no history of trauma or infection in the maxillofacial region. No abnormalities were found on blood or urine analysis. Based on these findings, the diagnosis of an active peripheral osteoma was suspected. Using the CT data and Mimics software® (version 23.0, Materialise, Leuven, Belgium), we created a three-dimensional (3D) model of the mandible (Figure 3) to facilitate an explanation to the patient. Resective surgery using an intraoral approach was planned. A fused deposition modeling 3D printer (da Vinci Mini w Plus, XYZ printing, Taiwan) and a thermoplastic resin (polylactic acid filament) were used to prepare the model.

On June 23, 2021, the entire tumor, including the portion that demonstrated Tc-99m uptake, was resected under general anesthesia. The myoprojection was temporarily dissected (Figure 4(a)), and the bone was repositioned and fixed with an absorbent plate (Super FIXSORB®) (Figure 4(b)). The excised mass measured 13×12.0×10.0mm with a weight of 2.7 g (Figure 4(c)). On histologic examination, osteomas are composed of dense, mature, predominantly lamellar bone. The osteoma was diagnosed an actively growing lesion ("hot") with radionuclide bone imaging, interosseous spaces composed of fibrous, fibrovascular, and lined by osteoblasts within a well-vascularized moderately cellular fibrous stroma (Figure 5). The case presented here was diagnosed as a compact osteoma because of its characteristic microscopical features, radiographic findings, and clinical features. Immediately after the operation, there was a slight trismus with no other complications. There were few functional changes and minimal temporomandibular joint dysfunction. The patient was followed-up for 5 months, and no recurrence was noted.

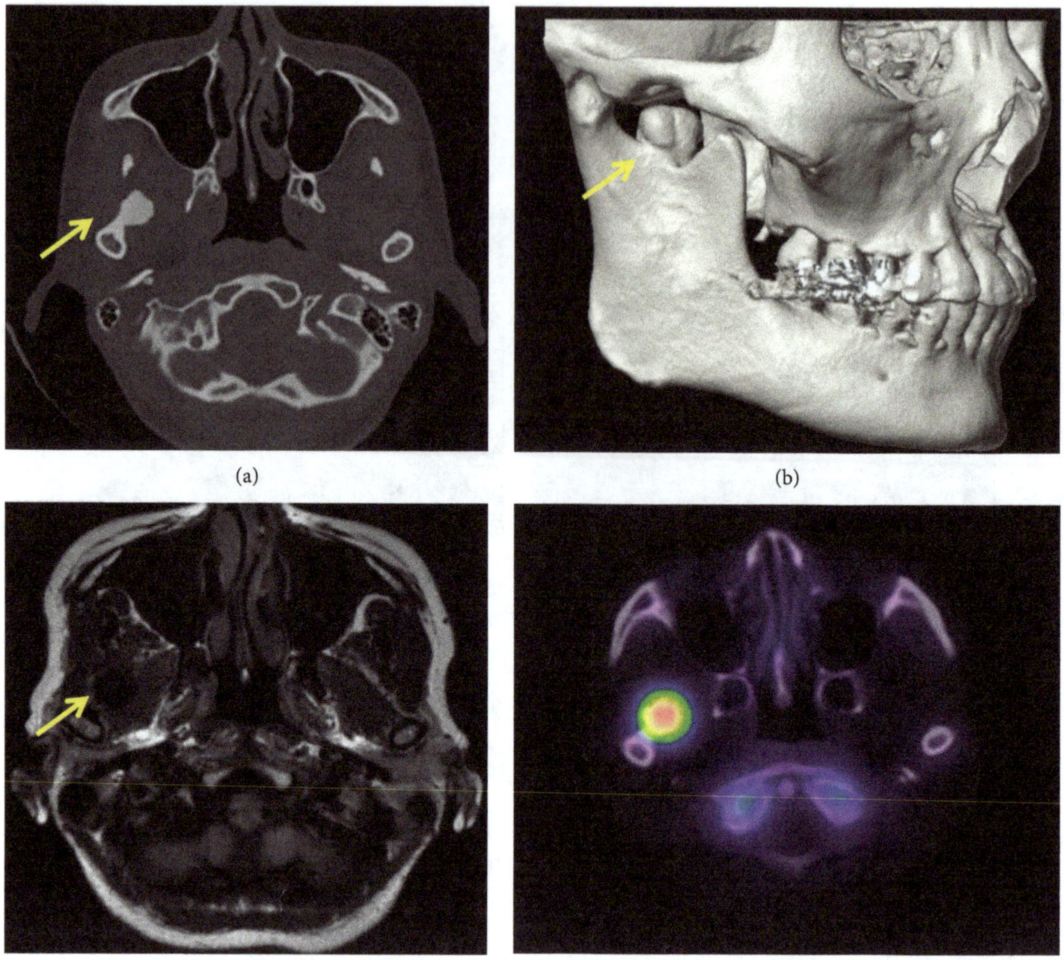

(a) (b) (c) (d)

FIGURE 2: Preoperative examination. (a) Computed tomography showed a 13.3×12.8×10.0mm sized lesion showing Hounsfield units (HU) equivalent to that of the mandible, arising from the right mandibular notch. The CT values of osteoma ranged from 1480 to 1580 HU. (b) 3D-CT showed osteoma was found in the right mandibular notch. (c) Magnetic resonance imaging showed uniform hypointense trabecular bone, and there was no continuity of fat signals in the bone marrow, suggesting exclusion of the lateral pterygoid muscle because of bone lesions. (d) Radioisotope imaging showed significant uptake of Tc-99m by the osteoma in the right mandibular notch.

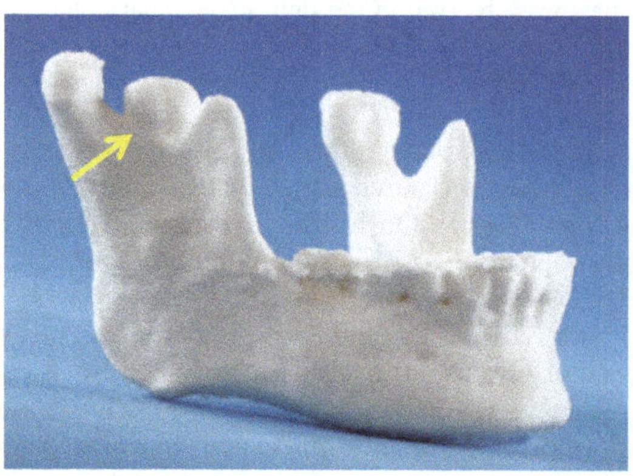

FIGURE 3: Three-dimensional model of the mandible. We created a three-dimensional model of the mandible to facilitate an explanation to the patient resection surgery using an intraoral approach was planned.

3. Discussion

Peripheral osteomas, also known as periosteal osteomas, most frequently involve the craniofacial bones and are the most common benign tumors of the paranasal sinuses. Peripheral osteomas of the jawbones are however uncommon [2]. The origin of peripheral osteoma onset is unknown, and it has been suggested that it results from a reaction to trauma and infection [2]. However, there was no history of infection or trauma in the present case. The osteoma may have slowly developed during the age of 21–26 years after the cessation of mandibular growth and development of secondary sexual characteristics. Surgery is considered for large, deforming osteomas [1, 6]. In the present case, surgical resection was considered owing to the progressive nature of the lesion confirmed by RI.

Only eight cases of osteomas in the mandibular notch have been reported so far [1, 6–10], and the present case is the ninth (Table 1). In the previous cases, the patients' age ranged from 16 to 78 years, with a male-to-female ratio of

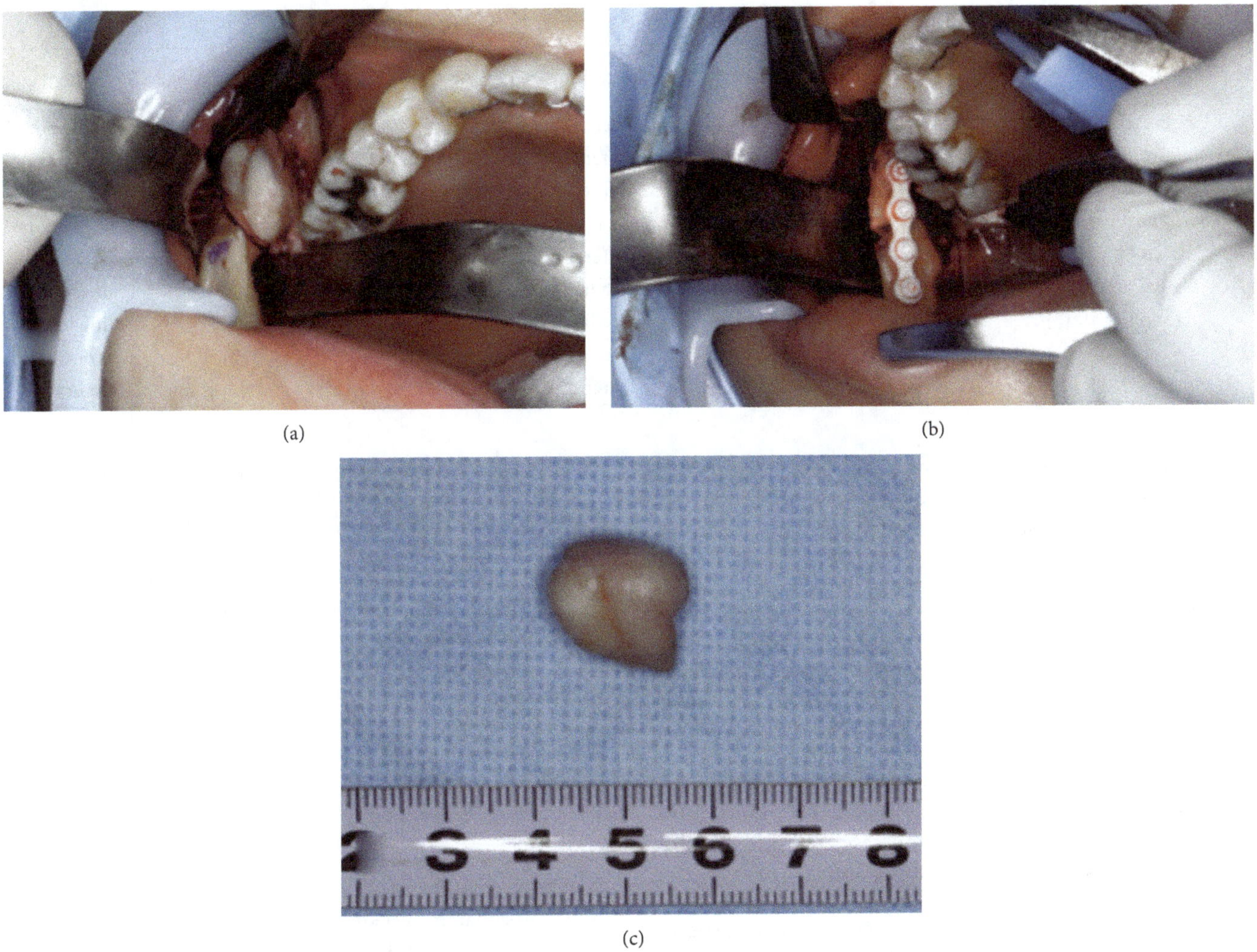

FIGURE 4: Intraoperative view. (a) The lesion was exposed by an intraoral approach. (b) The myoprojection was temporarily dissected, and the bone was repositioned and fixed with an absorbent plate. (c) Excised osteoma.

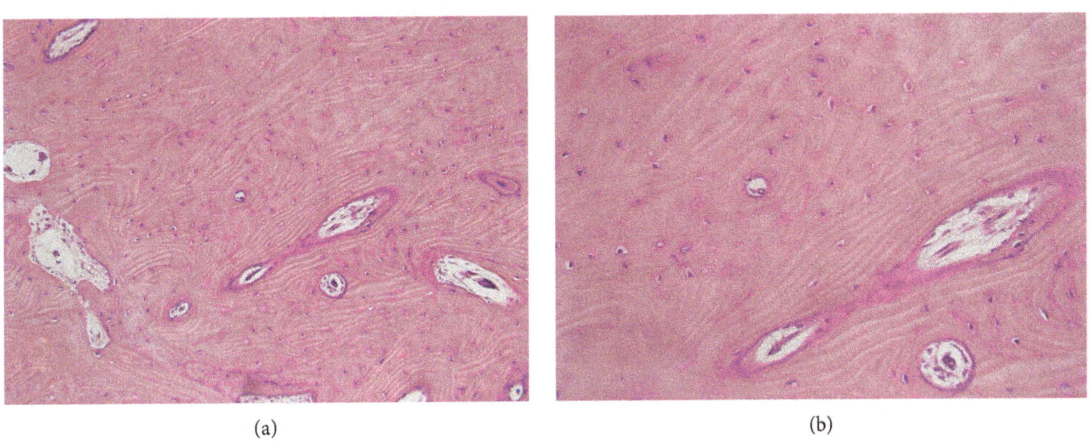

FIGURE 5: The histopathology of the peripheral osteoma. (a) Microscopic features of peripheral osteoma (hematoxylin-eosin, original magnification ×200). (b) Microscopic features of peripheral osteoma (hematoxylin-eosin, original magnification ×400).

1 : 3.5. The location of the osteoma was medial in four cases, lateral in four cases, and medial and lateral in one case. The lesion developed in the right mandibular notch in five cases and in the left mandibular notch in four cases. The patients displayed symptoms of swelling in four cases and pain in two, with no symptoms in three cases. Of

Table 1: Reported cases of peripheral osteoma in the mandibular notch.

No.	Reference	Year of publication	Age (years)	Sex	Location	Side	Size (in mm)	Symptoms	Treatment
1	Present case	2021	38	Female	Medial	Right	15×14×10	Pain	Surgery (intraoral)
2	*Nakayama* et al. [3]	2021	69	Female	Lateral	Left	25×20×15	Swelling	Surgery (extraoral)
3	*Bocchialini* et al. [1]	2018	37	Female	Medial and lateral	Left	15×13×11	Pain	Surgery (intraoral)
4	*Sasidharan* et al. [6]	2015	52	Female	Lateral	Left	30×25×20	Swelling	Surgery (intraoral)
5	*Rao* et al. [7]	2013	16	Female	Lateral	Right	30×30	Swelling	Surgery (intraoral)
6	*Iwai* et al. [4]	2013	78	Female	Medial	Right	36×35×30	None	Follow-up
7	*Sekerci* et al. [8]	2011	59	Male	Medial	Right	Not available	None	Follow-up
8	*Schulze* [9]	2008	73	Female	Medial	Left	30×30×27	Pain	Unknown
9	*Bessho* et al. [10]	1987	26	Male	Lateral	Right	34×29×17	Swelling	Surgery

the five surgically treated cases of osteoma, four were intraoral approaches. This is the first case to use RI to confirm the dynamic state of the osteoma; RI is therefore useful for diagnosing osteomas.

In addition, a 3D model was created based on the preoperative CT data using a fused deposition modeling 3D printer and a thermoplastic resin (polylactic acid filament). The 3D model is useful for preoperative patient education and surgical planning. In this case, because a 3D model was created only for the mandible, the surgery of the maxillary tuberosity and maxillary teeth was restricted, and it was difficult to predict. Among the reports of osteomas in the mandibular notch, there were descriptions of intraoral surgery in four cases. In the present case, considering the patient's aesthetics, we approached the lesion intraorally.

Currently, the number of reported cases of peripheral osteoma in the mandibular notch is small, and many aspects of this entity remain unclear, including the treatment method and prognosis. Further accumulation and examination of cases are expected.

4. Conclusions

We encountered a case of an active peripheral osteoma in the mandibular notch, which has rarely been reported in the literature. A dynamic diagnosis of peripheral osteoma was made possible using composite imaging. It was easy to obtain anatomical orientation in the surgical field through preoperative surgical simulation using a 3D model. An osteoma in the mandibular notch can be resected by an intraoral approach, in which case it is desirable to reposition the myoprojection.

References

[1] G. Bocchialini, A. B. Bolzoni Villaret, S. Negrini, A. Tironi, L. Salvagni, and A. Castellani, "The first case of osteoma of the mandibular notch located both medially and laterally and treated with a transoral endoscopy assisted approach. A case report," *International Journal of Surgery Case Reports*, vol. 49, pp. 70–73, 2018.

[2] I. Kaplan, S. Calderon, and A. Buchner, "Peripheral osteoma of the mandible: a study of 10 new cases and analysis of the literature," *Journal of Oral and Maxillofacial Surgery*, vol. 52, no. 5, pp. 467–470, 1994.

[3] A. Nakayama, R. Abe, M. Takahashi, H. Yamada, and Y. Takeda, "Peripheral osteoma in an unusual region of the mandible: a case report," *Oral and Maxillofacial Surgery Cases*, vol. 7, no. 1, article 100207, 2021.

[4] T. Iwai, T. Izumi, J. Baba, J. Maegawa, K. Mitsudo, and I. Tohnai, "Peripheral osteoma of the mandibular notch: report of a case," *Iranian Journal of Radiology*, vol. 10, no. 2, pp. 74–76, 2013.

[5] C. T. Chen and K. Adriane, "Endoscopic resection of a mandibular body and condylar osteoma," *Minimally Invasive Therapy & Allied Technologies*, vol. 17, no. 5, pp. 323–325, 2008.

[6] A. Sasidharan, A. Gohil, S. Koshy, and A. K. Gupta, "Bony tumour in an unusual location on the mandible," *Indian Journal of Plastic Surgery*, vol. 48, no. 2, pp. 200–203, 2015.

[7] S. Rao, S. Rao, and D. S. R. Pramod, "Transoral removal of peripheral osteoma at sigmoid notch of the mandible," *Journal of Maxillofacial and Oral Surgery*, vol. 14, Suppl. 1, pp. 255–257, 2015.

[8] A. E. Sekerci, H. Sahman, E. T. Ertas, and Y. Sisman, "An unusual peripheral osteoma of the mandibular notch: a case report with computed tomography evaluation," *Oral Radiology*, vol. 27, no. 1, pp. 78–82, 2011.

[9] D. Schulze, "Radiographic diagnostics: osteoma of the left mandibular notch," *Quintessence International*, vol. 39, no. 8, pp. 702-703, 2008.

[10] K. Bessho, K. Murakami, T. Iizuka, and T. Ono, "Osteoma in mandibular condyle," *International Journal of Oral and Maxillofacial Surgery*, vol. 16, no. 3, pp. 372–375, 1987.

8

Medication-Related Osteonecrosis of the Jaw Spontaneously Occurred in a Patient with Chronic Myelogenous Leukemia Only by Imatinib: A Report of a Rare Case

Makiko Okubo-Sato, Kenji Yamagata, Satoshi Fukuzawa, Kazuhiro Terada, Fumihiko Uchida, Naomi Ishibashi-Kanno, and Hiroki Bukawa

Department of Oral and Maxillofacial Surgery, Institute of Clinical Medicine, Faculty of Medicine, University of Tsukuba, 1-1-1 Tennodai, Tsukuba, Ibaraki 305-8575, Japan

Correspondence should be addressed to Kenji Yamagata; y-kenji@md.tsukuba.ac.jp

Academic Editor: Giuseppe Alessandro Scardina

The prevalence of medication-related osteonecrosis of the jaw (MRONJ) associated with molecular-targeted therapies such as bevacizumab and sunitinib has been constantly increasing in recent years. MRONJ frequently occurs after invasive dental procedures such as tooth extraction in patients currently or with a previous history of receiving antiresorptive agents including bisphosphonates and/or denosumab. Here, we report a rare case of spontaneously occurring MRONJ of the mandible in a 52-year-old Japanese woman with chronic myelogenous leukemia (CML) who was administered imatinib for 9 years. She had never been treated with antiresorptive agents, and her MRONJ developed spontaneously. Although there have been few reports of MRONJ related to imatinib, our case reported here indicates that imatinib may be capable of causing spontaneous MRONJ.

1. Introduction

Medication-related osteonecrosis of the jaw (MRONJ) is a severe adverse drug effect related to antiresorptive agents, and the number of reports of MRONJ cases associated with molecular-targeted therapies including antibody drugs and tyrosine kinase inhibitors (TKIs) has been increasing [1, 2]. Most cases are related to the administration of antiresorptive medications, such as bisphosphonates and receptor activator of nuclear factor κB ligand (RANKL) inhibitors, and precipitating events, such as tooth extraction, which may significantly increase the risk of developing MRONJ. Meanwhile, frequently reported agents among molecular-targeted therapies associated with MRONJ are bevacizumab [3, 4], sunitinib [5], sorafenib [6], everolimus [7], temsirolimus [3], and aflibercept [8].

Imatinib mesylate (Glivec®) is a TKI with specificity for the BCR–ABL protein resulting from the t(9, 22)-derived Philadelphia chromosome, platelet-derived growth factor receptors (PDGFRs), and c-kit. It is administered in patients with chronic myelogenous leukemia (CML), acute lymphocytic leukemia, and c-kit-positive gastrointestinal stromal tumor (GIST) [9]. The documented adverse effects of imatinib are nausea, vomiting, edema, tumor necrosis, muscle cramps, hematologic side effects, cardiovascular side effects, hepatic side effects, nephrotoxicity, and dermatologic side effects (such as skin rashes, pruritus, and petechiae); however, little is known about MRONJ [10]. The present report describes a very rare case of spontaneous MRONJ related to only imatinib in the absence of antiresorptive agents.

2. Case Report

A 52-year-old Japanese woman was referred to our department in July 2018. She complained of exposed bone with contact pain in the right mandible that had persisted for 6 months. She started using an oral antimicrobial mouthrinse, and the exposed bone was eliminated several times by her general practitioner, but her condition did not improve. She was diagnosed with CML in 2008 and administered only imatinib (400 mg daily) continuously with no apparent side effects. There was no other past medical history, and she had never received antiresorptive agents or undergone radiotherapy in the head and neck region. Clinical examination showed that the exposed bone measured approximately 5 mm on the lingual surface of the mandibular tori around the right premolars (Figure 1). Purulent discharge, swelling, tooth mobility, and percussion pain were not observed, and her oral hygiene was favorable. Although there were no significant findings on panoramic radiography (Figure 2(a)), computed tomography showed a separated sequestrum measuring approximately 25 mm, and magnetic resonance imaging indicated abnormal intramedullary signal intensity in the right mandible (Figures 2(b) and 2(c)). She was clinically diagnosed with MRONJ stage II. In November 2018, sequestrectomy and removal of the mandibular tori were performed under general anesthesia because of her vomiting reflex. Histopathological examination revealed necrotic lamellar bone with empty lacunae, bacterial aggregates, and an absence of neoplastic cells (Figure 3). Her postoperative course was uneventful, and at the 2-year follow-up, she was stable with no signs of MRONJ recurrence (Figures 4(a) and 4(b)).

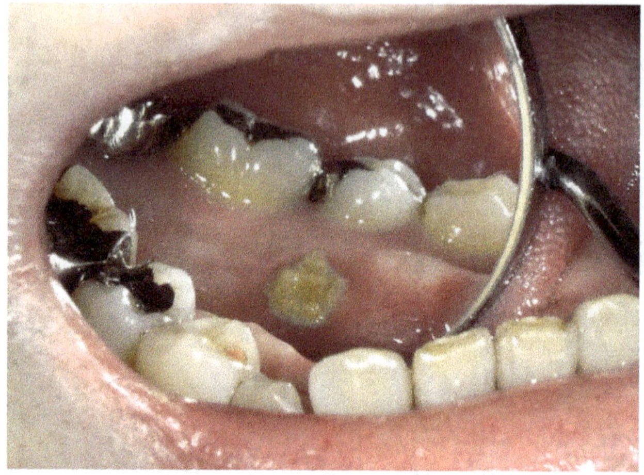

FIGURE 1: Examination of the oral cavity. Intraoral examination revealed bone exposure measuring approximately 5 mm on the lingual surface of the mandibular tori around the second premolar.

3. Discussion

In 2014, the American Association of Oral and Maxillofacial Surgeons (AAOMS) suggested that some cases of osteonecrosis of the jaw have been observed in patients with cancer following treatment with angiogenic inhibitors (bevacizumab), TKIs (sunitinib, sorafenib), and mammalian target of rapamycin (mTOR) inhibitors (sirolimus). The committee remains concerned about a similar potential risk associated with several other medications within the same drug class that have a similar mechanism of action [11]. Bevacizumab, sunitinib, and sorafenib inhibit vascular endothelial growth factor- (VEGF-) mediated angiogenesis and ultimately delay wound healing, which play relevant roles in the onset of MRONJ. Inhibition of mTOR, VEGF expression, and angiogenesis are also depressed [12].

Imatinib inhibits PDGFR and c-kit, which are both related to angiogenesis, and some reports have indicated that imatinib may partly reduce VEGF expression through the inhibition of these factors [13, 14]. Apart from its vascular effects, imatinib directly affects bone remodeling. The inhibition of c-fms and c-kit signaling by imatinib may decrease osteoclast number and activity. Imatinib also inhibits the proton-generating activity of carbonic anhydrase II and suppresses bone resorption [15]. In addition, the inhibition of PDGFR signaling in osteoblasts inhibits the production of macrophage colony-stimulating factor and RANKL, which are essential for osteoclast genesis, and decreases osteoblast proliferation [16]. Therefore, imatinib treatment should be included as a potential risk factor for developing MRONJ because of its inhibitory effects on angiogenesis and bone remodeling. Our patient had never received antiresorptive agents and spontaneously developed MRONJ, as suggested by the aforementioned mechanism.

There are only three reports describing MRONJ related to imatinib (Table 1). Nicolatou-Galitis et al. [17] reported a case of MRONJ that developed after tooth extraction in a woman with CML receiving imatinib for 19 months. Four years prior, she had received chemotherapy and rituximab for non-Hodgkin's lymphoma, as well as alendronate and one injection of zoledronate for osteoporosis. MRONJ was treated but recurred following an injection of denosumab. Mohamed et al. [18] reported a patient with chronic lymphocytic leukemia (CLL) treated with imatinib for 13 months. The patient was administered alendronate for 119 months, followed by denosumab for 5 months until 5 months before tooth extraction, which was a trigger for MRONJ. The last case reported by Viviano et al. [19] involved a patient with MRONJ after 22 months of receiving imatinib for a GIST. Although the patient had never received antiresorptive agents, a tooth was extracted prior to the patient developing MRONJ. Two of the three reported cases of MRONJ due to imatinib involved the administration of antiresorptive agents. Our case is the second case of MRONJ caused only by imatinib and is the first case of spontaneous development without any surgical invasion. Although the exposed bone was on the mandibular tori, which is usually considered an anatomical risk factor of mechanical stimulation, the patient had no clear history of trauma involved in the pathogenesis, such as wearing dentures and chewing hard foods. AAOMS (2014) recommended conservative treatments for patients

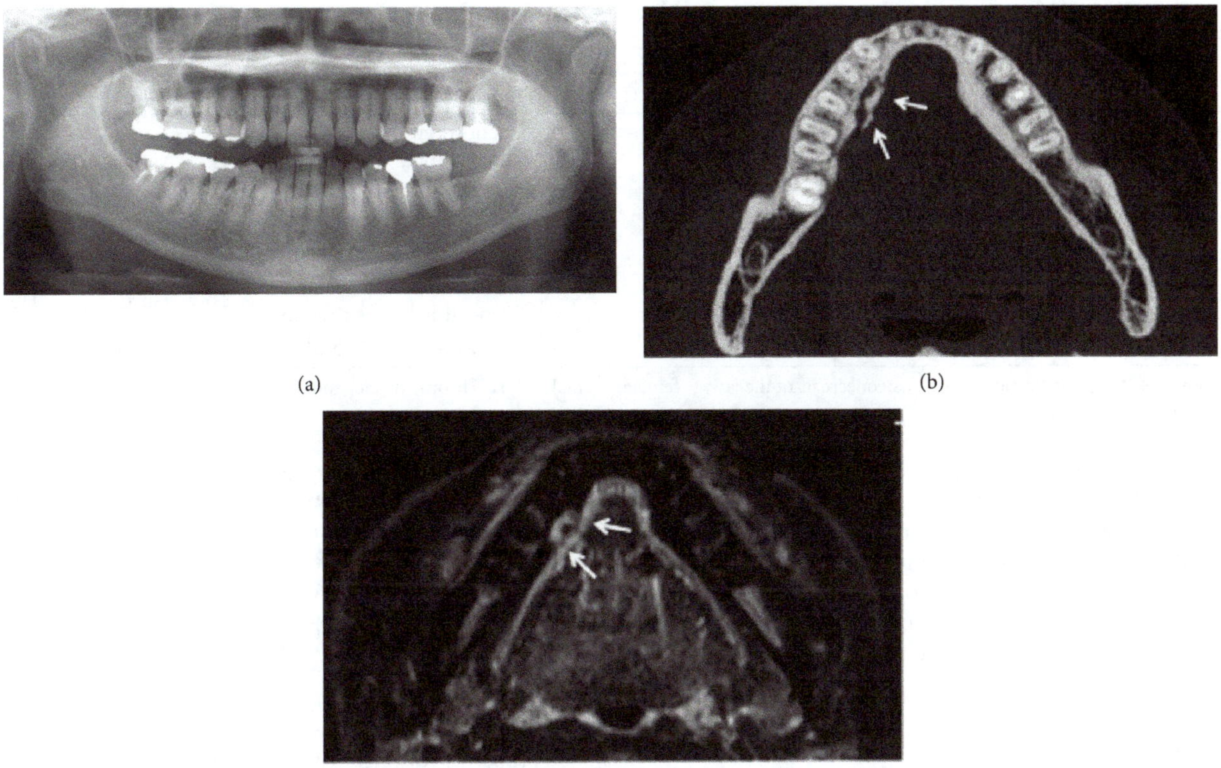

(a) (b)

(c)

FIGURE 2: Imaging findings. (a) Panoramic radiography showed no obvious bone destruction or marginal and apical periodontitis. (b) Axial computed tomography depicted a sequestrum measuring approximately 25 mm (arrow). (c) Axial magnetic resonance short T1 inversion recovery imaging showed abnormal intramedullary signal intensity (arrow) on the lingual side of the right lower premolar.

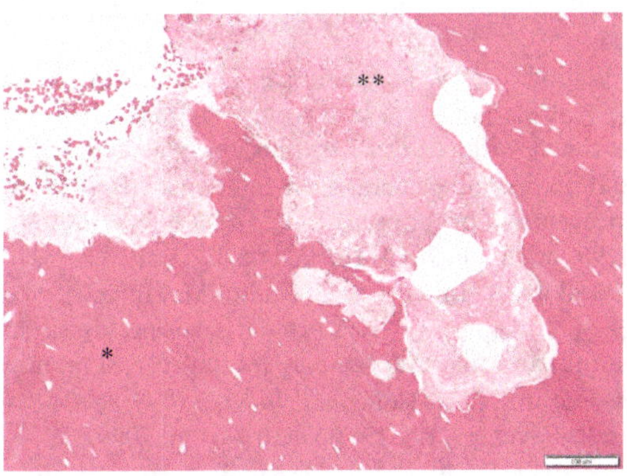

FIGURE 3: Microscopic findings. Histopathological examination revealed necrotic lamellar bone with empty lacunae (asterisk) and bacterial aggregates (double asterisk) (hematoxylin and eosin staining ×200 magnification).

with stage II MRONJ. However, the symptom of some patients with stage II and III do not respond to conservative treatments and reported that surgical management recently had a good prognosis [19]. The Position Paper 2017 of the Japanese Allied Committee on Osteonecrosis of the Jaw also recommended surgical treatments for stage II ONJ [20]. In our case, the patient continued to use antimicrobial mouthrinse but her condition did not improve. Therefore, we selected surgical treatment.

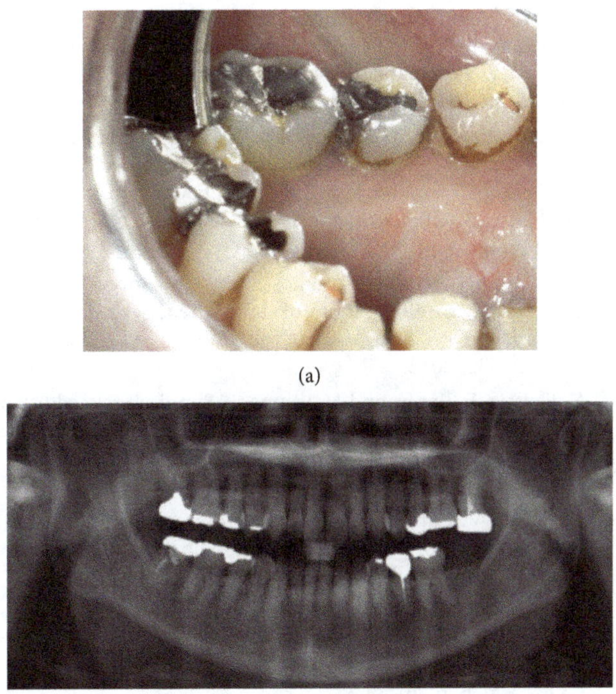

(a)

(b)

FIGURE 4: Follow-up oral examination 2 years after the surgery. (a) Follow-up observation revealed complete soft tissue healing with no signs of refractory osteonecrosis and exposed bone. (b) Panoramic radiography was also clear.

Table 1: Reported MRONJ cases related to imatinib [17–19].

No.	Study (yr)	Age (yr)/gender	Disease	Period of imatinib treatment (mo)	Antiresorptive agent	Trigger event	Stage	Treatment	Clinical outcome
1	Nicolatou-Galitis et al. (2013) [17]	71/M	CML	19	Alendronate Zoledoronate Denosumab	Tooth extraction	II	Antibiotic	Improved
2	Viviano et al. (2017) [19]	72/M	GIST	22	None	Tooth extraction	II	Antibiotic	Unknown
3	Mohamed et al. (2018) [18]	81/F	CLL	13	Alendronate Denosumab	Tooth extraction	II	Surgery	Healed
4	Present case (2020)	52/F	CML	111	None	None	II	Surgery	Healed

Abbreviations: MRONJ: medication-related osteonecrosis of the jaw; F: female; M: male; CML: chronic myelogenous leukemia; GIST: gastrointestinal stromal tumor; CLL: chronic lymphocytic leukemia.

To the best of our knowledge, we present the first case of spontaneous MRONJ attributed to the chronic use of imatinib with no history of receiving antiresorptive agents. The dental and medical communities must be aware that even if there are no apparent risk factors of MRONJ, the condition may develop in patients treated only with imatinib, and long-term monitoring and care are required.

References

[1] S. L. Ruggiero, T. B. Dodson, J. Fantasia et al., "American Association of Oral and Maxillofacial Surgeons position paper on medication-related osteonecrosis of the jaw–2014 update," *Journal of Oral and Maxillofacial Surgery*, vol. 72, no. 10, pp. 1938–1956, 2014.

[2] O. Nicolatou-Galitis, M. Kouri, E. Papadopoulou et al., "Osteonecrosis of the jaw related to non-antiresorptive medications: a systematic review," *Supportive Care in Cancer*, vol. 27, no. 2, pp. 383–394, 2019.

[3] A. R. Santos-Silva, G. A. Belizário Rosa, G. De Castro Júnior, R. B. Dias, A. C. Prado Ribeiro, and T. B. Brandão, "Osteonecrosis of the mandible associated with bevacizumab therapy," *Oral Surgery, Oral Medicine, Oral Pathology, Oral Radiology*, vol. 115, no. 6, pp. e32–e36, 2013.

[4] R. N. Hopp, J. Pucci, A. R. Santos-Silva, and J. Jorge, "Osteonecrosis after administration of intravitreous bevacizumab," *Journal of Oral and Maxillofacial Surgery*, vol. 70, no. 3, pp. 632–635, 2012.

[5] Y. Fleissig, E. Regev, and H. Lehman, "Sunitinib related osteonecrosis of jaw: a case report," *Oral Surgery, Oral Medicine, Oral Pathology, Oral Radiology*, vol. 113, no. 3, pp. e1–e3, 2012.

[6] F. Garuti, V. Camelli, L. Spinardi, L. Bucci, and F. Trevisani, "Osteonecrosis of the jaw during sorafenib therapy for hepatocellular carcinoma," *Tumori*, vol. 102, pp. S69–S70, 2016.

[7] D. Yamamoto, Y. Tsubota, T. Utsunomiya et al., "Osteonecrosis of the jaw associated with everolimus: a case report," *Molecular and Clinical Oncology*, vol. 6, no. 2, pp. 255–257, 2017.

[8] H. Mawardi, P. Enzinger, N. McCleary et al., "Osteonecrosis of the jaw associated with ziv-aflibercept," *Journal of gastrointestinal oncology*, vol. 7, no. 6, pp. E81–E87, 2016.

[9] S. Dulucq and M. Krajinovic, "The pharmacogenetics of imatinib," *Genome Medicine*, vol. 2, no. 11, pp. 1–8, 2010.

[10] H. Joensuu, J. C. Trent, and P. Reichardt, "Practical management of tyrosine kinase inhibitor-associated side effects in GIST," *Cancer Treatment Reviews*, vol. 37, no. 1, pp. 75–88, 2011.

[11] N. A. Valente, S. Chatelain, F. Alfonsi, C. Mortellaro, and A. Barone, "Medication-related osteonecrosis of the jaw," *The Journal of Craniofacial Surgery*, vol. 30, no. 4, pp. 1095–1101, 2019.

[12] H. A. Lane, J. M. Wood, P. M. J. McSheehy et al., "mTOR inhibitor RAD001 (everolimus) has antiangiogenic/vascular properties distinct from a VEGFR tyrosine kinase inhibitor," *Clinical Cancer Research*, vol. 15, no. 5, pp. 1612–1622, 2009.

[13] J. Litz and G. W. Krystal, "Imatinib inhibits c-kit-induced hypoxia-inducible factor-1α activity and vascular endothelial growth factor expression in small cell lung cancer cells," *Molecular Cancer Therapeutics*, vol. 5, no. 6, pp. 1415–1422, 2006.

[14] G. Vlahovic, Z. N. Rabbani, J. E. Herndon, M. W. Dewhirst, and Z. Vujaskovic, "Treatment with Imatinib in NSCLC is associated with decrease of phosphorylated PDGFR- β and VEGF expression, decrease in interstitial fluid pressure and improvement of oxygenation," *British Journal of Cancer*, vol. 95, no. 8, pp. 1013–1019, 2006.

[15] S. Parkkila, A. Innocenti, H. Kallio, M. Hilvo, A. Scozzafava, and C. T. Supuran, "The protein tyrosine kinase inhibitors imatinib and nilotinib strongly inhibit several mammalian α-carbonic anhydrase isoforms," *Bioorganic & medicinal chemistry letters*, vol. 19, no. 15, pp. 4102–4106, 2009.

[16] K. Vandyke, S. Fitter, A. L. Dewar, T. P. Hughes, and A. C. W. Zannettino, "Dysregulation of bone remodeling by imatinib mesylate," *Blood*, vol. 115, no. 4, pp. 766–774, 2010.

[17] O. Nicolatou-Galitis, E. Razis, D. Galiti, E. Vardas, F. Tzerbos, and S. Labropoulos, "Osteonecrosis of the jaw in a patient with chronic myelogenous leukemia receiving imatinib - a case report with clinical implications," *Forum of Clinical Oncology*, vol. 4, no. 4, pp. 29–33, 2013.

[18] H. A. M. Mohamed, C. E. N. Nielsen, and M. Schiodt, "Medication related osteonecrosis of the jaws associated with targeted therapy as monotherapy and in combination with antiresorptives. A report of 7 cases from the Copenhagen Cohort," *Oral Surgery, Oral Medicine, Oral Pathology, and Oral Radiology*, vol. 125, no. 2, pp. 157–163, 2018.

[19] M. Viviano, M. Rossi, and S. Cocca, "A rare case of osteonecrosis of the jaw related to imatinib," *Journal of the Korean Asso-*

ciation of Oral and Maxillofacial Surgeons, vol. 43, no. 2, pp. 120–124, 2017.

[20] Japanese Allied Committee On Osteonecrosis Of The Jaw, T. Yoneda, H. Hagino et al., "Antiresorptive agent-related osteonecrosis of the jaw: position paper 2017 of the Japanese Allied Committee on osteonecrosis of the jaw," *Journal of Bone and Mineral Metabolism*, vol. 35, no. 1, pp. 1–14, 2017.

9

A Conservative Approach to Surgical Management of Root Canal Perforation

Régis Augusto Aleixo Alves, André Luiz Gomide Morais, Thábata Frederico Izelli, Cyntia R. A. Estrela, and Carlos Estrela

Department of Stomatology Sciences, Federal University of Goiás, Goiânia, Brazil

Correspondence should be addressed to André Luiz Gomide Morais; gomide100@gmail.com

Academic Editor: Giuseppe Alessandro Scardina

This study describes a conservative approach to surgical management of root canal perforation in maxillary lateral incisors. A patient was referred for retreatment of a maxillary lateral incisor. Her chief complaint was discomfort in the buccal mucosa. Periapical radiography showed radiopaque material consistent with sealing material inside the root canal. A CBCT scan was acquired and revealed a gutta-percha cone outside the root canal, from the middle third to beyond the root apex. The imaging examination showed that the pulp cavity had not been affected. Thus, we took the clinical alternative of surgically managing the perforation by sealing with MTA, thereby avoiding endodontic treatment, and followed up with only clinical and radiographic control. At the two-year follow-up, after the surgical procedure to remove the extruded filling material, we observed bone tissue formation and positive response to pulp tests, without any clinical signs or symptoms. Root perforation is considered an unpleasant error in an operative procedure. Once a perforation is properly diagnosed, located, and sealed with biomaterial, a favorable prognosis is often achieved. MTA offered good sealing of the perforation, with promising results. Decision-making using the CBCT scan enabled us to adopt a conservative approach and favored more reliable treatment predictability.

1. Introduction

Root perforation results in communication between the root canal system and the external tooth surface [1]. When completing the last steps of the endodontic therapeutic protocol, all care must be taken to avoid accidents that may risk losing teeth [2].

In clinical practice, pathological perforations are frequent. Iatrogenic root perforations may occur at any time in root canal treatment, during access cavity opening, root canal preparation, or post preparation. All these procedural operative errors may lead to treatment failure [3–6].

In this respect, previous planning for root canal treatment becomes essential, particularly clinical and radiographic examination. Operative procedures prior to access cavity preparation involve removal of all carious tissue, restoration of defects, and weakening of the dentin structure, actions which could change the coronal references. Careful analysis of the coronary chamber based on 3-dimensional imaging exams, well-planned selection of a drill compatible with the coronary volume, and good lighting and magnification are essential procedures, because they favor visualization of the cavity during coronary opening, and prevent unpleasant accidents [2, 6].

The advent of new technologies incorporated into imaging exams in endodontics, such as cone beam computed tomography (CBCT) [7–9], have impacted the outcome of root canal treatment. Better diagnostic accuracy across several clinical conditions [8–12] and better predictability in the decision-making process in clinical practice have allowed establishing more conservative therapeutic protocols. In this respect, the present study describes a conservative approach to surgical management of root canal perforation in a maxillary lateral incisor.

2. Case Presentation

An 11-year-old female patient in good general health sought treatment at the Public Dental Specialty Center, Brazil, with

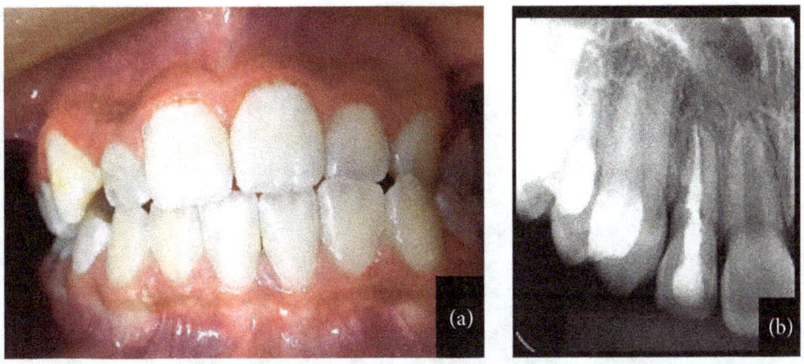

(a) (b)

Figure 1: (a, b) Buccal gingival tissue of the maxillary lateral incisor reveals normal clinical features. Initial periapical radiography shows sealing material in the pulp cavity.

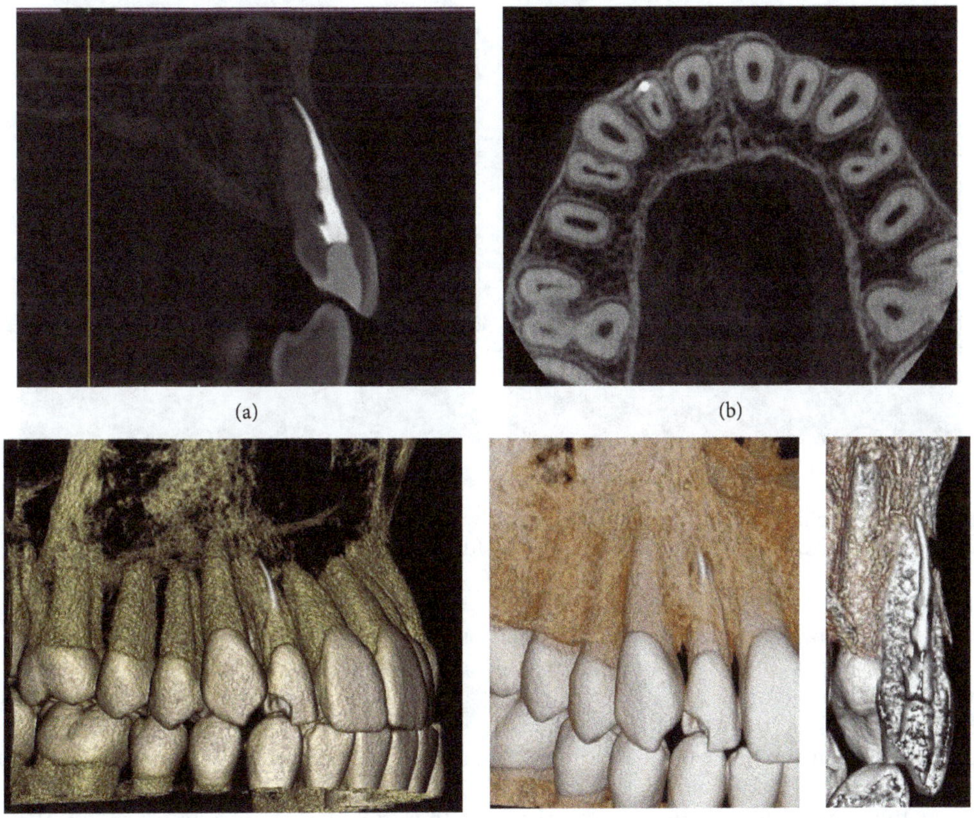

(a) (b)

(c) (d) (e)

Figure 2: CBCT scans (a–e) and 3D reconstructions show sealing material out of the channel, extruded by root perforation in the middle third of the root canal.

the chief complaint of mild discomfort in the buccal mucosa of the maxillary lateral incisor. The patient and the caregiver reported that endodontic treatment was carried out on this tooth 1 year prior, owing to a history of dental traumatism with coronary fracture.

Clinical examination revealed no signs of swelling, fistula, or change in the tooth color (Figure 1(a)). No pain was manifested in the percussion tests, but moderate pain was reported during palpation of the buccal mucosa. Pulp tests were performed in all maxillary anterior teeth using Endo-Frost (Roeko-Wilcos, Rio de Janeiro, RJ, Brazil), which suggested the presence of vital pulp tissue, including tooth #7. The periapical radiography revealed no periapical radiolucency and showed filling material apparently inside the root canal, a situation incompatible with the positive response of the pulp vitality test (Figure 1(b)). Thus, a cone beam computed tomography scan (PreXion, San Mateo, CA, USA) was obtained to improve image interpretation and achieve a more reliable diagnosis. Both sagittal and axial planes revealed a root perforation in the middle third of the

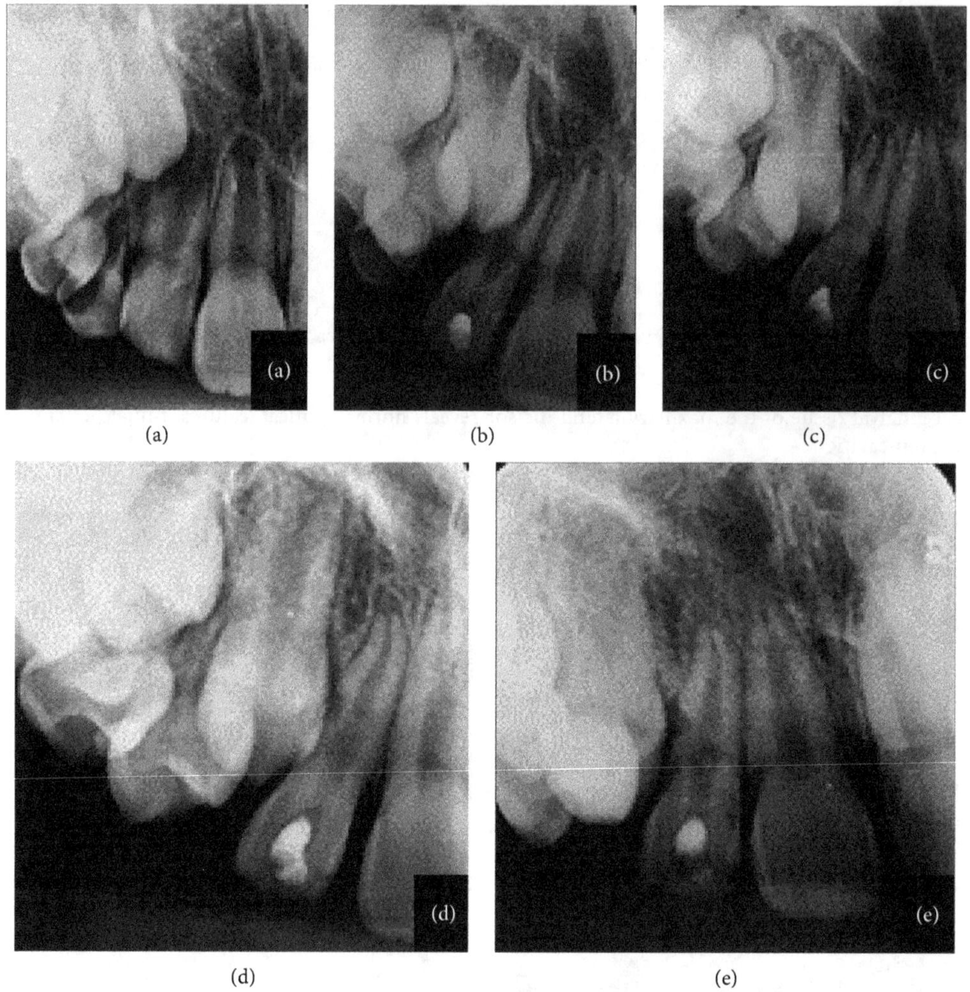

FIGURE 3: (a–e) 26-month radiographic follow-up: periapical radiography before endodontic access and root perforation (a); maxillary lateral incisor with evidence of coronal access (b); follow-up at 14 (c) and 20 (d) months; evidence of complete rhizogenesis (e).

buccal surface, with no evidence of invasion of the root canal space. In addition, the tooth showed signs of normality, with complete closure of the root apex and without apical periodontitis, characterizing the physiological process of rhizogenesis (Figures 2(a)–2(e)). Seeking to ensure that the most appropriate decision would be made, the colleague responsible for the case was asked to provide us with all the radiographs taken between the start of the treatment until the supposed root canal filling. Our request was promptly met and allowed us to perform the chosen surgical technique more confidently. Previous radiographs requested of the patient revealed that the rhizogenesis process was evolving naturally without any complications, despite the root perforation. One hypothesis is that the first professional who started treating the incomplete rhizogenesis saw that the root apex was completely closed and concluded the endodontic treatment without realizing that the sealing he had performed was actually outside the root canal. Radiographic follow-up over time revealed that the root had developed naturally, given that the pulp tissue was healthy (Figures 3(a)–3(e)).

Based on the radiographic aspect of the patient's history, and the favorable condition of pulp vitality, a conservative surgical approach was considered the best choice. Surgery was limited to removal of the extruded gutta-percha and subsequent sealing of the root perforation without any endodontic intervention.

Once the treatment plan was established, the patient signed an informed consent form agreeing to undergo the study procedures. A 2% lidocaine solution containing 1 : 100000 adrenaline (DFL, Rio de Janeiro, RJ, Brazil) was administered as local anesthesia for the right infraorbital nerve, followed by the surgical phase, initiated by making a semilunar incision. After the surgical flap was made, the root perforation was located, and the extruded gutta-percha was exposed (Figures 3(a) and 3(b)). Removal of the extruded gutta-percha was performed with heat condensers, and the cavity was sealed with white MTA (Angelus Ltda, Londrina, Brazil) (Figures 4(a)–4(e)). The suturing was done with nonabsorbable monofilament nylon. The final aspect of the radiographic exam conducted immediately after surgery may cause confusion, because it suggests that the canal was filled below the working limit, owing to the limitations of two-dimensional exams. After seven days, the patient returned to remove the suture, and 10 days following the surgery, the mucosal wound healed completely. In a subsequent follow-up two years after the periapical surgery (Figures 5(a)–5(d)), a

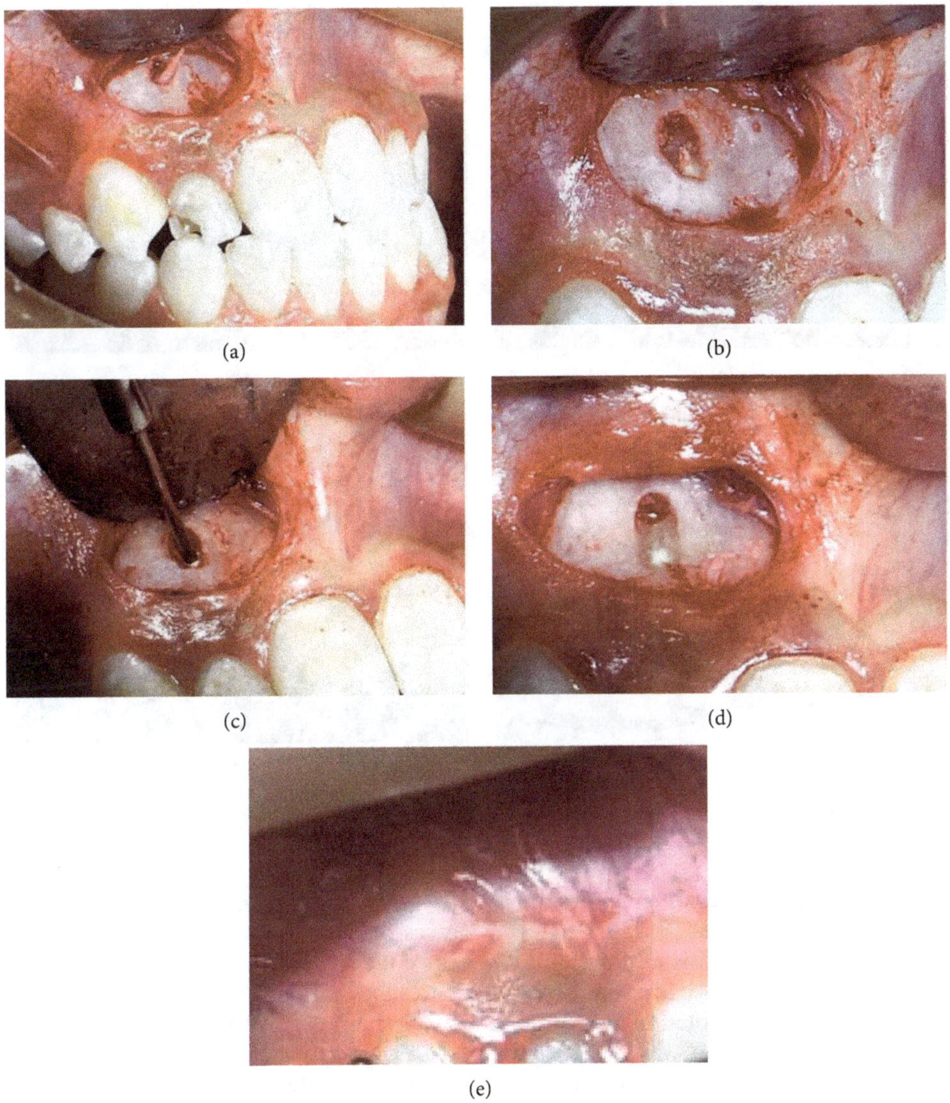

FIGURE 4: (a–e) Surgical procedure for removal of extruded gutta-percha and sealing with MTA; one year after the surgery, showing the gingival tissue in the buccal area, with normal characteristics.

new CBCT scan was obtained, and bone repair was observed in the root perforation area, as well as aspects of normality at the periapical level (Figure 3(e)). Clinically, the patient remains asymptomatic with no signs of inflammation in the gingival mucosa and is responding positively to the pulp vitality tests. The patient was informed of the required continuation of follow-up and control appointments.

3. Discussion

Root perforations may occur at any time during root canal treatment and require preventive measures, so that unpleasant accidents of this nature can cease to become a risk factor for tooth loss. The consequences of root perforation may result in an inflammatory response associated with periodontal tissue and alveolar bone destruction [6].

Diagnosis of the perforation is usually made by clinical investigation and imaging exams. After the advent of cone beam computed tomography (CBCT), anatomical alterations and pathological conditions not identified by way of conventional radiographic examinations became clearly evidenced and could be measured by volumetric study, a feature offered by CBCT. The accuracy in detecting apical periodontitis using CBCT is significantly greater than that of panoramic and periapical radiographs [9–12].

Periapical radiography offers information on two planes and cannot perform three-dimensional reconstruction. This represents an important limitation that can compromise decision-making and prognosis, mainly in cases of buccal and lingual root perforation, in which overlapping structures can hide the pathological area.

Root perforation caused by an operative procedure error represents the vast majority of cases and may be associated with lack of professional ability and factors related to anatomy and dental position, the presence of pulp calcifications, extensive caries, and the presence of intracanal posts [6, 13, 14]. The prognosis is related to treatment time and the size and location of the perforation. The success rates are higher

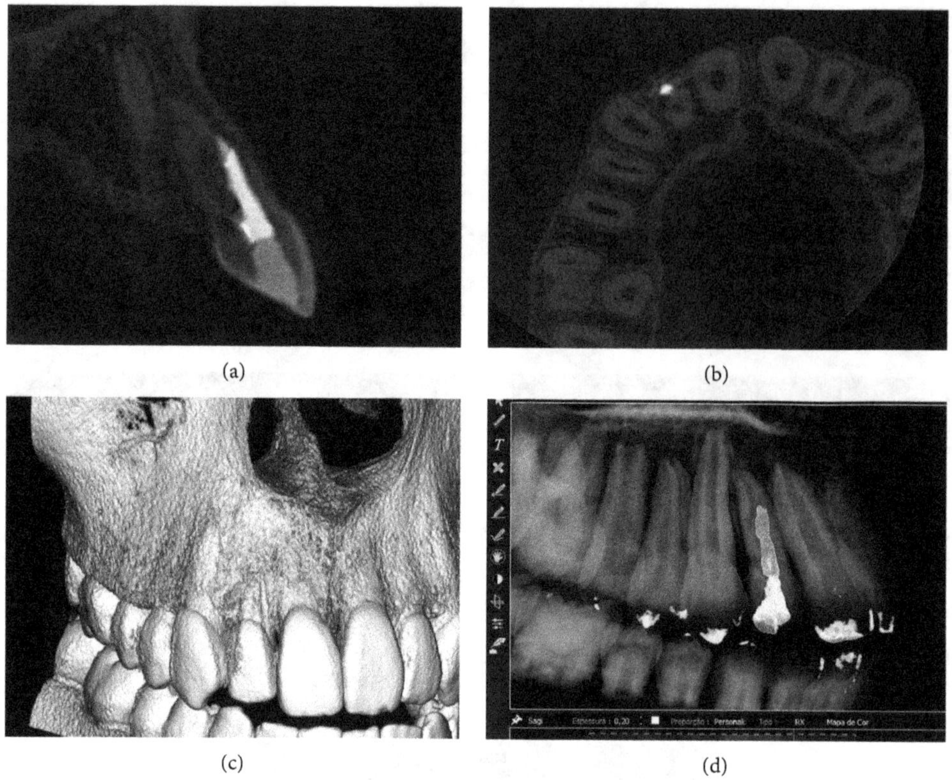

Figure 5: (a–d) CBCT scan and 3D reconstructions two years after the surgery show healing process of the buccal bone and absence of signs of inflammation in the root apex.

in situations of immediate repair or cases of small perforations located in the coronal or apical thirds [3, 4, 6].

Given these characteristics, the prognosis for this clinical case would have been unfavorable, since the iatrogenic procedure was caused by a drill driven in high rotation in the middle third of the root, and the perforation was sealed only years later. However, after a two-year follow-up, the prognosis was very favorable, especially considering the positive response of pulp vitality. The good response seen in this case may have been related to the patient's age and the great pulp regeneration capability of immature teeth [15], associated with conservative management.

In the present clinical case, the conservative management of the root perforation, by avoiding the conventional treatment of the root canal, allowed the root to develop without any complications. Furthermore, image monitoring showed that the root was developing according to the classic pattern of physiological apical closure (continuity of longitudinal and transversal growth of the root without decreasing the size of the tooth) (Figures 2(a)–2(e)). This is unlike cases treated with apexification (resulting in less thick dentin walls and apical closure induced by intracanal medication and ultimately producing reduced root dimensions) [13–16].

In regard to the imaging tests, the use of CBCT scans has brought numerous benefits to endodontics. Because CBCT is a dynamic examination, and images can be viewed in axial, sagittal, and coronal sections, the possibility of navigation represents an excellent resource that significantly improves diagnosis and planning [7–12]. This type of technology has become quite common among endodontists, especially in cases of nonsurgical retreatment and presurgical planning, since it saves time and effort during canal treatment procedures, by searching for canals or discovering why a previous treatment has failed [2, 17].

However, the production of beam hardening artifacts can hinder the interpretation of the images and consequently compromise the diagnosis and decision-making in complex cases. More recently, software packages have been developed [8] to aid in resolving or at least in reducing these limitations observed in viewing the exams. The e-Vol DX (CDT, São José dos Campos, Brazil) is a new CBCT software package capable of changing volume parameters, such as thickness and slice intervals, correcting data, applying image filters, and manipulating brightness and contrast. Compared to other software packages, its main advantages include compatibility with all current CBCT scanners, ability to export DICOM data, access to a more comprehensive brightness and contrast library, customized slice thickness adjustment, adjustable custom sharpness, advanced noise reduction algorithm that improves image quality, predefined image filters, dedicated endodontic volume rendering filters able to enlarge the image by 1000x (3D reconstructions) without loss of resolution, and automatic customization of image parameters for better standardization and improved research procedures [8].

In this clinical case, the CBCT images were crucial in determining the suitable diagnosis and establishing a favorable interventive surgical plan. The sealer material appeared inside the root canal in the periapical radiography but was found to have been extruded by root perforation on the buccal surface of the tooth in the CBCT images, with destruction of the bone cortex. Measurements of the exact location of the root perforation could be made, thus enabling a conservative surgical approach to be performed with minimal damage to the gingival and bone tissues, and ensuring a better postoperative outcome and favorable prognosis for the patient. In the two-year follow-up, e-Vol DX software tools enabled viewing the repair in great detail at the surgical intervention site.

Root perforation represents a significant iatrogenic error, committed especially by professionals less experienced in endodontics, but is a procedural error that may also be made by professionals with greater expertise. Anomalies in dental development such as C-shaped canals, *dens invaginatus*, taurodontism, root fusion, root dilaceration, giro version, microdontia, and palatogingival grooves, as well as physiological endodontic conditions, such as calcified/curved canals and pulp stones, are factors that may jeopardize the endodontic treatment and make it susceptible to iatrogenic maneuvers [2, 17].

4. Conclusions

The use of modern technological tools and professional updating are attitudes that contribute to improving diagnosis and decision-making and that characterize the recommended conduct for both prevention and management of procedural errors, to ultimately offer better predictability of root canal treatment.

References

[1] American Association of Endodontists, *Glossary of Endodontic Terms*, American Association of Endodontists, Chicago, 9th edition, 2016.

[2] C. Estrela, J. D. Pécora, C. R. A. Estrela et al., "Common operative procedural errors and clinical factors associated with root canal treatment," *Brazilian Dental Journal*, vol. 28, no. 2, pp. 179–190, 2017.

[3] Z. Fuss and M. Trope, "Root perforations: classification and treatment choices based on prognostic factors," *Endodontics & Dental Traumatology*, vol. 12, no. 6, pp. 255–264, 1996.

[4] R. S. Roda, "Root perforation repair: surgical and nonsurgical management," *Practical Procedures & Aesthetic Dentistry*, vol. 13, pp. 467–472, 2001.

[5] I. Tsesis and Z. Fuss, "Diagnosis and treatment of accidental root perforations," *Endodontic Topics*, vol. 13, no. 1, pp. 95–107, 2006.

[6] C. Estrela, D. A. Decurcio, G. Rossi-Fedele, J. A. Silva, O. A. Guedes, and A. H. Borges, "Root perforations: a review of diagnosis, prognosis and materials," *Brazilian Oral Research*, vol. 32, article e73, suppl 1, 2018.

[7] Y. Arai, E. Tammisalo, K. Iwai, K. Hashimoto, and K. Shinoda, "Development of a compact computed tomographic apparatus for dental use," *Dento Maxillo Facial Radiology*, vol. 28, no. 4, pp. 245–248, 1999.

[8] M. R. Bueno, C. Estrela, B. C. Azevedo, and A. Diogenes, "Development of a new cone-beam computed tomography software for endodontic diagnosis," *Brazilian Dental Journal*, vol. 29, no. 6, pp. 517–529, 2018.

[9] M. R. Bueno, C. Estrela, J. A. P. Figueiredo, and B. C. Azevedo, "Map-reading strategy to diagnose root perforations near metallic intracanal posts by using cone beam computed tomography," *Journal of Endodontia*, vol. 37, no. 1, pp. 85–90, 2011.

[10] C. Estrela, M. R. Bueno, C. R. Leles, B. Azevedo, and J. R. Azevedo, "Accuracy of cone beam computed tomography and panoramic and periapical radiography for detection of apical periodontitis," *Journal of Endodontia*, vol. 34, no. 3, pp. 273–279, 2008.

[11] C. Estrela, M. R. Bueno, B. C. Azevedo, J. R. Azevedo, and J. D. Pécora, "A new periapical index based on cone beam computed tomography," *Journal of Endodontia*, vol. 34, no. 11, pp. 1325-1331, 2008.

[12] C. Estrela, M. R. Bueno, A. H. De Alencar et al., "Method to evaluate inflammatory root resorption by using cone beam computed tomography," *Journal of Endodontia*, vol. 35, no. 11, pp. 1491-1497, 2009.

[13] R. S. Roda and B. H. Gettleman, "Nonsurgical retreatment," in *Cohen's Pathways of the Pulp*, K. M. Hargreaves and L. H. Berman, Eds., pp. 324–386, Elservier, St. Louis, 11th edition, 2016.

[14] S. Friedman, "Retreatment of failures," in *Principles and Practices of Endodontics*, R. E. Walton and M. Torabinejad, Eds., pp. 336–353, WB Saunders, Philadelphia, 2nd edition, 1996.

[15] A. Diogenes and N. B. Ruparel, "Regenerative endodontic procedures: clinical outcomes," *Dental Clinics of North America*, vol. 61, no. 1, pp. 111–125, 2017.

[16] R. Bose, P. Nummikoski, and K. Hargreaves, "A retrospective evaluation of radiographic outcomes in immature teeth with necrotic root canal systems treated with regenerative endodontic procedures," *Journal of Endodontia*, vol. 35, no. 10, pp. 1343–1349, 2009.

[17] M. Alrahabi, M. S. Zafar, and N. Adanir, "Aspects of clinical malpractice in endodontics," *European journal of dentistry*, vol. 13, no. 3, pp. 450–458, 2019.

10

Computer-Controlled Local Anesthesia Complication: Surgical Retrieval of a Broken Dental Needle in Noncooperative Autistic Paediatric Patient

Damian Chybicki, Małgorzata Lipczyńska-Lewandowska, Gaja Torbicka, and Anna Janas-Naze

Department of Oral Surgery, Central Clinical Hospital, Medical University of Lodz, Poland

Correspondence should be addressed to Damian Chybicki; damian.chybicki@gmail.com

Academic Editor: Michael J. Wahl

The article describes an unusual case of retrieval of 8 mm fragment of a broken 30-gauge 21 mm dental needle in a 6 y.o. noncooperative autistic male patient. The needle of a computer-controlled local anesthesia device was broken during an attempt to administer local anesthetic, in order to perform conservative treatment of teeth 55 and 54 by a pedodontist. Despite the fact that the patient was under nitrous oxide sedation, an unexpected movement of the patient occurred and resulted in needle breakage. Due to the lack of patient cooperation, the surgical retrieval of a broken needle was performed under general anesthesia as part of one-day surgery procedures. The purpose of the article is to emphasize careful decision-making in proper choice of dental instruments during treatment of noncooperative paediatric patients even under sedation and to suggest dentists to carry out treatment of such patients under general anesthesia.

1. Introduction

Autistic disorder is categorized in the *DSM-IV* (*Diagnostic and Statistical Manual of Mental Disorders, 4th Edition*), and it is characterized by abnormal emotional, social behavior, and linguistic development [1, 2]. The interest in autism has grown tremendously over the past twenty years. Knowledge and awareness of this disorder grow in all areas of public life, among parents and health professionals.

Skillful dental treatment without pain is one of the basic principles of treating children in a dental office, especially those with behavioral disorders. This is an essential step towards obtaining and maintaining cooperation [3]. Children are very sensitive to unpleasant sensations in the dentist's chair, which determines their future attitude to treatment. Fear of dental treatment is common in children and affects 6% to 42% of young patients. This psychological condition can completely eliminate the child's willingness to cooperate with the dentist [4]. Various techniques, both pharmacological and nonpharmacological, have been developed to alleviate this negative attitude (e.g., distracting the child, atraumatic restorative techniques, and local anesthesia with a camouflaged syringe) [4, 5].

Local anesthesia has a significant role in pain control and the success of dental procedures. Although local anesthesia is intended to completely eliminate the pain during treatment, the traditional techniques of its administration are painful for the patients [6].

However, paradoxically, patients often fear pain caused by anesthetic injections more than pain from dental treatment itself [7]. Fear/anxiety-related behavior has long been recognized as the most difficult aspect of patient management and can undermine adequate dental care, especially in children [8]. Despite careful anesthetic procedures, dental local anesthesia can cause pain for a variety of reasons, for example, soft tissue damage during penetration of the oral mucosa by the needle, pressure, temperature and low pH of the anesthetic solution, and pain from the characteristics of the drug [7].

Several techniques have been introduced in order to reduce pain caused by the administration of local anesthesia, for example, topical anesthesia, distraction method, warming the anesthetic solution, regulation of the injection rate, buffering anesthetic agent, counterirritation, and local precooling with refrigerant spray [3]. Among the above-mentioned methods, topical anesthesia is the most widely used for reducing pain associated with needle insertion [3].

Computer-controlled anesthetic delivery systems have been developed in an attempt to attenuate or overcome patients' fear and anxiety of local anesthesia required prior to invasive procedures. According to the manufacturers of these electronic devices, it provides a precise injection flow rate and allows controlling the pressure exerted according to tissue resistance and density variations [8]. All these features are aimed at eliminating unpleasant sensations during the application of local anesthesia.

Both demanding cases and patients often present themselves to the dentist specialist, for treatment that requires highly specialized methods. One of these methods is nitrous oxide sedation. Nitrous oxide is a colorless gas with a sweetish taste so it is pleasant for children. It is an effective analgesic and anxiolytic agent that causes depression and euphoria in the central nervous system with negligible effects on the respiratory and cardiovascular system. For some patients, especially noncooperative children, the feeling of loss of control could be a problem, some patients find the nasal mask imprisoning and have the feeling of not breathing well [9]. This situation may result in unexpected and sudden movement of the patient and complications such as described in the article.

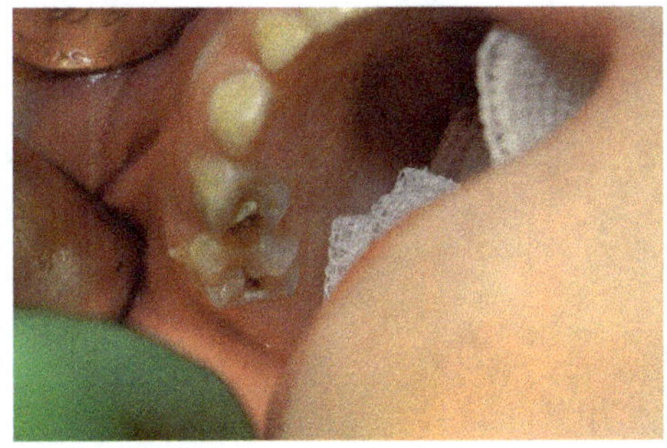

FIGURE 1: Intraoral view of operative region. Even though the needle is visible on the radiograph, it is not possible to firmly locate it intraorally.

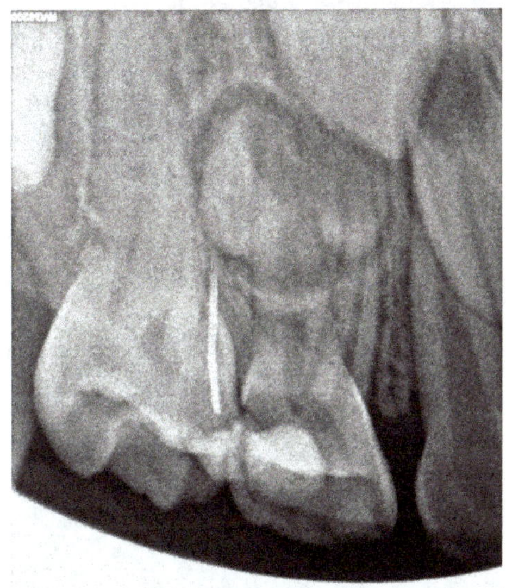

FIGURE 2: The periapical radiograph shows the exact location of a broken tool between teeth 55 and 54.

2. Case Report

A 6-year-old patient, suffering from a mild form of autism, who does not require any medications, was referred by a pedodontist to the Department of Oral Surgery, Medical University of Lodz, for removal of a broken needle from a computer-controlled local anesthesia device. The local anesthesia was performed a day before, due to a necessary conservative treatment of teeth 55 and 54. The circumstances of this situation were as follows: at first, the patient was sedated with nitrous oxide through a nasal mask; the next step was to administer local anesthetic with a computer-controlled local anesthesia device. The purpose was to eliminate, as much as possible, unpleasant sensations associated with appointment in a dental office and dental treatment. During administration of local anesthetic, unexpected movement by the patient occurred, which resulted in 30-gauge and 21 mm needle breakage and, consequently, total loss of the patient's cooperation. On the day of the patient's appointment in our Department, extraoral examination showed no pathologies. Intraoral examination revealed no symptoms of mucosa inflammation in the operative region; also, the broken needle was not visible. Teeth 54 had caries on its occlusal and distal surfaces, and tooth 55 had caries on its occlusal and mesial surfaces (Figure 1).

Based on clinical examination and radiological evaluation (Figure 2), the treatment plan included designing the correct surgical access to interproximal space between teeth 54 and 55 and retrieval of the broken needle. After presenting the parents with a detailed plan and obtaining mandatory permissions, the preoperative recommendations, medications, and laboratory blood tests were ordered (complete blood count, APTT), and the surgery was scheduled.

Under general anesthesia (short-term intravenous anesthesia with use of combination of 50 mg of propofol and 20 μg of fentanyl with monitoring the saturation and heart rate), a sulcular incision along the gingival margin of teeth 55 and 54 was performed with scalpel blade No. 15 (Swann-Morton, Sheffield, England), and the flap was reflected with the Molt 9 periosteal elevator (Kohler Medizintechnik, Stockach, Germany) (Figure 3).

The needle was removed from periodontal ligament space with a dental applicator (Figures 4 and 5).

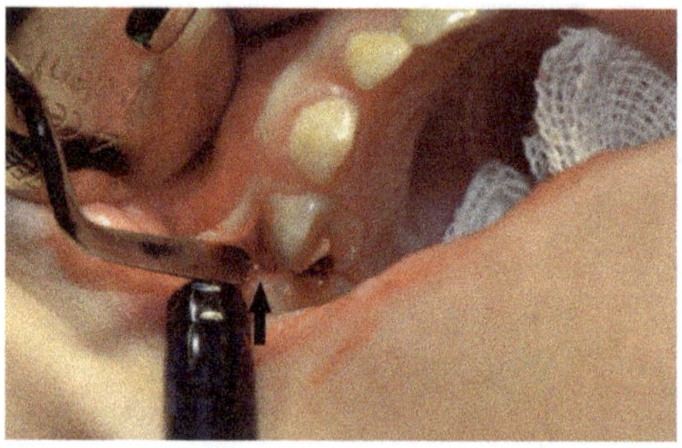

Figure 3: The broken needle is visible (black arrow) in periodontal ligament space of tooth 55 after flap reflection.

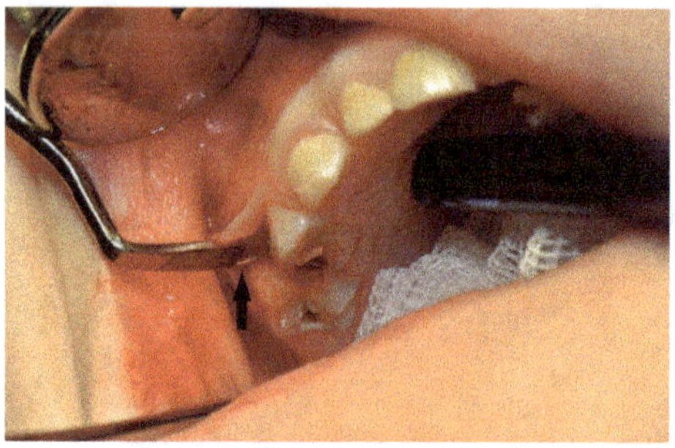

Figure 4: Surgical retrieval of a broken needle (black arrow).

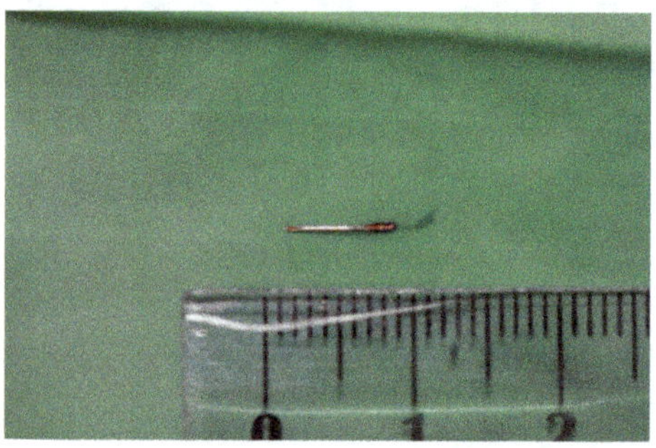

Figure 5: Removed needle, approximately 8 mm long.

The flap was repositioned, and simple interrupted sutures were performed (Novosyn 4/0, B. Braun, Germany). The patient regained consciousness in the recovery room and was discharged home. Postoperative antibiotic (150 mg of clindamycin every 8 hours) and analgetic (150 mg of ibuprofen depending on the needs, but not more than three times a day) were prescribed.

Follow-up examination was performed the day after surgery. Proper healing of the wound was observed, with no edema of the operative region and no pain. Sutures were left for spontaneous dissolution. Two weeks after surgery, the wound was completely healed. The patient did not report any complaints.

3. Discussion

Patients with autism should be treated with appropriate caution as their behavior in a dental office cannot be fully predicted; moreover, the oral health care of such patients can be complicated as they sometimes are not able to describe complaints about any dental problems they may be experiencing [2]. All these circumstances require a dentist to be flexible in their approach to such a patient, as well as to select the appropriate treatment tools for dental procedures. The main purpose is to eliminate pain, vibrations, and acoustic stimuli, which can worry an autistic patient.

Local anesthesia is the most common form of pain control in dentistry. Several different measures and various techniques and devices are used to attain local anesthesia in the mouth. Some of these methods, such as periodontal ligament injection, are unique to dentistry. Pain can occur during a variety of dental interventions, which involve dental surgery or stimulation of the dental pulp by cutting dentine. Common dental treatments performed in children causing pain, which can be prevented by using local anesthetic, include the placement of restorations and extraction of teeth [10].

Administration of local anesthesia is one of the most feared dental procedures by the patient. The pain perceived during local anesthesia administration in children is mitigated by various methods such as application of topical anesthetics [3], camouflaging of the syringe [5], distraction with audiovisual glasses [11], and counterstimulation. Vibration, pressure application, and precooling are different types of counterstimulatory measures to reduce pain perception during local anesthesia administration [12]. The new generations of dental anesthesia devices, which are designed to minimize unpleasant sensations during administration of local anesthetic, are computer-controlled local anesthesia devices. The flow of injection is adjusted to, among others, tissue resistance so the patient does not feel the expansion of anesthetic solution. Both children and adult patients can benefit from the advantages of these devices [8, 13]. Since the introduction of computer-controlled local anesthetic delivery systems, studies have compared its effectiveness to traditional methods of local anesthesia. Some of the cases found in literature have compared the pain of injection with the computer-assisted injection system to a conventional needle. Results from a majority of studies have favored the computer-assisted injection system [6].

However, despite all these measures, sometimes the dentist fails to achieve a satisfactory level of cooperation with a young patient. Then, it is possible to use nitrous oxide (laughing gas), to relax a stressed child and perform dental treatment with due care. During sedation, the reduction of physiological and psychological responses of the patient to surgery is obtained, without a loss of consciousness, collaboration, and protective reflexes; it is used to treat moderately anxious patients and allows for a calm and relaxed patient during therapy, with anterograde amnesia [9].

In extreme cases, when any cooperation with the child is impossible, the only solution is treatment under general anesthesia as it was described in this case report. This kind of treatment requires the presence of an anesthesiologist and the recovery room after dental procedure for the patient to regain consciousness. General anesthesia is defined as a controlled state of drug-induced loss of consciousness during which patients cannot be aroused, even by painful stimuli, and lose their protective reflexes. Independent ventilatory function is frequently inadequate, and cardiovascular function may be impaired [14, 15]. The indisputable advantage of treatment under general anesthesia is that almost every patient can undergo it, which means that, regardless of age and cooperation, it is possible to achieve therapeutic success.

In this case report, breakage of a 30-gauge 21 mm needle resulted from sudden movement of the patient. However, such complications can also be observed in adults whose behavior is calm. Other causes of needle breakage include bending the needle before injection, placing it in the tissues up to its base, and using needles with a diameter inappropriate for the anatomical situation [16]. The latter factor is of exceptional importance, as it results from the desire to minimize the pain of the injection, although it has been proven that the pain caused by the injection does not depend on the diameter of the needle. In addition, thinner needles are prone to cause more pain because the pressure applied on the syringe is much greater with a small gauge needle, so it is advisable to use a 27-gauge 21 mm needle, instead of a 30-gauge 21 mm needle, for young patients who have low pain threshold [17].

This article presents a case of a broken dental needle as a foreign body. Other foreign bodies that may be encountered in the oral cavity theoretically include almost all tools used by the dentist. There are cases that describe iatrogenic breakages of dental instruments during mandibular third molar surgeries: dental root elevator embedded into a subgingival caries of second mandibular molar [18], elevator tip, broken and buried in soft tissues [19], breakage of high-speed handpiece bur [20]. Patients themselves can also place various objects in the mouth that can break, especially into the canals of the teeth, as well as into interproximal spaces. Examples of these situations may be tips of metallic compasses, stapler pin, copper strip, and sewing needles [21].

Removal of foreign bodies from the oral cavity is very important as they can lead to chronic inflammation with the formation of fistulas and abscesses [21]. When breakage of any instrument occurs, the most important is communication between the patient and the dentist so the patient is aware of the condition of his body. If the dentist is not able to remove the separated instrument, then the patient should be referred to a more specialized medical center.

4. Conclusions

Dental treatment of autistic children should be carried out in specialized centers by experienced pedodontists. This is due to the fact that it is impossible to predict the child's behavior in various situations taking place in the dental office. As presented in this article, treatment in sedation with nitrous oxide, despite the child's initial cooperation, may result in serious complications such as needle breakage in oral tissues. It should be considered whether in cases of behavioral disorders such as autism treatment under general anesthesia is the most suitable option for the patient.

References

[1] U. Jaganathan, "Autism disorder (AD): an updated review for paediatric dentists," *Journal of Clinical and Diagnostic Research: JCDR*, vol. 8, no. 2, pp. 275–279, 2014.

[2] S. Chandrashekhar and J. S. Bommangoudar, "Management of autistic patients in dental office: a clinical update," *International Journal of Clinical Pediatric Dentistry*, vol. 11, no. 3, pp. 219–227, 2018.

[3] A. Vafaei, M. Rahbar, R. Dadkhah, B. Ranjkesh, and L. Erfanparast, "Children's pain perception and behavioral feedback during local anesthetic injection with four injection site preparation methods," *Maedica*, vol. 14, no. 4, pp. 343–349, 2019.

[4] C. El Hachem, M. K. Kaloustian, F. Cerutti, and N. R. Chedid, "Metallic syringe versus electronically assisted injection system: a comparative clinical study in children," *European Journal of Paediatric Dentistry*, vol. 20, no. 4, pp. 320–324, 2019.

[5] A. M. Melwani, I. Srinivasan, J. V. Setty, D. R. Murali Krishna, S. S. Pamnani, and D. Lalitya, "A clinical comparative study between conventional and camouflaged syringes to evaluate behavior and anxiety in 6-11-year-old children during local anesthesia administration-a novel approach," *Journal of Dental Anesthesia and Pain Medicine*, vol. 18, no. 1, pp. 35–40, 2018.

[6] M. I. Al-Obaida, M. Haider, R. Hashim et al., "Comparison of perceived pain and patients' satisfaction with traditional local anesthesia and single tooth anesthesia: a randomized clinical trial," *World Journal of Clinical Cases*, vol. 7, no. 19, pp. 2986–2994, 2019.

[7] E.-J. Kwak, N.-S. Pang, J.-H. Cho, B.-Y. Jung, K.-D. Kim, and W. Park, "Computer-controlled local anesthetic delivery for painless anesthesia: a literature review," *Journal of Dental Anesthesia and Pain Medicine*, vol. 16, no. 2, pp. 81–88, 2016.

[8] A. M. Queiroz, A. B. Carvalho, L. L. Censi et al., "Stress and anxiety in children after the use of computerized dental anesthesia," *Brazilian Dental Journal*, vol. 26, no. 3, pp. 303–307, 2015.

[9] L. Fiorillo, "Conscious sedation in dentistry," *Medicina*, vol. 55, no. 12, p. 778, 2019.

[10] G. S. George, A. Morgan, J. Meechan et al., "Injectable local anaesthetic agents for dental anaesthesia," *The Cochrane Database of Systematic Reviews*, vol. 7, article CD006487, 2018.

[11] M. Nunna, R. K. Dasaraju, R. Kamatham, S. K. Mallineni, and S. Nuvvula, "Comparative evaluation of virtual reality distraction and counter-stimulation on dental anxiety and pain perception in children," *Journal of Dental Anesthesia and Pain Medicine*, vol. 19, no. 5, pp. 277–288, 2019.

[12] S. P. Tirupathi and S. Rajasekhar, "Effect of precooling on pain during local anesthesia administration in children: a systematic review," *Journal of Dental Anesthesia and Pain Medicine*, vol. 20, no. 3, pp. 119–127, 2020.

[13] T. D. Yogesh Kumar, J. B. John, S. Asokan, P. R. Geetha Priya, R. Punithavathy, and V. Praburajan, "Behavioral response and pain perception to computer controlled local anesthetic delivery system and cartridge syringe," *Journal of the Indian Society of Pedodontics and Preventive Dentistry*, vol. 33, no. 3, pp. 223–228, 2015.

[14] H. Oubenyahya and N. Bouhabba, "General anesthesia in the management of early childhood caries: an overview," *Journal of Dental Anesthesia and Pain Medicine*, vol. 19, no. 6, pp. 313–322, 2019.

[15] C. G. Hicks, J. E. Jones, M. A. Saxen et al., "Demand in pediatric dentistry for sedation and general anesthesia by dentist anesthesiologists: a survey of directors of dentist anesthesiologist and pediatric dentistry residencies," *Anesthesia Progress*, vol. 59, no. 1, pp. 3–11, 2012.

[16] H. Mohammed, N. Shallik, M. Barsoum et al., "Dental needle foreign body in the neck: a case report," *Journal of Dental Anesthesia and Pain Medicine*, vol. 20, no. 2, pp. 83–87, 2020.

[17] J.-s. You, S.-G. Kim, J.-S. Oh, H.-I. Choi, and M.-K. Jih, "Removal of a fractured needle during inferior alveolar nerve block: two case reports," *Journal of Dental Anesthesia and Pain Medicine*, vol. 17, no. 3, pp. 225–229, 2017.

[18] J. Miranda-Rius, L. Brunet-Llobet, E. Lahor-Soler, O. Mrina, and A. Ramírez-Rámiz, "Dental root elevator embedded into a subgingival caries: a case report," *BMC Research Notes*, vol. 8, no. 1, p. 60, 2015.

[19] S. M. Balaji, "Burried broken extraction instrument fragment," *Annals of Maxillofacial Surgery*, vol. 3, no. 1, pp. 93-94, 2013.

[20] S. Matsuda, H. Yoshimura, H. Yoshida, and K. Sano, "Breakage and migration of a high-speed dental hand-piece bur during mandibular third molar extraction: two case reports," *Medicine*, vol. 99, no. 7, article e19177, 2020.

[21] S. Passi and N. Sharma, "Unusual foreign bodies in the orofacial region," *Case Reports in Dentistry*, vol. 2012, Article ID 191873, 4 pages, 2012.

11

Maxillary Sinus Natural Killer/T-Cell Extranodal Lymphoma Mimicking a Dentoalveolar Abscess

Erika Antonia dos Anjos Ramos,[1] Luciana Munhoz,[1] Basílio Almeida Milani,[2] Tomás Zecchini Barrese,[3] Stephanie Kenig Viveiros,[1] and Emiko Saito Arita[1]

[1]*Department of Stomatology, School of Dentistry, University of São Paulo, 2227 Lineu Prestes Avenue, 05508-000 São Paulo, SP, Brazil*
[2]*Department of Maxillofacial Surgery, Hospital Municipal do Campo Limpo, 1661 Estrada da Itapecerica, 05835-005 São Paulo, Brazil*
[3]*Department of Pathological Sciences, School of Medicine, Santa Casa de Sao Paulo School of Medical Sciences, 61 Dr. Cesário Motta Junior Street, 01221-020 São Paulo, SP, Brazil*

Correspondence should be addressed to Erika Antonia dos Anjos Ramos; erika.antonia.ramos@usp.br

Academic Editor: Ricardo Alves Mesquita

Extranodal natural killer/T-cell lymphoma (ENKL) is an aggressive and infrequent malignant neoplasm. Early sinonasal ENKL clinical symptomatology is often not specific which can mimic several clinical odontogenic processes such as dentoalveolar abscesses. A 41-year-old female was referred to our institution due to facial pain with skin rash, fever, and intraoral swelling in the left side of the maxillary region. Computed tomography (CT) revealed a soft tissue hypodense area in the left side with bone discontinuity in anterior and lateral maxillary sinuses. Initial laboratorial tests showed no alterations on hemogram, coagulation profile, and immune phenotype ($CD3^+/CD4^+$). However, the lesion progressed fastly showing an evident growth, so it was decided that an intraoral biopsy should be performed. The diagnosis was sinonasal ENKLs. This case is an example that the rare T-cell lymphoma can mimic an odontogenic lesion, thus puzzling the clinician. Fortunately, the rapid growth of the lesion prompted the correct diagnosis and early treatment.

1. Introduction

Extranodal natural killer/T-cell lymphoma (ENKL) is an infrequent malignant neoplasm [1] that arises primarily from the natural killer cell [2] and accounts for 15% of all non-Hodgkin lymphomas located in the nasal fossae and maxillary sinuses [3]. The sinonasal ENKL location is unusual [4]. Formerly, the lesion was not recognized as a neoplastic process, and it was named "malignant centrofacial granuloma," [4] "lethal midline granuloma," or angiocentric lymphoma, due to its necrotizing and invasive evolution features [2].

Sinonasal ENKL presents as a highly aggressive neoplasm [2], which is characterized by the progressive destruction of the midline facial and/or nasal structures [3, 5] and eventually also may affect the orbit by contiguity [3]. Early sinonasal ENKL clinical symptomatology is often not specific and may include headache, facial pain, nasal congestion, and fever [1]. Although most of the sinonasal ENKL patients exhibit locoregional disease, systemic involvement may be present [5].

Due to the anatomical proximity with oral cavity and paranasal sinuses, ENKL can affect intraoral elements, which can mimic several clinical odontogenic origin entities, including inflammatory and infectious diseases, such as dentoalveolar abscesses [6].

Accordingly, the objective of this report is to describe the main clinical, radiographic, and histologic characteristics of a

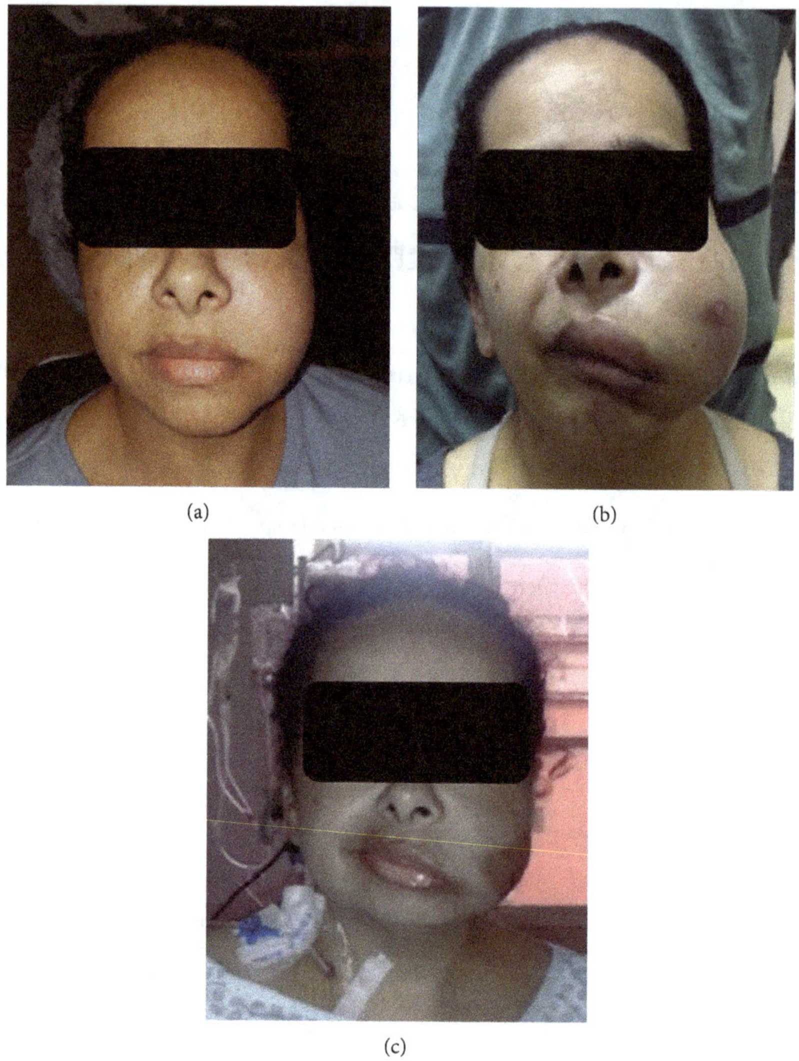

Figure 1: From left to right: (a) exhibits patient facial aspect at the first consultation, note the slight bulging in the left side of the face; (b) demonstrates the lesion fast progress by showing the evident lesion growth in 3 weeks; (c) shows lesion shrink after 4 weeks of chemotherapy.

sinonasal ENKL case in the maxillary sinuses, first diagnosed as an odontogenic abscess due to its early clinical features. Furthermore, the aggressive lesion development is also illustrated in tomographic examinations performed in different short time interval moments.

2. Case Report

A 41-year-old Caucasian woman noticed left cheek swelling and pain in corresponding upper premolars and molars and attended to a consultation in the Oral and Maxillofacial service at Hospital Municipal do Campo Limpo (São Paulo, Brazil). Her medical history revealed a previously ischemic cerebrovascular accident and continuous use of anticoagulants but no other past disease.

Extraoral examination showed no lymphadenopathy or paresthesia but an evident swelling in the left cheek (Figure 1(a)) with a hardened consistency. The patient mentioned she noticed the symptoms for a period of time higher than a week. Intraorally, she showed severe periodontal disease and pain during vertical/horizontal percussion tests. Pulp vitality could not be determined at this point, due to the severity of pain presented during teeth percussion tests. Buccoalveolar sulcus bulging and a floating tumefaction in the left upper molar root region were observed. Although the first diagnostic hypothesis was dental abscess, due to the unusual duration of the tumefaction, the patient was then referred to imaging examinations (multislice computed tomography—MCT). However, due to the presence of an intraoral floating tumefaction and dental origin symptomatology, drainage was performed, and antibiotic treatment was prescribed.

Despite of accomplishing imaging examinations as requested in the first consultation, the patient only came back to the Oral and Maxillofacial service after three weeks, when she felt paresthesia and severe pain in her left face. Figure 1(b) exhibits the patient left face swelling aspect at this moment. Due to the increase in painful symptomatology and evident speedy lesion development, the patient was immediately hospitalized, and a new CT examination was

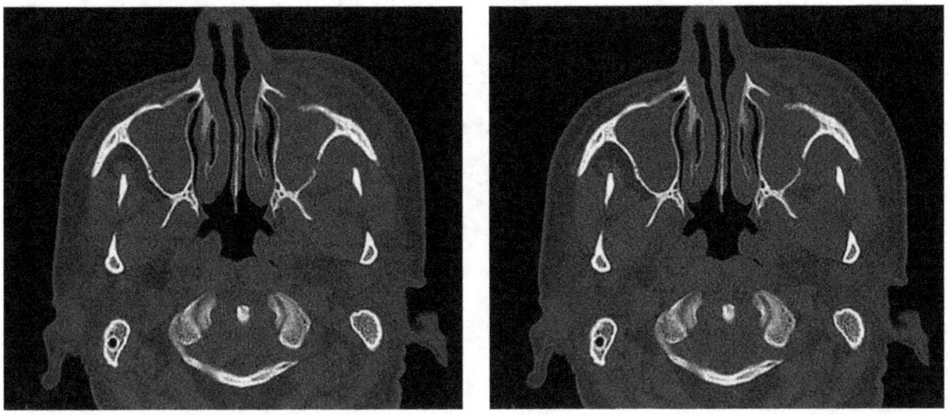

(a) (b)

FIGURE 2: First consultation examination. (a) The axial MCT scan shows a soft-tissue mass anterior to the maxillary sinus, left side, and sinus anterior and lateral wall bone erosion. (b) Coronal MCT scan exhibits nasal cavity involvement by soft-tissue mass, as well as sinus lateral wall bone destruction.

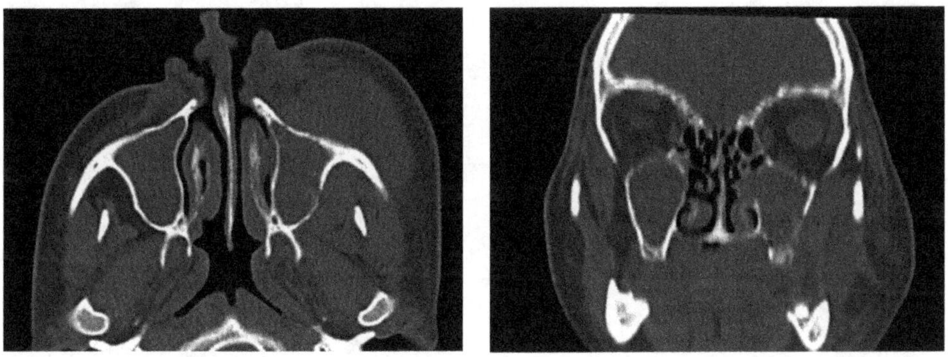

(a) (b)

FIGURE 3: MCT examination 3 weeks after the first consultation. (a) Axial MCT scan, note the prominent increasing of extensive soft tissue. In (b), the nasal cavity involvement is even more evident when compared to the first consultation imaging examination.

performed, as well as routine and biochemical blood test examinations. Intraoral floating was now absented.

No alterations were verified in the patient hemogram, coagulation tests, and immune phenotype ($CD3^+/CD4^+$) examinations, as well as blood tests for hormones, especially the parathyroid hormone.

2.1. Imaging Evaluations. Noncontrast-enhanced, high resolution MCT with 16 slices (Toshiba Activion, Medical Systems Corporation, Japan) was used for MCT imaging. Acquisition imaging parameters were 0.5 mm slice thickness, 1.0 mm *Spacing* Between Slices, 250 mm field of view, 120 kV peak, and 250 mA. The first consultation MCT axial slices revealed a soft tissue hypodense area in the left side, comprising the maxillary sinus area and bone discontinuity in the anterior and lateral maxillary sinus wall (Figure 2(a)) orbital cavity floor. Frontal slices showed discrete nasal cavity involvement (Figure 2(b)).

The second consultation MCT axial slices revealed that the soft tissue hypodense area in the left side increased in size, with greater nasal cavity involvement and bone destruction than Figure 2.

At this point, the main diagnostic hypothesis was osteosarcoma, sinonasal diffuse large B-cell lymphoma, parathyroid brown tumor, and extranodal malignant lymphoma, particularly maxillary ENKL. The hypothesis of dentoalveolar abscess was disregarded: floating tumefaction might be coincidentally previously present due to the periodontal disease severe status.

2.2. Histopathological Results/Histopathology. A biopsy was taken from the lesion (oral cavity) and sent to the hospital's pathology department. The histopathological examination with hematoxylin and eosin (H&E) showed a diffuse proliferation of small to medium-sized atypical lymphocytes with areas showing an angiocentric pattern effacing the normal architecture of the oral mucosa. Mild epithelium tropism and espongiosis were observed (Figures 4(a) and 4(b)). Focal areas of ulceration and necrosis were also seen. Trial immunohistochemical and in situ hybridization reactions were made (Figures 4(c)–4(i)). The findings were consistent with ENKL. As part of staging, a bone marrow biopsy was done, and no abnormalities were found.

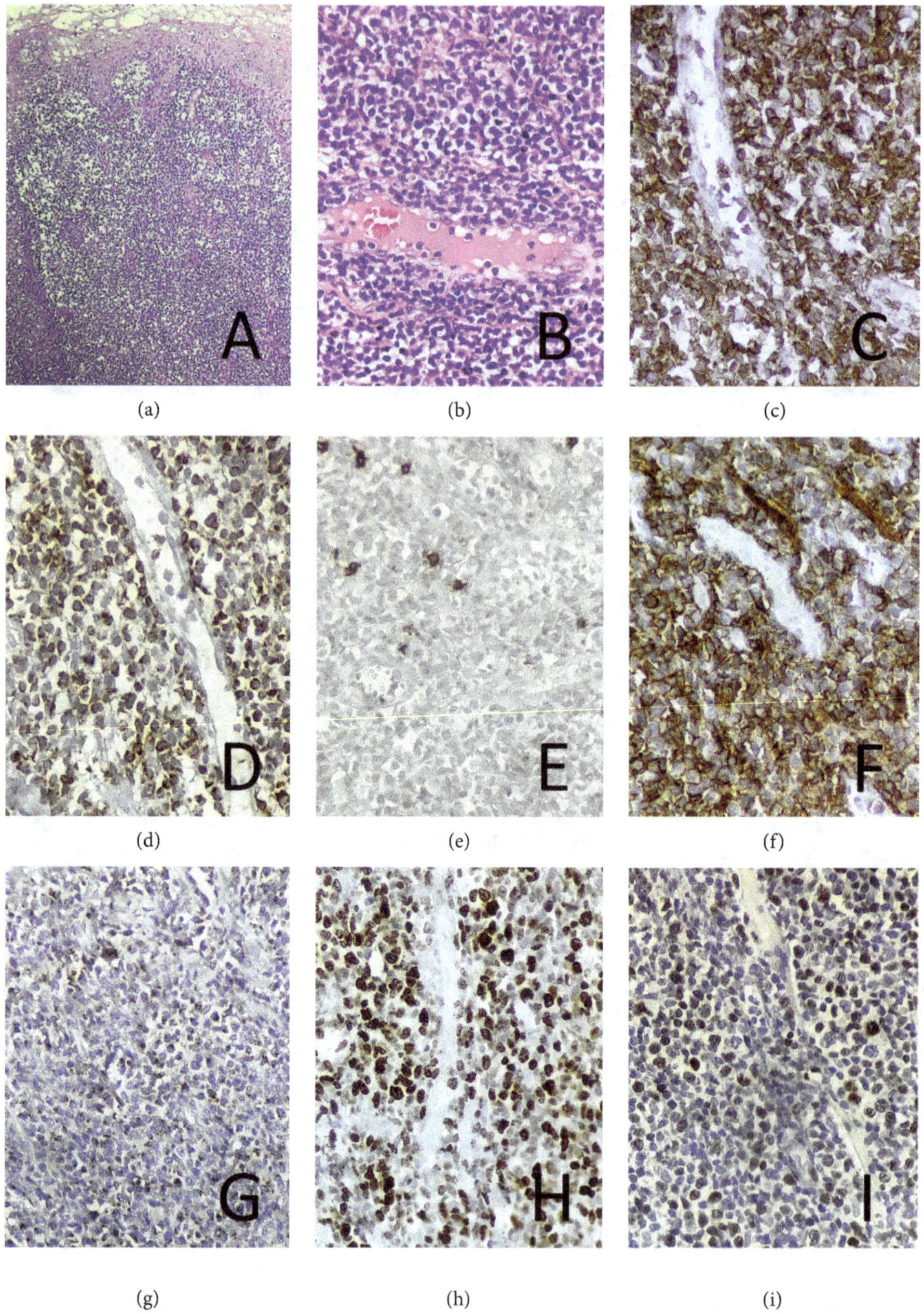

FIGURE 4: Histopathological features: in (a), the histologic section from the lesion biopsy sample shows a diffuse and permeative infiltrate of small to medium-sized atypical lymphocytes (H&E, ×100); in (b), an evident angiocentric and angiodestructive growth pattern is represented (H&E, ×400). Immunohistochemical and in situ hybridization reactions: in (c), the neoplastic cells show immunopositivity for CD45 (×400); in (d), immunopositivity (partial/weak) for CD3 (×400); in (e), immunonegativity for CD20 (×400); in (f), immunopositivity for CD56 (×400); in (g), immunopositivity (cytoplasmic granules) for TIA1 (×400); in (h), Ki67 index (×400); and in (i), positive nuclear labeling for in situ hybridization for EBV (×400).

2.3. Treatment. Before the diagnostic definition, the patient was treated with one cycle of CHOP (cyclophosphamide, doxorubicin, vincristine, and prednisolone). Once the diagnosis was established, the AspaMetDex (L-asparaginase, methotrexate, and dexamethasone) regimen was started, but no response was observed after two cycles of chemotherapy; on the contrary, the lesion became larger, and the acute inflammatory signs turned more evident. Facing this, the DICE (dexamethasone, isofosfamide, cisplatin, and etoposide) regimen and local radiotherapy (30 Gy) were started. After two cycles, the lesion presented a significant reduction, but her general condition deteriorated and was associated with mucositis and persistent neutropenia. Before even starting another cycle, five months after the diagnosis, the patient passed away.

3. Discussion

Although malignant lymphomas are also considered opportunistic neoplasms as they usually affect immunocompromised patients [7], in the present case, there were no history, blood laboratory results, or signs that suggested compromised immunity, as previously described in the literature [1].

Sinonasal ENKL is an aggressive and speedy evolution lesion [1]. Our case confirms this, demonstrating the fast disease progress clinically observed in three weeks and at MCT. Furthermore, due to the anatomical proximity with the oral cavity, sinonasal ENKL may compromise intraoral structures and, eventually, in the presence of a concomitant odontogenic disease, mimic infectious diseases [6], such as dentoalveolar abscesses, as specified in the case described. Lymphomas and infectious diseases may present similar MCT images, mainly during the early disease stage, such as the slight bone destruction [6]. Furthermore, clinical symptoms such as mobile teeth, gingival enlargement, oral masses, and swelling next to the oral cavity as chief complaints may lead clinicians to misdiagnose lymphomas as dentoalveolar abscesses [8] in an initial consultation which may delay the final diagnosis.

Imaging features in MCT often shows infiltrative or permeative bony discontinuity, with different destruction degrees [9]; in our case, evident destruction of sinonasal walls was also observed. The presence of the partially preserved sinus wall for the most extensive tumor involvement, as noticed in Figure 3, is also a usual characteristic of sinonasal lymphomas [9], although sinus wall bone erosion can be the result of other aggressive neoplasm [10]. Extensive soft-tissue mass can be observed in sinonasal ENKLs [10] particularly with lesion progression.

The differential diagnosis should include malignant maxillary tumors, such as sinonanasal undifferentiated and nasopharyngeal carcinoma [1], or other midline ulcerative destructive lesions [3], squamous cell carcinoma [9, 10], oral manifestations of Wegner's granulomatosis [1, 4, 10], primary orbit tumors [3], malignant melanoma, adenoid cystic carcinoma [10], and sinonasal diffuse large B-cell lymphomas, which have similar characteristics when compared to sinonasal ENKLs [2]. In the present case, the leading diagnosis hypothesis after imaging examination evaluation was sinonasal ENKL mainly due to the bony wall destruction noticed and concomitant right and left maxillary sinus opacification, resembling to another case previously described, in which sinonasal ENKL has also mimicked an odontogenic origin infection, delaying the final diagnosis [6].

Outcomes for sinonasal malignancies, enclosing ENKL, have improved recently [2]; nonetheless, prognosis is still relatively poor [2, 4], particularly to patients who have systemic disease [5, 6], and even worse in the case of recurrence [5]. Early precise disease diagnosis for any maxillofacial malignant lymphoma is crucial to achieve better treatment results [1, 11, 12].

Overall, paranasal sinus malignant lymphomas usually present nonspecific early clinical symptomatology [2, 12]. The dental professional can play a valuable role in the diagnosis of patients with sinonasal malignancies which warrants immediate referral to an appropriate specialist when the combination of patient clinical signs arouses suspicion, mainly due to the fact that the mucosa of paranasal sinuses is not accessible as the oral mucosa for further inspection [12].

Notwithstanding, considering the aforementioned nonspecific signals and symptoms, the final diagnosis of the sinonasal ENKLs is achieved by histological and immunohistochemical evaluations [1, 6]. The histological features of ENKLs are usually the same no matter the site affected. The lesions tend to have a diffuse and permeative infiltration of atypical lymphocytes that can be small, medium-sized, large, or anaplastic. The neoplastic cells can be accompanied by a mixture of inflammatory cells. An angiocentric and angiodestructive growth pattern is often present. Besides, this entity frequently shows extensive necrotic areas and ulceration, and multiple biopsies may be required until representative material is acquired. Fortunately, and due to the dimensions of the tumor described here, one single biopsy was enough to the diagnosis. Typically, the immunophenotype of ENKT is CD45 positive, surface CD3 negative, CD2 positive, CD5 negative, and, although not specific, CD56 positive. Cytotoxic molecules such as granzyme B, TIA1, and perforin are positive. The diagnosis virtually requires the presence of EBV, and the most reliable way to demonstrate it is the *in situ* hybridization for EBER, since immunostaining for LMP1 is frequently negative [13].

Treatment for ENKL is mainly dependent on the disease stage at the diagnosis and, although controversial [13], the histologic subtype [2] and is not as yet well codified [4]. Radiotherapy and chemotherapy may be applied [4], but it has often unsatisfactory results [5, 6]. Unfortunately, in our case, the patient have not had a satisfactory response by the moment this manuscript was written.

In conclusion, sinonasal ENKL is an infrequent aggressive disease that can resemble to odontogenic origin diseases, which can delay the diagnosis. Imaging examinations are essential to guide diagnostic hypotheses; however, histological and immunohistochemical examinations are essential in the diagnosis process. The speedy neoplasm progress of this malignant disease was illustrated in this report by the CT examinations performed in distinct moments, with short time interval.

References

[1] N. Nikolaos, P. Grigorios, K. Konstantinos et al., "Extranodal nasal-type NK/T-cell lymphoma of the palate and paranasal sinuses," *American Journal of Case Reports*, vol. 13, pp. 79–85, 2012.

[2] P. M. Dubal, R. Dutta, A. Vazquez, T. D. Patel, S. Baredes, and J. A. Eloy, "A comparative population-based analysis of sinonasal diffuse large B-cell and extranodal NK/T-cell lymphomas," *Laryngoscope*, vol. 125, no. 5, pp. 1077–1083, 2015.

[3] A. Hervás-Ontiveros, E. España-Gregori, P. Hernández-Martínez, F. J. Vera-Sempere, and M. Díaz-Llopis, "Orbital involvement by non-Hodgkin lymphoma NK T cells," *Archivos de la Sociedad Española de Oftalmología*, vol. 89, no. 11, pp. 450–453, 2014.

[4] M. Hmidi, M. Kettani, A. Elboukhari, N. Touiheme, and A. Messary, "Sinonasal NK/T-cell lymphoma," *European Annals of Otorhinolaryngology, Head and Neck Diseases*, vol. 130, no. 3, pp. 145–147, 2013.

[5] C. C. Li, H. F. Tien, J. L. Tang et al., "Treatment outcome and pattern of failure in 77 patients with sinonasal natural killer/T-cell or T-cell lymphoma," *Cancer*, vol. 100, no. 2, pp. 366–375, 2004.

[6] T. Yamada, K. Mishima, A. Ota et al., "A case of ATLL (adult T-cell leukemia/lymphoma) mimicking odontogenic infection," *Oral Surgery, Oral Medicine, Oral Pathology, Oral Radiology, and Endodontology*, vol. 109, no. 6, pp. e51–e55, 2010.

[7] E. Zapater, J. V. Bagán, F. Carbonell, and J. Basterra, "Malignant lymphoma of the head and neck," *Oral Diseases*, vol. 16, no. 2, pp. 119–128, 2010.

[8] L. Ardekian, A. Rachmiel, D. Rosen, I. Abu-El-Naaj, M. Peled, and D. Laufer, "Burkitt's lymphoma of the oral cavity in Israel," *Journal of Cranio-Maxillofacial Surgery*, vol. 27, no. 5, pp. 294–297, 1999.

[9] H. Kato, M. Kanematsu, H. Watanabe, S. Kawaguchi, K. Mizuta, and M. Aoki, "Differentiation of extranodal non-Hodgkins lymphoma from squamous cell carcinoma of the maxillary sinus: a multimodality imaging approach," *SpringerPlus*, vol. 4, no. 1, p. 228, 2015.

[10] G. C. Ooi, C. S. Chim, R. Liang, K. W. T. Tsang, and Y. L. Kwong, "Nasal T-cell/natural killer cell lymphoma: CT and MR imaging features of a new clinicopathologic entity," *AJR American Journal of Roentgenology*, vol. 174, no. 4, pp. 1141–1145, 2000.

[11] L. Munhoz, F. P. M. Marsan, and E. S. Arita, "Radiographic enlargement of mandibular canal as an extranodal primary non-Hodgkin's lymphoma early sign in an asymptomatic patient," *Case Reports in Dentistry*, vol. 2017, Article ID 9193165, 4 pages, 2017.

[12] G. W. Bell, B. B. Joshi, and R. I. Macleod, "Maxillary sinus disease: diagnosis and treatment," *British Dental Journal*, vol. 210, no. 3, pp. 113–118, 2011.

[13] S. H. Swerdlow, E. Campo, N. L. Harris et al., *World Health Organization Classification of Tumors of Haematopoietic and Lymphoid Tissues*, IARC Press, Lyon, 5th edition, 2017.

12

A Suggested Approach of Managing Excessive Maxillary Gingival Display in Terminal Dentition

Daniel Saad,[1,2] **Celine Moukarzel**,[1] **Naim El Haddad**,[1] **and Anthony Rizk**[1]

[1]*Postgraduate Department, MOI, Faculty of Dentistry, Goethe University, Frankfurt, Germany*
[2]*Private Practice, Beirut, Lebanon*

Correspondence should be addressed to Daniel Saad; saadaniel@gmail.com

Academic Editor: Anastasios Markopoulos

The aim of this paper is to report a suggested approach for the management of excessive maxillary gingival display with terminal dentition. A segmental osteotomy of the maxillary process was performed, and the latter used as grafting material for lateral sinus augmentation that was performed simultaneously. Following the graft maturation period, implants were inserted and rehabilitated with a fixed dentogingival prosthesis. Consequently, the mandible was prosthetically restored following the new occlusal plane dictated by the rehabilitated maxilla. Clinically, the procedure showed a drastic improvement in the patient's appearance, eliminating the excessive gingival display. Radiologically, it led to a vertical translation of the maxillary process level in an apical direction. Nevertheless, the resected process used as grafting material was noticed to have a suboptimal behavior as long as it showed increased intrasinusal resorption, barely sufficient for a regular implant accommodation. The described therapy concept seems to be a plausible approach when it comes to manage excessive maxillary gingival displays in edentulous patients or those presenting a terminal dentition. However, at the time of sinus augmentation, authors recommend to graft a mixture of resected maxillary process and a bone substitute material, in order to get more stable results.

1. Introduction

Nowadays, social media prevalence interferes with every aspect of one's life. Many bloggers and social media influencers are dictating the way of living by keeping up a stylish lifestyle. Consequently, a person's perfect appearance is becoming a must in society. Hence, dentists are increasingly solicited to maintain their patients' glamourous smiles whereas the business of laminate veneers and smile makeovers is flourishing.

One of many stigmas encountered while smiling is what is commonly known as "gummy smile." A "gummy smile" refers to an unpleasant excessive maxillary gingival display while smiling. Its clinical correction starts by establishing the right diagnosis in order to find the appropriate treatment. First, an exhaustive facial examination is necessary to determine the facial and lateral proportions and symmetry, as well as the smile line, gum exposure, and lip length. Afterward, an intraoral examination is required for the teeth anatomy, the bite plane, and the periodontal state [1].

Determining the etiology of the excessive gingival display is the next step in the management of such cases. Herein will be presented several diagnoses implicated in the latter.

The first diagnosis is drug and plaque-induced gingival hypertrophy. In this case, gingival inflammation due to plaque or medical treatments—immunosuppressant drugs such as cyclosporine, antiepileptic drugs such as phenytoin, and calcium channels blockers such as nifedipine [2]—can induce a hyperplastic-overgrown gingiva covering the maxillary crowns, hence, causing excessive gingival display. Maintaining impeccable oral hygiene may be the treatment of choice; however, surgical intervention can be indicated in specific cases.

Another mechanism for excessive gum display is originated from an altered passive eruption. In fact, teeth eruption is divided into 2 stages. The first, known as active eruption, consisting of the tooth migration to the occlusal plane, whereas the second stage, known as passive eruption, is due to the migration of the gingiva apically to uncover the tooth. When the passive eruption is altered, the gingiva will still cover the tooth, thus causing shorter clinical crowns and in some cases excessive gingival display. Colset et al. [3] classified the altered passive eruption into two types each having two subtypes:

(i) Type 1-A: normal distance between cementoenamel junction (CEJ) and alveolar crest with an excessive amount of keratinized tissue and it can be treated by gingivectomy

(ii) Type 1-B: CEJ and alveolar crest at the same level with excessive amount of keratinized tissue, it can be treated by gingivectomy and osseous reduction

(iii) Type 2-A: normal distance between CEJ and alveolar crest with a normal amount of keratinized tissue, it can be treated by apically positioned flap

(iv) Type 2-B: CEJ and alveolar crest at the same level with a normal amount of keratinized tissue, it can be treated by osseous reduction and apically positioned flap

Furthermore, a third cause would be vertical maxillary excess (VME). VME can be defined as a disproportional growth of the maxilla in the vertical direction, which could lead to a long face syndrome [4]. VME is generally associated with an open bite; however, when associated with a normal bite, an excessive gingiva display would hence be covering the incisal edge of the canines [5]. Garber and Salama classified VME into 3 degrees:

(i) Degree 1: excessive gingival display of 2-4 mm and it can be treated by orthodontic intrusion, crown lengthening, or botulinum toxin injection

(ii) Degree 2: excessive gingival display of 4–8 mm and it can be treated by [6] lip stabilization technique or orthognathic surgery

(iii) Degree 3: excessive gingival display of more than 8 mm and can only be treated by orthognathic surgery

A fourth etiology is a short or hypermobile lip. In fact, short upper lips with less than 15 mm of distance between the lower border of the upper lip and the subnasale [7], or hypermobile lips caused by excessive contractions of the lip elevator muscles, can induce an excessive gingival display. This condition may be treated by the lip stabilization technique [6]. When there is a gingival exposure of 1 to 3 mm, an injection of botulinum toxin is preferred every 6 months to limit the lip elevator activity.

Treatment of excessive gingival display requires a multidisciplinary approach to achieve successful aesthetic and functional results. While the treatment of gummy smile for dentulous patients represents some challenges, albeit more obstacles are encountered with edentulous patients, in order to achieve desirable outcomes.

Complete edentulous upper jaws can be rehabilitated by either conventional removable dentures, or by means of implant-supported prostheses. In the latter, it consists either of a removable implant-supported denture with extended vestibular flanges or a flange-free cross-arch fixed implant-retained prosthesis with (hybrid design) or without (crown design) pink ceramic [8]. Consequently, in order to decide on the optimal therapeutic option regarding the prosthetic design, a diligent complex and multifactorial treatment planning should be considered, which takes into account the volume of the hard and the soft tissue to be compensated, as well as the emergence profile of the future prosthetic teeth along with their vertical, horizontal, and sagittal positions, and provides at once an adequate lip support and balanced facial harmony [8, 9]. Within this scope, a benchmark article [8] addressing this matter was published in 2013 where authors tried to establish a comprehensive decision-making tree with regards to implant-supported prosthesis selection based on the aforementioned patient's clinical characteristics. The published work documented exhaustively different clinical situations of deficient edentulous maxillae. What it did not address is the situations where edentulous maxillae are prominent and excessively visible when smiling.

This paper describes an implant-supported prosthetic rehabilitation of an excessively prominent maxillary process with terminal dentition.

2. Case Presentation

In February 2018, one female patient stepped into the private clinic for a complete oral rehabilitation after years of neglected oral care. The patient, who is 58 years old, was seeking for a global dental care and a solution for her excessive gingival display. Intraoral examination revealed a terminal maxillary dentition. Radiographic examination showed an impacted canine #23. In the mandible, apart the present natural anterior teeth, radiologic examination showed the presence of three restored implants on the right side and failed bridge over hopeless teeth on the patient's left side. Extraoral examination revealed a VME reflected by an excessive gingival display at smiling, showing unpleasantly the whole maxillary process all the way up to the tuberosities (Figure 1).

The following treatment plan was agreed on;

Maxilla: extraction of the remaining teeth with alveolar segmental reduction along with a bilateral sinus floor elevation, followed by a maxillary rehabilitation by means of a Toronto prosthesis [10] retained by 6 implants also known as abutment-hybrid overdenture.

Mandible: crowning of the anterior teeth, restoring the left side by implant-supported bridge, and a new set of crowns over the present implants on the right.

Treatment began by rehabilitating the maxilla:

First, segmental alveolar osteotomy was performed on the right hemimaxilla to remove the vertical maxillary excess using Piezosurgery-touch (Mectron, Cherasco, Italy). The intervention carried out at once a lateral sinus floor elevation, where resected maxillary crest after being crushed, was grafted inside the sinus. Simultaneously, an implant (Duravit 3P, B&B Dental Implant Company, Bologna, Italy) was inserted in the region of the right canine. Then, the buccal

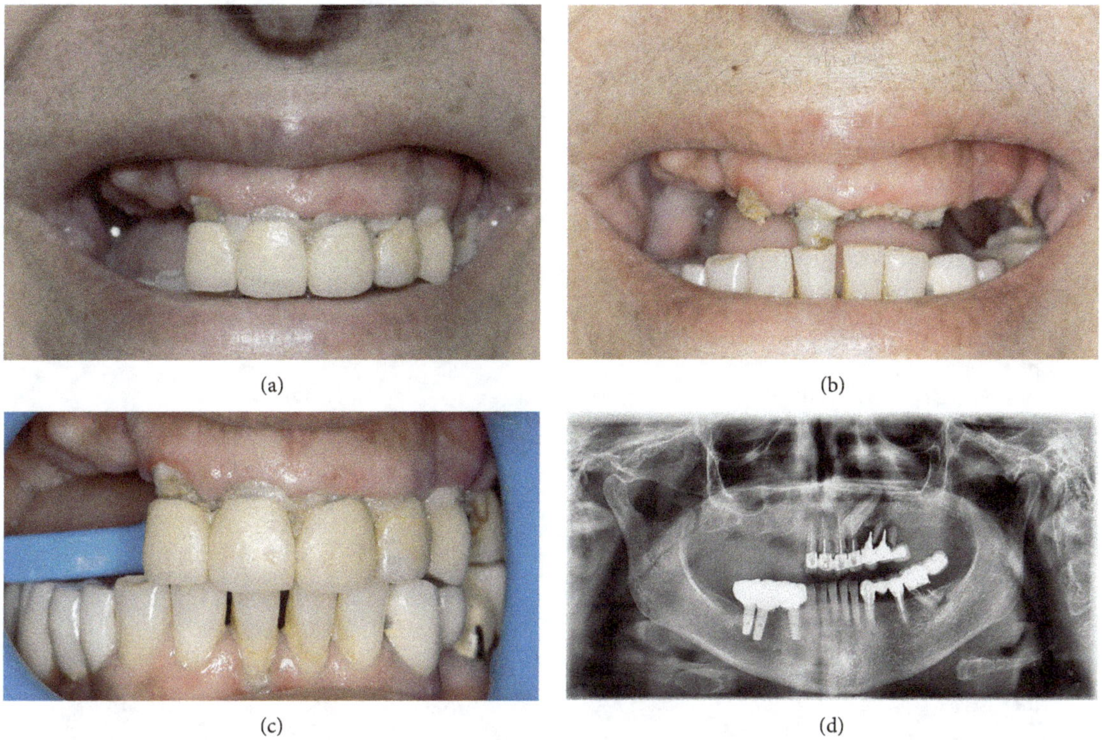

FIGURE 1: Baseline: (a–c) clinical situation of the patient at the baseline. (d) Radiological situation at the baseline.

flap was repositioned apically to preserve the keratinized mucosa (Figure 2).

Two weeks later, a similar procedure was performed on the left hemimaxilla along with the extraction of the impacted canine. Here, the implant (Duravit EV, B&B Dental Implant Company, Bologna, Italy) was inserted partially in the canine socket, which was filled with the crushed resected alveolar process. The right maxillary subantral space was packed first with bovine xenograft (Ti-Oss, Gyeonggi-do, South Korea) towards the back and then filled with the remaining autogenous resected ridge anteriorly (Figure 3).

After a 2-week healing period, serving as temporary prosthesis during the maturity phase of the grafted sinuses, a removable denture was delivered which was retained by the two inserted implants through their respective transitional implant overdenture attachments (OT equator, Rhein83, Bologna, Italy) (Figure 4).

6 months later, two implants (Duravit EV, B&B Dental Implant Company, Bologna, Italy) were inserted in each of the sinuses and left submerged for a two-month period (Figure 5).

After 2 months, an open tray impression of the maxilla with its six osseointegrated implants was taken using polyether impression material (Impregum, 3M, Minneapolis, USA), then the poured master cast was scanned with the respective scanbodies in place. Appropriate multiunit abutment was selected for 5 out of the 6 implants, and that for the ease of insertion of the future prosthesis. Consequently, an intermediate Chrome-Cobalt bar was 3D printed using Selective Laser Melting (SLM) technology (SISMA spa, Vicenza, Italy) to check intraorally the passivity fit, which was found to be satisfactory. A diagnostic wax setup using resin denture teeth was then built over the intermediate bar and tried-in intraorally for functional and esthetic evaluation as well as patient approval. The occlusal plane was set parallel to the Camper plane, regardless of the occlusal curve of the mandibular dentition. Then, the diagnostic setup was scanned in-lab, and the final framework of the mesostructure and of its individual crowns was virtually designed.

The mesostructure and the 8 posterior individual crowns' frameworks were 3D printed (SLM) in Chrome-Cobalt alloy, while 6 anterior individual crowns were milled out of zirconia for improved esthetics.

The mesostructure was then manually veneered with gingival pink porcelain (VC gingiva, Creation Willi Geller International GmbH, Meiningen, Austria), while the crowns were built-up with veneering ceramic (Creation Willi Geller International GmbH, Meiningen, Austria), ending up into a hybrid prosthesis. The said prosthesis was screwed-in safely directly over one implant and indirectly through the 5 underlying multiunit abutments, and the individuals crowns cemented on its top subsequently (Figure 6).

The mandible underwent a more straightforward treatment plan, which is out of the scope of this report. Concisely, the roots of the teeth #34, #36, and #37 were extracted; then, a flap was raised showing buccal bone deficiency. 3 implants (Rootform, ROOTT, Trate AG, Baech, Switzerland) were inserted along with autogenous horizontal bone augmentation following the principles of the split bone block technique [11]. The bony plates were fixed using titanium microscrews (Conmet LLC , Moscow, Russia). The whole augmentation was then covered by a synthetic resorbable membrane (Tisseos, Biomedical Tissues, Nantes, France). Two months later, implants on both sides were restored prosthetically, with

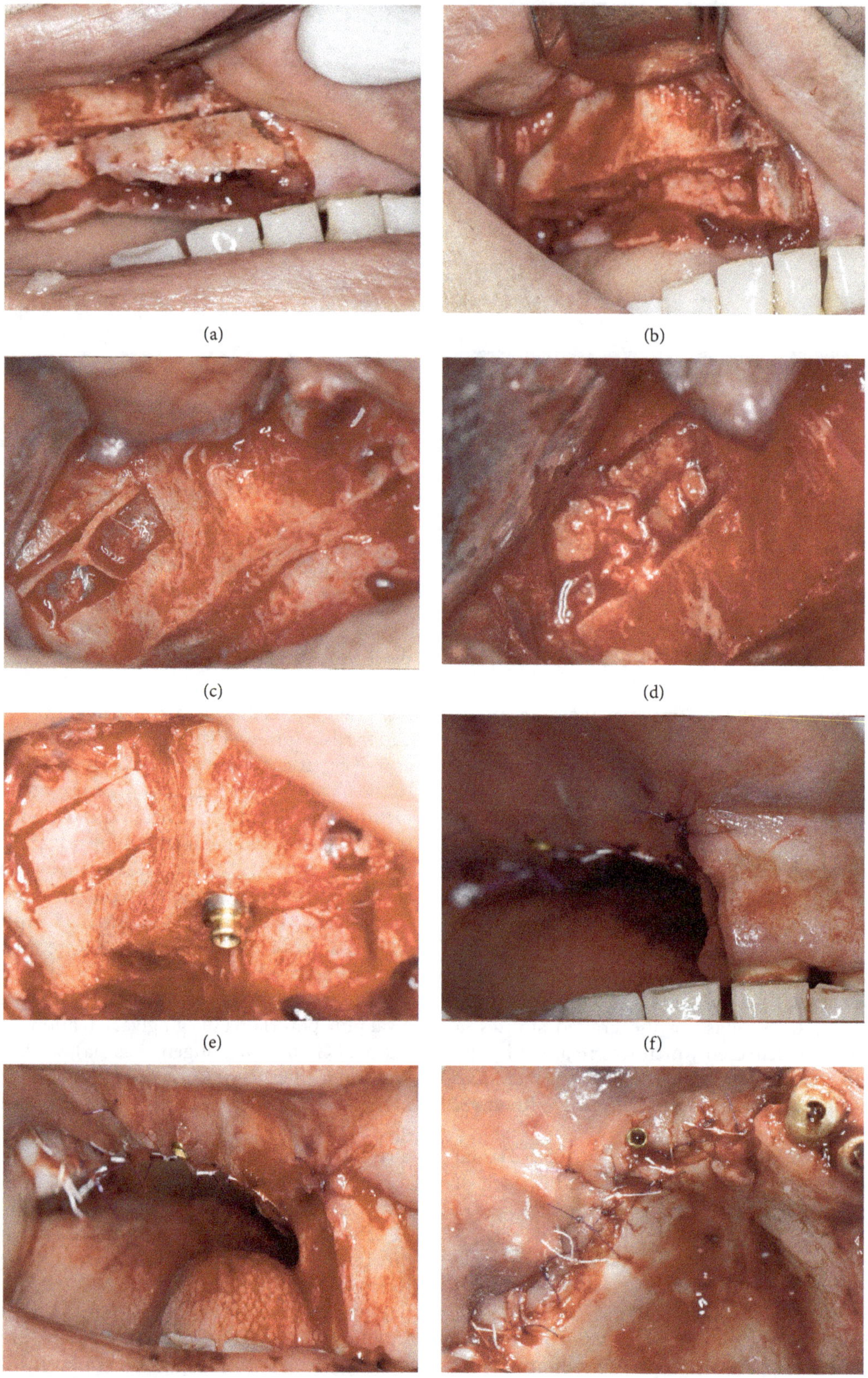

(a) (b) (c) (d) (e) (f) (g) (h)

FIGURE 2: Left hemimaxilla: (a, b) segmental osteotomy of the alveolar process. (c) Lateral window approach during left maxillary sinus floor elevation. (d) Crushed resected alveolar process grafted inside the sinus. (e) Picture showing lateral bony window placed back and implant inserted in the canine region. (f–h) Respectively: frontal, lateral, and occlusal view of the postoperative clinical situation immediately after suturing.

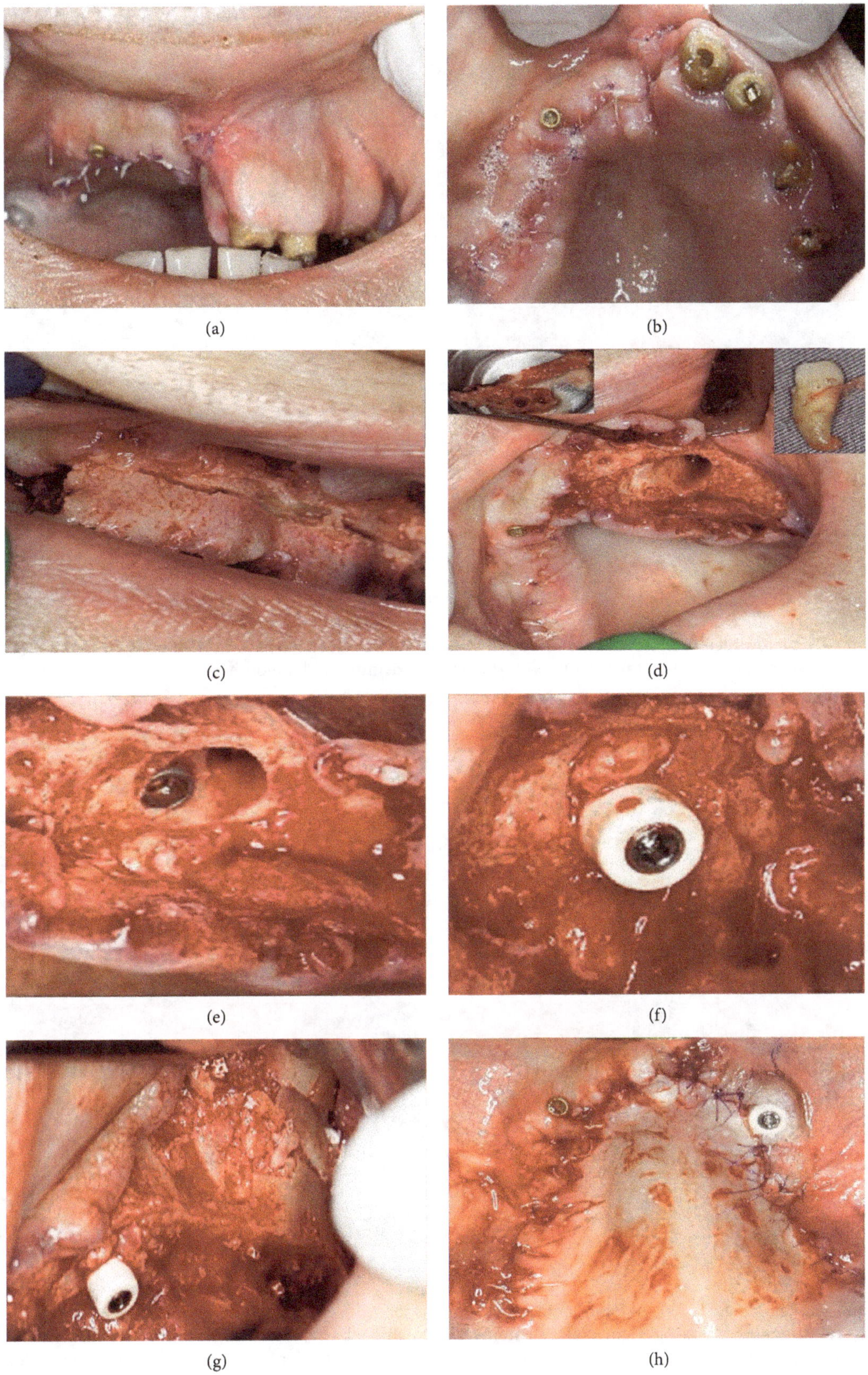

FIGURE 3: Right hemimaxilla: (a, b) clinical situation 2 weeks following left hemimaxilla resection and immediately before proceeding with the right hemimaxilla. (c) Segmental osteotomy of the right hemimaxilla. (d) Impacted canine extraction. (e) Implant insertion in the remaining canine socket. (f) Jumping space filled with autogenous resected alveolar process. (g) Sinus floor elevation. (h) Occlusal view of the postoperative clinical situation.

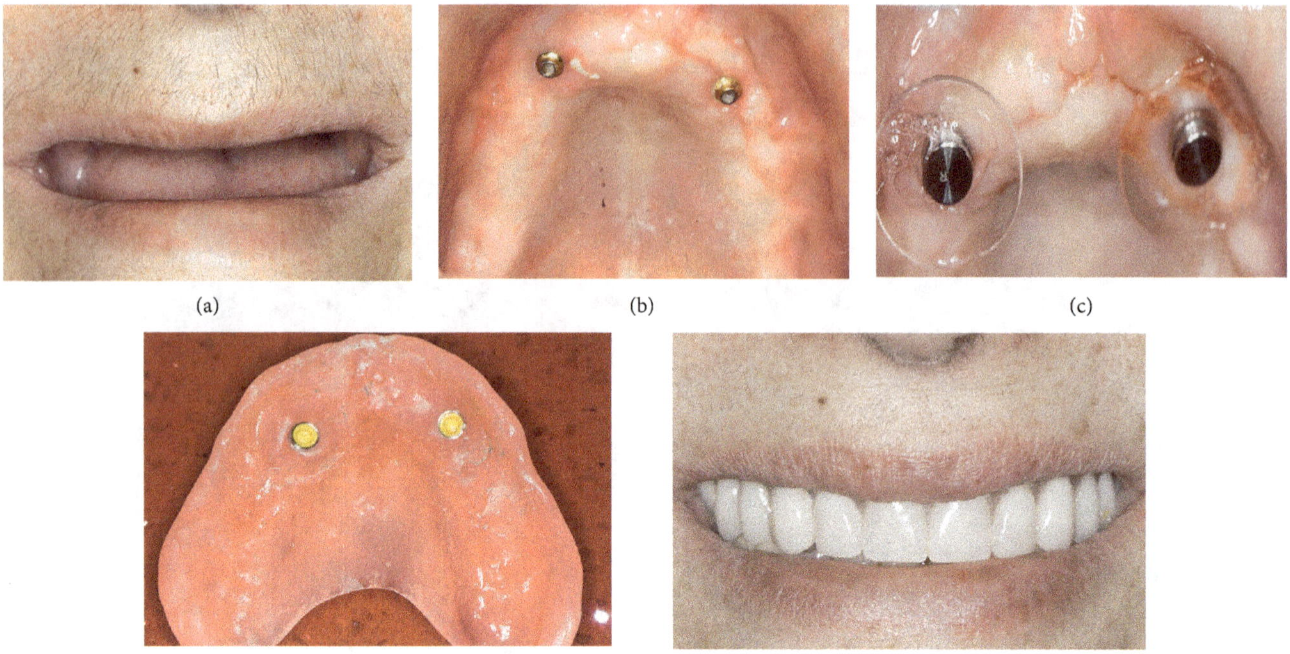

(a) (b) (c) (d) (e)

FIGURE 4: Temporization, 2-3 weeks following right hemimaxilla segmental resection: (a) maximum smile showing the successfully eliminated gingival display. (b) Occlusal view of the healed maxilla with two protruding implant overdenture attachments. (c) Respective housings mounted over the overdenture attachments to be picked-up in the denture intrados by a relining procedure. (d) Denture ready to be seated over the attachments. (e) Patient new smile with the retained denture in the mouth.

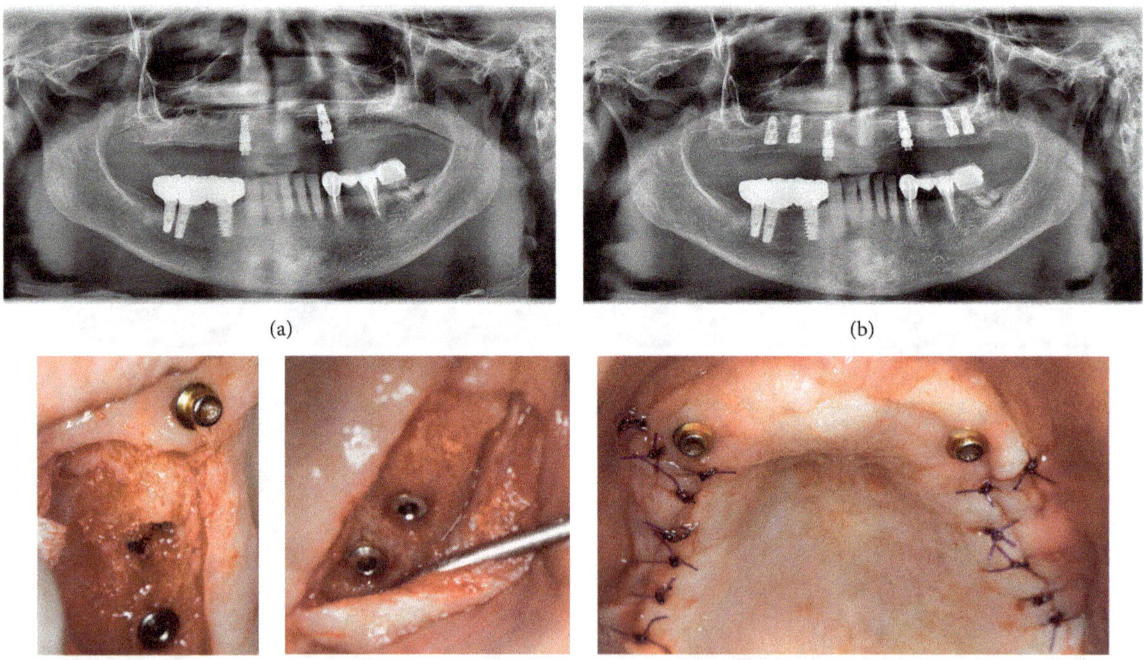

(a) (b) (c) (d) (e)

FIGURE 5: Following sinus graft maturation: (a) Panoramic x-ray 6 months following segmental osteotomy along bilateral sinus augmentation. (b) Panoramic x-ray, 8-months following segmental osteotomy along with bilateral sinus augmentation, and 2 months after implant placement in the sinuses region. (c, d) Two implant placement per each sinus 6-months following bilateral sinus floor elevation. (e) Occlusal view of the maxilla immediately after implant placement and flaps suturing.

porcelain fused to metal crowns taking into consideration an adequate vertical dimension. The anterior teeth underwent a root canal treatment and received 6 splinted zirconia crowns (Figure 7).

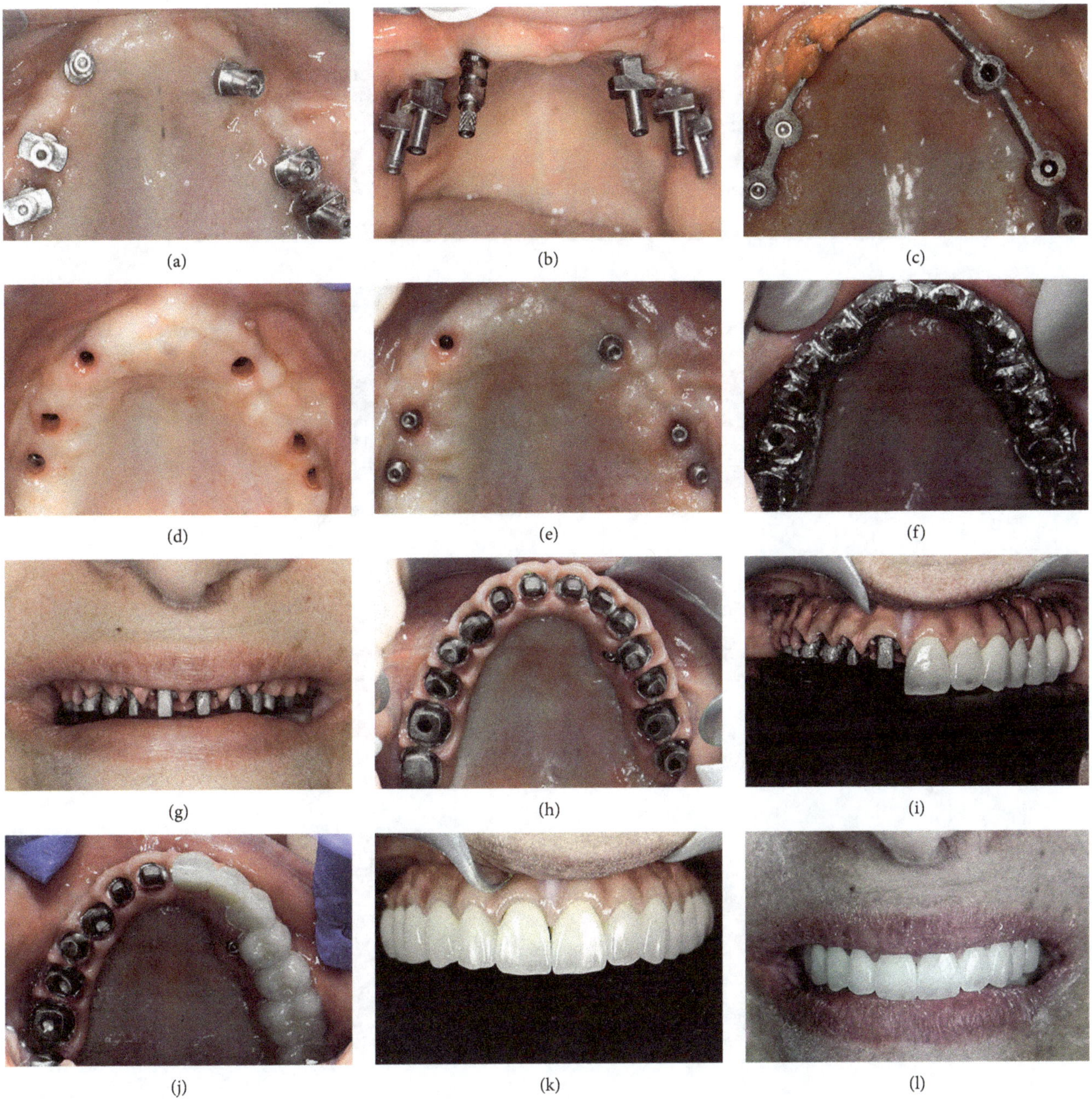

Figure 6: Final rehabilitation of the maxilla: (a, b) Pictures of the impression copings over their respective implants. (c) Passivity fit check using a milled bar. (d) Occlusal view of the maxilla with abutments off. (e) Occlusal view of the maxilla showing five straight multiunit abutments mounted over their respective implants. (f) Try-in of the final milled mesostructure. (g, h) Try-in of the mesostructure after it was layered with pink ceramic. (i, j) Try-in of the individual crowns over the mesostructure. (k, l) Maxillary work completed.

3. Results

Clinically, the procedure showed a drastic improvement in the patient's appearance, eliminating the excessive gingival display. Radiologically, it led to a clear vertical translation of the maxillary process level in an apical direction (Figure 8). Nevertheless, the resected process used as grafting material was noticed to have a suboptimal behavior as long as it showed increased intrasinusal resorption rate, barely sufficient for a regular implant accommodation.

4. Discussion

As discussed earlier, little is reported about managing excessive gingival display in edentulous patients. Generally, tooth loss is accompanied by an unavoidable alveolar resorption [9]. This phenomenon, in the posterior region, is usually followed by a sinus pneumatization [12, 13]. Both facts contribute in leaving a minimal posterior ridge height, which impede a proper implant placement in this particular region.

In case of excessive gingival display, when the alveolar vertical reduction is an option, in order to minimize the

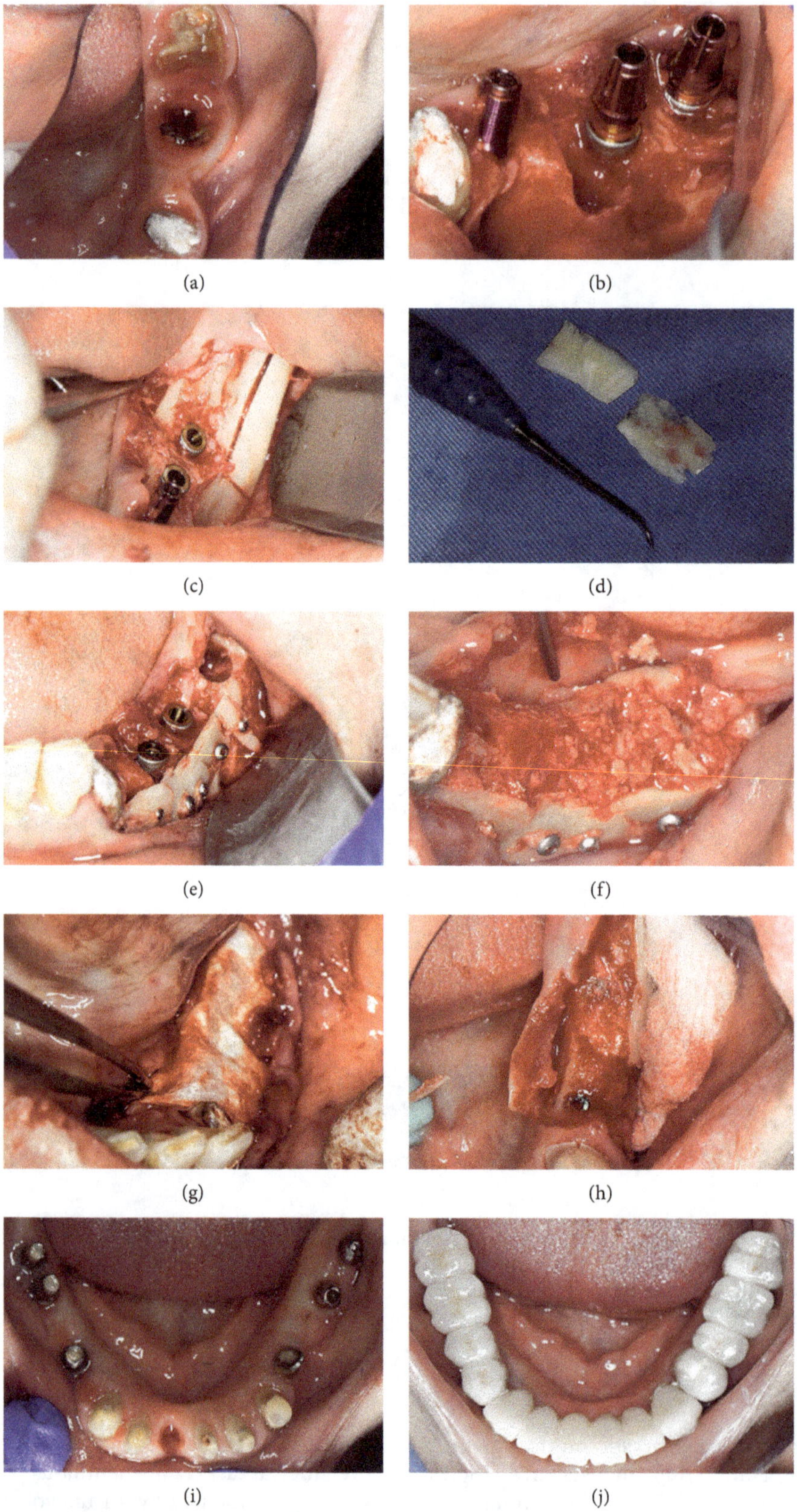

Figure 7: Mandible: (a) Baseline situation of the left hemimandible. (b) Three implants insertion in position #34, #36, and #37. (c) Autogenous bone block harvesting from the external oblique line. (d) Harvested block split in two. (e) Bone block fixation in the recipient site. (f) Autogenous bony particulates filled in the medullary zone. (g) Coverage of the augmentation area by a membrane. (h) Situation at uncovery, 2 months after the augmentation procedure. (i) Abutments and prepared teeth ready to receive their crowns. (j) Mandibular work completed showing the bridges in place.

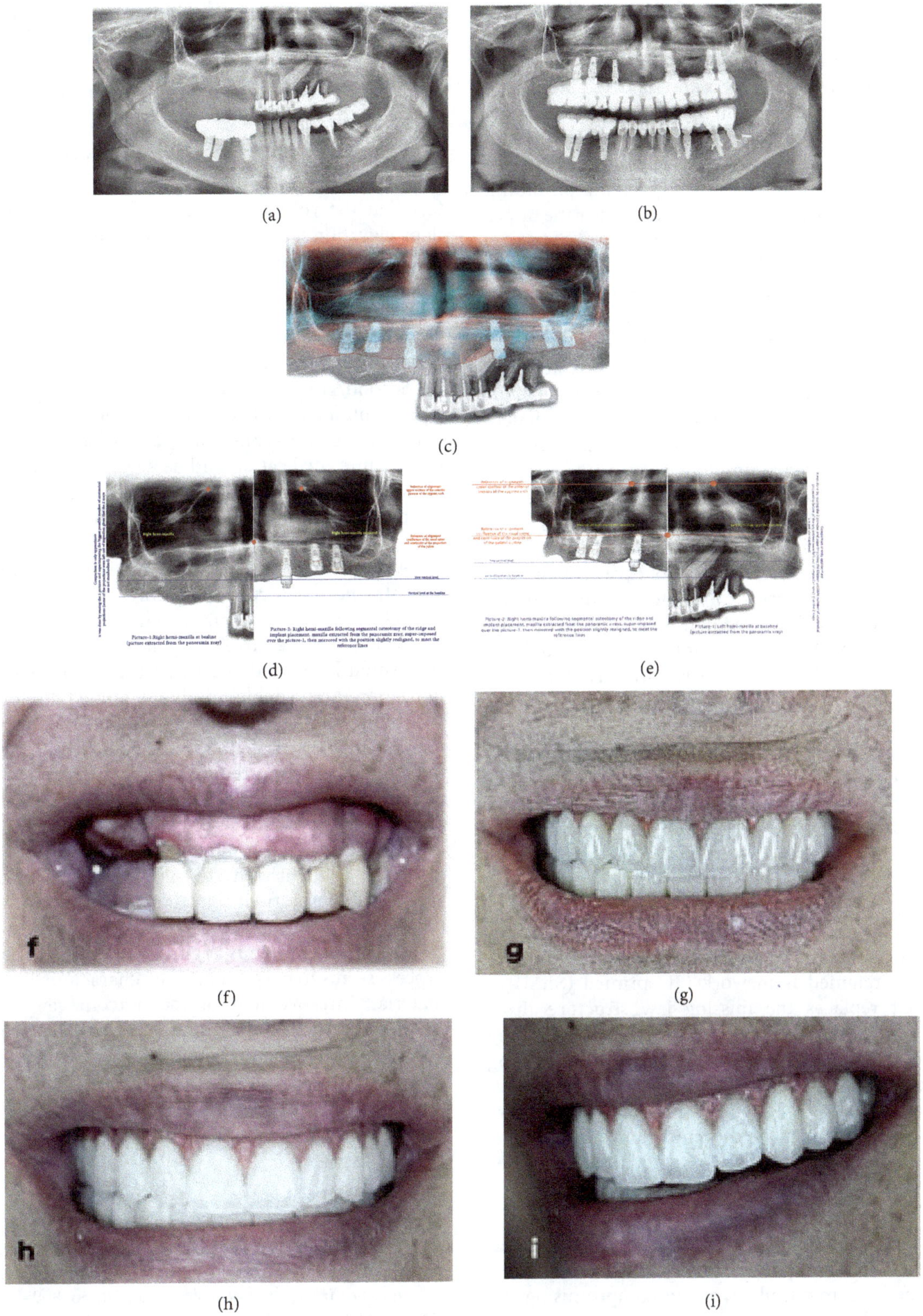

FIGURE 8: Comparisons. (a, b) Panoramic x-rays at the baseline and after case completion, respectively. (c) 2 overlayed maxillary x-rays, extracted from their respective panoramic (before and after segmental osteotomy) and superimposed to show the approximate difference between the baseline and the actual vertical level of the maxillary process. (d, e) Comparison between the baseline and after osteotomy showing the vertical translation of the maxilla in an upward direction. (f, g) Pictures revealing maximum smile at the baseline and after case completion, respectively. (h, i) Additional pictures showing the final outcome.

gummy smile, one may shave off totally the maxillary sinus floors, especially if they are enough pneumatized.

In the present case, and according to their planning, authors reduced the alveolar process and rendered intentionally the case from an excessive gummy smile to a class B situation as per the classification of Avrampou et al. [8], then managed the case accordingly by a fixed hybrid prosthesis.

The rationale behind that was mostly relying on hiding the future mucosal-prosthesis junction away under the upper lip, not to be seen on the maximal smile, as well as giving the required vertical space to fit in the components of the Toronto Bridge, while providing enough room to accommodate a certain height of pink ceramic. On the other hand, ridge reduction was limited by the remaining osseous capital in the anterior region and by the sinuses laterally. Anteriorly, in the canine region, care was taken to leave a vertical height of at least 10 mm in order to insert properly and immediately two regular implants. Posteriorly, since limited by the sinuses, the latter were grafted simultaneously by the resected autogenous material in order to achieve a minimal subantral ridge height able to receive endosseous implants.

Segmental maxillary ostectomy is discussed scarcely in the literature, as a modality of treatment of excessive gingival display [14–16]. Nevertheless, to the extent of the authors' knowledge, the protocol described in this paper is being proposed for the first time: While correcting the gummy smile by segmental osteotomy, the sinus floor elevation is performed concomitally, taking advantage of the resected autogenous alveolar bone that is used as grafting material.

The treatment lasted over a period of a whole year, from osteotomy with sinus floor elevation, throughout the graft maturity, then osseointegration period of the delayed inserted implants, followed by the prosthetic workflow till the final prosthesis delivery, and lastly the mandibular rehabilitation.

Concerning the maxillary prosthetic design, it was opted to rehabilitate the six maxillary implants with a Toronto prosthesis, which consists of a staged fixed prosthesis comprising a screw-retained framework (3D printed (SLM) in this case) that replaces the missing jaw structure. It is designed in a way to be layered with pink material imitating the gum from which emerges a sort of abutment mimicking the prepared teeth as in conventional fixed prosthodontics. As a second stage, come the individual crowns that are intended to be seated over the aforementioned abutments, forming a complex cemented/screw-retained prosthetic construction with the following main advantages:

(i) Ease of retrievability [10] of the concerned parts in case of maintenance in an event of a repair of chipped ceramic while avoiding compromising the framework, provided that the crowns are cemented with a temporary cement, and the underlying mesostructure is screw-retained

(ii) Achievability of desired esthetics of the individual crowns regardless of the screw access openings situated in the underlying screw-retained framework [17]

(iii) Improved metal framework fitting over the implants, related to the reduced number of repeated porcelain firing over the framework itself, which is responsible for metal shrinkage and a further misfit [18]

Speaking about the drawbacks of the whole procedure:

First, concerning the surgical part, authors agree on the fact that the volume of the obtained bone following sinus floor elevation was hardly sufficient, except the areas where the xenogenic material was inserted, precisely and exclusively in the posterior part of the left maxillary sinus. This clearly reflects the inferiority of the autologous alveolar process grafted into the sinuses in terms of volume stability, an evidence barely reported in the literature [19].

Second, regarding the prosthetic design, despite the aforementioned assets of the abutment-hybrid overdenture, it remains a time-consuming and costly prosthetic option that requires dedication and perseverance of the dental technician, especially when adapting the peripheral porcelain of the prosthetic teeth to that of the underlying screw-retained mesostructure.

At the time of this paper submission, the advent of digital dentistry has been revolutionizing all the aspects of dental medicine. And it is thought that these technologies would have enhanced the proactive planning of this particular case and would have rendered its surgical and prosthetic execution more predictable implying guided bone reductions, and the possibility of instant immediate loading by priorly manufactured provisionals of the guidedly inserted implants, thus significantly shortening the overall treatment period and patient chair time [20, 21].

In conclusion, the described therapy option turns out to be plausible, when it comes to managing an excessive gingival display in a patient with a terminal maxillary dentition. However, assiduous patient selection remains an utmost importance. Also, according to what was witnessed in the present case, regarding the sinus augmentations, the resected alveolar process seems to have suboptimal characteristics as a grafting material. Improvement of the outcome is thought to be achieved by mixing the autogenous alveolar process with a bone substitute biomaterial, to prevent the heavy postoperative intrasinusal graft resorption. In addition, nowadays' unmissable digital tools and 3D printing technologies would increase the predictability of the final outcome.

References

[1] N. Silberberg, M. Goldstein, and A. Smidt, "Excessive gingival display–etiology, diagnosis, and treatment modalities," *Quintessence International*, vol. 40, no. 10, pp. 809–818, 2009.

[2] N. Nakib and S. S. Ashrafi, "Drug-induced gingival overgrowth," *Disease-a-Month*, vol. 57, no. 4, pp. 225–230, 2011.

[3] J. G. Coslet, R. Vanarsdall, and A. Weisgold, "Diagnosis and classification of delayed passive eruption of the dentogingival junction in the adult," *The Alpha Omegan*, vol. 70, no. 3, pp. 24–28, 1977.

[4] S. A. Schendel, J. Eisenfeld, W. H. Bell, B. N. Epker, and D. J.

Mishelevich, "The long face syndrome: vertical maxillary excess," *American Journal of Orthodontics*, vol. 70, no. 4, pp. 398–408, 1976.

[5] D. A. Garber and M. A. Salama, "The aesthetic smile: diagnosis and treatment," *Periodontology*, vol. 11, no. 1, pp. 18–28, 1996.

[6] M. Bhola, P. Fairbairn, S. Kolhatkar, S. Chu, T. Morris, and M. De Campos, "LipStaT: the lip stabilization technique - indications and guidelines for case selection and classification of excessive gingival display," *The International Journal of Periodontics & Restorative Dentistry*, vol. 35, no. 4, pp. 549–559, 2015.

[7] I. Ahmad, "Anterior dental aesthetics: dentofacial perspective," *British Dental Journal*, vol. 199, no. 2, pp. 81–88, 2005.

[8] M. Avrampou, R. Mericske-Stern, M. B. Blatz, and J. Katsoulis, "Virtual implant planning in the edentulous maxilla: criteria for decision-making of prosthesis design," *Clinical Oral Implants Research*, vol. 24, Supplement A100, pp. 152–159, 2013.

[9] S. Hansson and A. Halldin, "Alveolar ridge resorption after tooth extraction: a consequence of a fundamental principle of bone physiology," *Journal of Dental Biomechanics*, vol. 3, 2012.

[10] J. Montero, C. Macedo de Paula, and A. Albaladejo, "The "Toronto prosthesis", an appealing method for restoring patients candidates for hybrid overdentures: a case report," *Journal of Clinical and Experimental Dentistry*, vol. 4, no. 5, pp. e309–e312, 2012.

[11] F. Khoury and T. Hanser, "Mandibular bone block harvesting from the retromolar region: a 10-year prospective clinical study," *International Journal of Oral & Maxillofacial Implants*, vol. 30, no. 3, pp. 688–697, 2015.

[12] A. Sharan and D. Madjar, "Maxillary sinus pneumatization following extractions: a radiographic study," *The International Journal of Oral & Maxillofacial Implants*, vol. 23, no. 1, pp. 48–56, 2008.

[13] M. C. Cavalcanti, T. E. Guirado, V. M. Sapata et al., "Maxillary sinus floor pneumatization and alveolar ridge resorption after tooth loss: a cross-sectional study," *Brazilian Oral Research*, vol. 32, article e64, 2018.

[14] O. T. Jensen, M. W. Adams, J. R. Cottam, S. M. Parel, and W. R. Phillips, "The All-on-4 shelf: Maxilla," *Journal of Oral and Maxillofacial Surgery*, vol. 68, no. 10, pp. 2520–2527, 2010.

[15] A. S. Bidra, J. R. Agar, and S. M. Parel, "Management of patients with excessive gingival display for maxillary complete arch fixed implant-supported prostheses," *The Journal of Prosthetic Dentistry*, vol. 108, no. 5, pp. 324–331, 2012.

[16] R. Calixto, F. Faleiros, E. Marangoni, F. Medeiros, A. Wady, and A. Paleari, "Surgical and prosthetic approach for oral rehabilitation of patient with excessive gingival display and gummy smile," *British Journal of Medicine & Medical Research*, vol. 21, no. 11, pp. 1–7, 2017.

[17] B. Uludag, O. Ozturk, G. Celik, and G. Goktug, "Fabrication of a retrievable cement- and screw-retained implant-supported zirconium fixed partial denture: a case report," *The Journal of Oral Implantology*, vol. 34, no. 1, pp. 59–62, 2008.

[18] J. Piermatti, "Using CAD-CAM technology for the full-mouth, fixed, retrievable implant restoration: a clinical report," *The Journal of Oral Implantology*, vol. 33, no. 1, pp. 23–27, 2007.

[19] W. Peng, I. K. Kim, H. Y. Cho et al., "Assessment of the autogenous bone graft for sinus elevation," *Journal of the Korean Association of Oral and Maxillofacial Surgeons*, vol. 39, no. 6, pp. 274–282, 2013.

[20] M. A. Pikos, C. W. Magyar, and D. R. Llop, "Guided full-arch immediate-function treatment modality for the edentulous and terminal dentition patient," *The Compendium of Continuing Education in Dentistry*, vol. 36, no. 2, 2015.

[21] F. Alzoubi, N. Massoomi, and A. Nattestad, "Bone reduction to facilitate immediate implant placement and loading using CAD/CAM surgical guides for patients with terminal dentition," *The Journal of Oral Implantology*, vol. 42, no. 5, pp. 406–410, 2016.

13

Concentrated Growth Factors as an Ingenious Biomaterial in Regeneration of Bony Defects after Periapical Surgery: A Report of Two Cases

Nivedhitha Malli Sureshbabu,[1] Kathiravan Selvarasu,[2] Jayanth Kumar V,[3] Mahalakshmi Nandakumar,[1] and Deepak Selvam[1]

[1]*Department of Conservative Dentistry and Endodontics, Saveetha Dental College, Saveetha Institute of Medical and Technical Sciences, Saveetha University, 162, Poonamallee High Road, Chennai, 600077 Tamil Nadu, India*
[2]*Department of Oral and Maxillofacial Surgery, Saveetha Dental College, Saveetha Institute of Medical and Technical Sciences, Saveetha University, 162, Poonamallee High Road, Chennai, 600077 Tamil Nadu, India*
[3]*Department of Oral Medicine and Radiology, Saveetha Dental College, Saveetha Institute of Medical and Technical Sciences, Saveetha University, 162, Poonamallee High Road, Chennai, 600077 Tamil Nadu, India*

Correspondence should be addressed to Nivedhitha Malli Sureshbabu; nivea16@hotmail.com

Academic Editor: Pia L. Jornet

The overall success of a periapical surgery is assessed in terms of regeneration of functional periradicular tissues. The regenerative potential of platelets has been well documented. This article describes the use of concentrated growth factors (CGF), a new family of autologous platelet concentrates, as a sole material for bone regeneration after periapical surgery. 32- and 35-year-old female patients diagnosed with Ellis Class IV, an open apex in 11 with apical periodontitis in 11 and 12 and previously root canal-treated 31 and 41 with a chronic apical abscess, respectively, were managed with endodontic surgery. Subsequent to apicectomy and retrograde filling, the CGF fibrin block and membrane were used before suturing. There was uneventful healing during the immediate post-op and the subsequent follow-up periods. CGF is produced by a differential centrifugation process that results in the formation of a denser fibrin matrix richer in growth factors than those observed in PRF. Reasonable osseous healing was seen as early as 6-month follow-up, thereby recommending the use of CGF as an alternative to bone grafts and membranes in extensive periapical lesions to enhance bone regeneration and to decrease the healing time.

1. Introduction

Periapical surgery is the treatment of choice for teeth with persistent apical periodontitis when the conventional nonsurgical method fails to achieve the principal objectives [1]. It has been predicted that the smaller defect heals around one year, whereas for the larger defects, the healing time may be more than two years [2]. However, recently, Lin et al. have demonstrated that the healing of periapical tissues is a "programmed event." More than the size of the lesion, it is the microenvironment consisting of the progenitor/stem cells, extracellular matrix, and bioactive molecules that plays a crucial role in tissue regeneration or scar formation during wound healing [3].

Platelet-rich plasma (PRP) and plasma rich in growth factors (PRGF) classified as the first generation of autologous platelet concentrates (APCs) have demonstrated promising results in the management of extensive periapical lesions, apicomarginal defects, and combined endo-perio lesions and also improved the quality of life of patients undergoing endodontic surgery [4]. However, both have several drawbacks like use of anticoagulant, artificial polymerization, and a time-consuming two-step centrifugation process.

Platelet-rich fibrin (PRF), considered as the second generation platelet concentrate and classified into L-PRF, A-PRF, i-PRF, CGF, PRFM, and Vivostat PRF [5]. A systematic review reported that APCs have a favourable effect on patients' quality of life and are supportive for bone regeneration after endodontic surgery [6].

Concentrated growth factor (CGF) is a newer second generation platelet concentrate that is prepared by centrifuging blood samples at alternating and controlled speeds using a special centrifuge. Differential centrifugation results in the formation of a denser fibrin matrix richer in growth factors than those observed in the PRF and PRP. To our knowledge, this is the first case report for the use of CGF alone in endodontic surgery. For describing the case reports, we have followed the checklist given in CARE guidelines (http://www.care-statement.org/) [7].

2. Case Presentation

2.1. Case Report 1. A 32-year-old female patient was referred to the Department of Conservative Dentistry and Endodontics with chief complaint of discolouration of the upper right front tooth (tooth 11) for the past 6 months. Past dental history revealed a traumatic fall 5 years ago which involved the upper front teeth for which no dental treatment was sought for. Recently, as the discolouration gradually worsened, the patient sought dental treatment to restore esthetics.

Intraoral clinical examination revealed a slightly discoloured 11 and chipping of the incisal edge with no presenting symptoms (Figure 1(a)). Both 11 and 12 responded negatively to the electric pulp tester (Gentle Pulse™ Pulp Vitality Tester, Parkell, USA) and elicited mild tenderness on percussion.

On radiographic examination (VistaScan Mini, UK), extensive periapical radiolucency involving the roots of 11 and 12 and an open apex of 11 was revealed (Figure 1(b)). CBCT for this case (Dentsply Sirona, Orthophos XG 3D) was taken at standardized settings (90 kV, 6 mA, 5 × 5.5 cm, 160 μm, and 14 s) to assess the exact location, size, and extent and proximity of the lesion to anatomical structures.

The preoperative measurements of the lesion as seen in CBCT in different planes can be seen in Figures 1(g), 1(i), 1(k). According to the CBCT-PAI scores, it was graded as a 5D lesion [8]. The score 5 indicates that the diameter of the periapical lesion is greater than 8 mm, and D represents destruction of the periapical cortical bone in the palatal region.

A tentative diagnosis of an Ellis Class IV fracture and open apex in 11 with apical periodontitis in 11 and 12 was made. The differential diagnosis could be a chronic periapical abscess, periapical cyst, and periapical granuloma. The treatment plan was root canal treatment for 11 and 12. The patient was informed about the risks and benefits of the procedure and a written consent was taken.

Under local anaesthesia (2% lignocaine in 1 : 200,000 dilution adrenaline, Neon Laboratories Ltd.) and rubber dam isolation, an access cavity was prepared in 11 and 12 with an Endo access bur (Dentsply Maillefer, Switzerland). The working length was determined with an apex locator (Propex Pixi, Dentsply Maillefer, Switzerland) and confirmed with radiograph. Cleaning and shaping was initiated with 45 K file (Mani, Inc. Japan), and apical preparation was performed till size 80 K file in 11. In 12, apical preparation was done till size 45 K file to full working length, after which step-back preparation was done till 80 K file. Routine root canal-shaping procedure was done along with copious irrigation using 3% sodium hypochlorite (VIP, Vensons, India) and final flush with 0.9% physiologic saline (acuLIFE, India). Calcium hydroxide medicament (RC Cal, Prime Dental Products, India) was placed thrice for a period of 1 week each. As the root canals exhibited persistent discharge of exudates and due to two prognostic factors (size of the lesion which was more than 10 mm and the thinning or destruction of the palatal bone) which were unfavourable for this case [9], periapical surgery was planned following the recommendation given by the Spanish Society of Oral Surgery (point 3: a radiotransparent lesion measuring over 8 to 10 mm in diameter).

The root canals were obturated a day before the surgery using custom-made roll cone technique for 11 and conventional cold lateral compaction technique for 12.

During surgery, after achieving adequate anaesthesia, a crevicular incision was placed from 22 to 14 with a vertical releasing incision on the mesial aspect of 14 to reflect a full thickness mucoperiosteal triangular flap. Cortical softening of the periapical bone was noted from regions 11 to 13. A bony window was created and thorough curettage was done (Figure 1(c)).

Apicoectomy was performed extending 3 mm into the canal space using no.702 tapered fissure burs (SS White burs) in 12. Apicoectomy was not done in 11 because of the presence of an open apex. Root end cavity preparation was done using zirconium nitride ultrasonic retro-tips (Dentsply Maillefer, Switzerland) in 11 and 12. Subsequently, retrograde filling was done with Mineral Trioxide Aggregate (MTA Angelus® Brazil) (Figure 1(d)). Later, the surgical site was prepared for placement of CGF fibrin gel and CGF membrane.

A standard, disposable, two 10 mL nonanticoagulant glass tubes and a matching centrifuge device (MEDIFUGE, Silfradent s.r.l., S. Sofia, Italy) were used. 20 mL of intravenous blood sample from the patient was placed in centrifuge tubes without anticoagulants and accelerated for 30 s, centrifuged at 2700 rpm for 2 min, 2400 rpm for 4 min, 2700 rpm for 4 min, and 3000 rpm for 3 min, and decelerated for 36 s to stop. All of these processes are adjusted automatically by "preprogramming" in the machine.

From the three layers formed, the uppermost platelet-deprived fraction was removed with a sterile syringe. The layer in the form of a fibrin gel containing the CGF was separated from the red blood cell layer. The prepared CGF fibrin gel was placed inside the surgical site and covered with CGF membrane. The layer in the form of a membrane containing the concentrated growth membrane was held with a hemostatic clamp and separated from the RBC layer by using microsurgical scissors. The CGF layer is then placed in a condensing disc and compressed to convert to CGF membrane. (Figures 1(e), 1(f)).

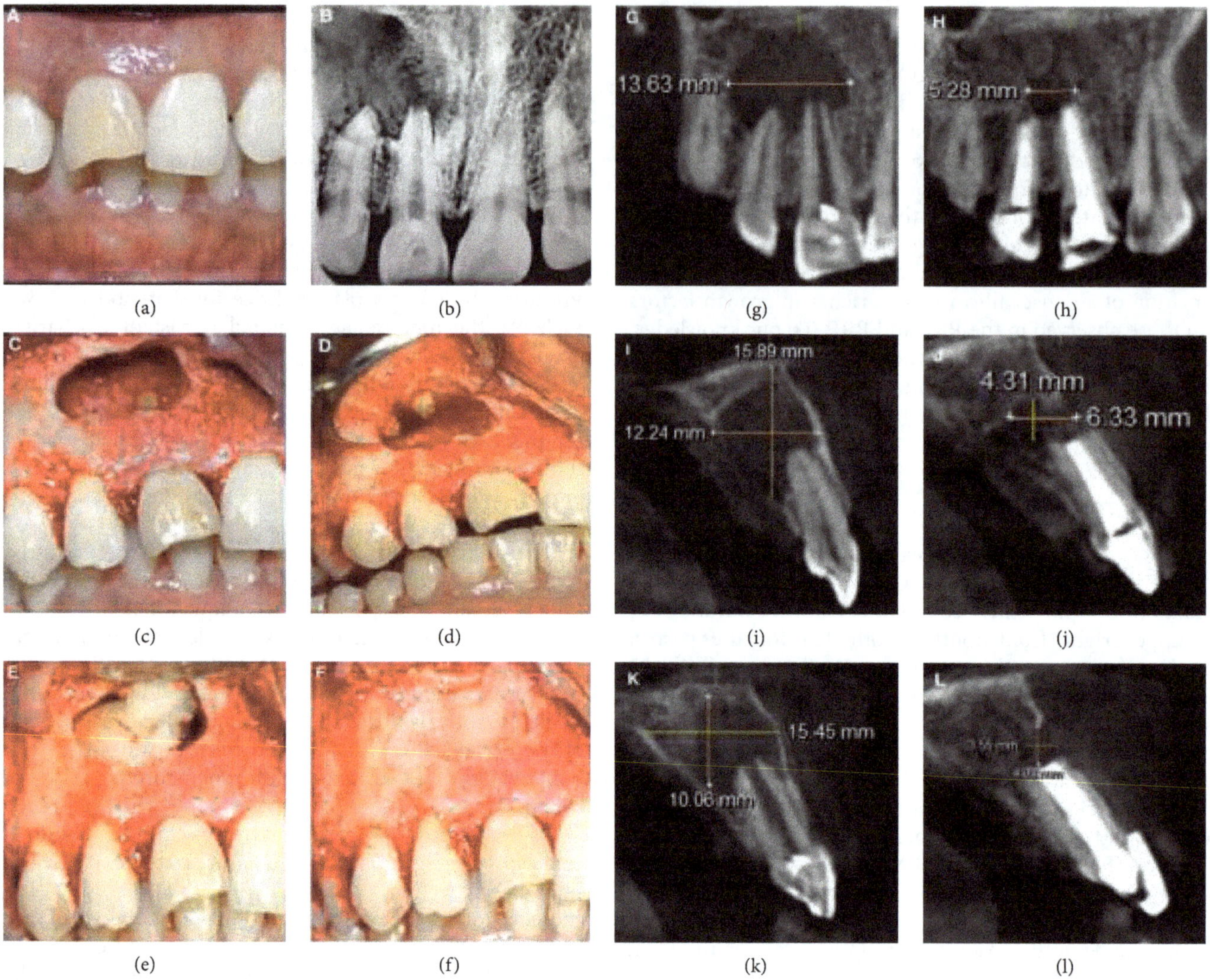

FIGURE 1: Preoperative clinical and surgical procedure and radiographic images: IOPA and CBCT images (Case Report 1). (a) Pre-op clinical photograph showing discoloured 11 with chipping of the incisal edge of the crown. (b) Preoperative IOPA showing the periapical lesion involving the apices of 11 and 12 and extending to the mesial margin of 13. (c) Complete curettage of the lesion and apicectomy done in 12. (d) Retrograde preparation and filling with MTA in 11 and 12. (e) CGF fibrin block placed in the bony cavity. (f) CGF membrane placed to cover the bone defect. (g) Pre-op CBCT image showing the lesion measurement in the coronal slice. (h) Post-op CBCT image showing the lesion measurement in the coronal slice. (i) Pre-op CBCT image showing the lesion measurement in sagittal slice corresponding to 12. (j) Post-op CBCT image showing the lesion measurement in sagittal slice corresponding to 12. (k) Pre-op CBCT image showing the lesion measurement in sagittal slice corresponding to 11. (l) Post-op CBCT image showing the lesion measurement in sagittal slice corresponding to 11.

Subsequent to CGF placement, the flap was closed with 3-0 vicryl sutures (Ethicon Inc. Piscataway, USA). Postoperative instructions were given and systemic antibiotics, analgesics, and supplemental 0.2% chlorhexidine mouthwash were prescribed.

The postoperative CBCT at 1-year follow-up showed satisfactory healing with evident reduction in lesion size as shown in Figures 1(h), 1(j), 1(l), and the patient was asymptomatic at all the recall periods, suggesting a successful treatment outcome. The patient is kept under review, to be followed up after 18 months, 24 months, and 36 months.

2.2. Case Report 2. A 35-year-old female patient reported mild swelling and pus discharge in the lower front region of the mouth for the past 2 months. Past dental history revealed trauma to lower anterior teeth 4 years ago, following which she underwent endodontic treatment. History suggested that there were multiple retreatments in the past for the current chief complaint.

On clinical examination, 31 was discoloured with mild swelling on the labial aspect (Figure 2(a)). Radiographic examination revealed a well-obturated 31 and 41 with large periapical radiolucency (Figure 2(b)). The CBCT-PAI score was 5D (Figures 2(g), 2(i), 2(k)). Based on the above findings, a diagnosis of previously root canal-treated 31 and 41 with a chronic apical abscess was made. History suggested that there were multiple retreatments in the past for the current chief complaint, with presenting complaint of recurring,

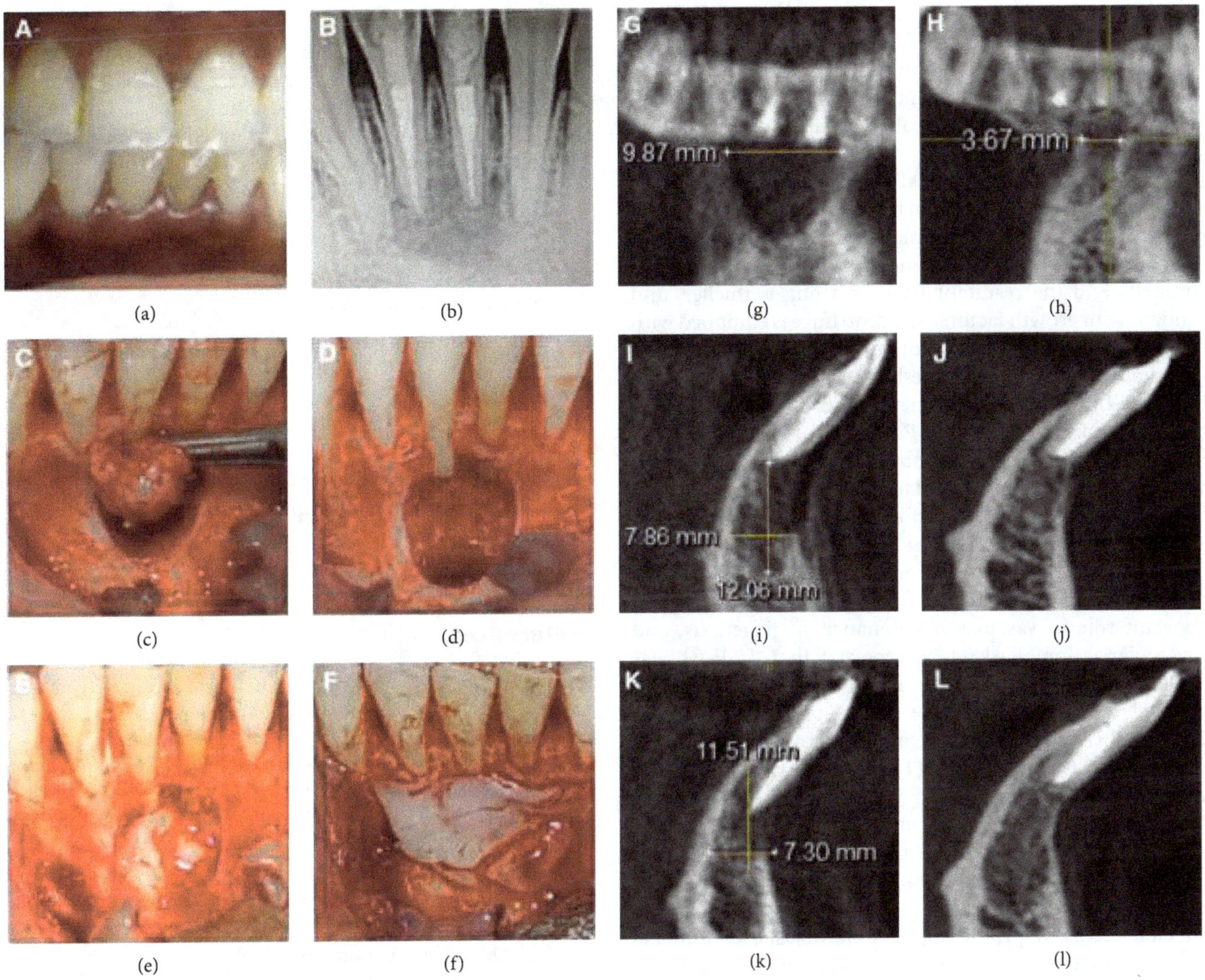

FIGURE 2: Preoperative clinical and surgical procedure and radiographic images: IOPA and CBCT images (Case Report 2). (a) Pre-op clinical photograph shows discoloured 31. (b) Preoperative IOPA showing the periapical lesion involving the apices of 11 and 12 and extending to the mesial margin of 13. (c) Complete curettage of the lesion. (d) Apicectomy done and MTA retrograde filling given in 31 and 41. (e) CGF fibrin-rich block placed in the bony defect. (f) CGF membrane placed before suturing of the flap. (g) Pre-op CBCT image showing the lesion measurement in the coronal slice. (h) Post-op CBCT image showing the lesion measurement in coronal slice. (i) Pre-op CBCT image showing the lesion measurement in sagittal slice corresponding to 41. (j) Post-op CBCT image showing the lesion measurement in sagittal slice corresponding to 41. (k) Pre-op CBCT image showing the lesion measurement in sagittal slice corresponding to 31. (l) Post-op CBCT image showing the lesion measurement in sagittal slice corresponding to 31.

intermittent swelling with pus discharge in the lower front region. And radiographic examination revealed adequate obturation and apical seal, with nonhealing chronic periapical radiolucency. The treatment plan of periapical surgery was decided in accordance with the indications given by the European Society of Endodontology, 2006 (point 3: presence of persisting periapical disease after root canal retreatment).

Under local anaesthesia, the full thickness trapezoidal mucoperiosteal flap was reflected with vertical releasing incisions taken from the mesial aspect of 43 and 33. The surgical site was flushed with sterile saline after thorough curettage of the lesion (Figure 2(c)). Following which, apicectomy and retrograde MTA filling were done (Figure 2(d)). The CGF preparation was similar as described in Case Report 1, and the prepared CGF was placed inside the surgical site and covered with CGF membrane (Figures 2(e), 2(f)). The flap was approximated with interrupted sutures. Follow-up CBCT at 1 year revealed complete healing with complete bone repair, evidently seen in coronal and sagittal views (Figures 2(h), 2(j), 2(l)).

At 1-year follow-up with CBCT, livewire segmentation using OSIRIX Version 9.5 (PIXMEO, Geneva, Switzerland) was done to delineate the lesion from the healthy bone. In case 1, the preoperative and postoperative volume calculations were $0.7862\,cm^3$ and $0.08\,cm^3$, respectively. The lesion size reduction was found to be 89.2%. In case 2, the preoperative and postoperative volume calculations were $0.1358\,cm^3$ and $0.0101\,cm^3$, respectively. The lesion size reduction was found to be 92.5%.

3. Discussion

Our case reports are unique in that CGF was produced using the recommended centrifuge, and it was used as a sole material to understand its exclusive role in repair and regeneration after periapical surgery.

During the preparation of APCs, the quality of the resultant product is greatly influenced by centrifugal characteristics like rotational speed (rpm), time (min), and centrifugation protocols. The centrifugation method for CGF is "preprogrammed" and the resultant CGF is stronger, thicker, and abundant with growth factors. The centrifuge is equipped with self-ventilation that prevents the temperature rise which helps to maintain the viability of enmeshed cells in the fibrin matrix. The dense three-dimensional network of the fibrin ensures slow release of growth factors. Park et al. affirmed that CGF consisted of thicker fibrinogen fibres per area unit and regular fibrinogen structures compared to PRF [10].

The presence of growth factors and leucocytes including also the few CD34+ circulating cells that are concentrated in a small volume is the probable reason for this success, since all the elements have been demonstrated to play an important role in vascular maintenance, angiogenesis, and neovascularization. Park et al. reported that TGF-β1 was released for one week whereas PDGF-BB for 3 weeks and identified that VEGF was one and a half times more in CGF than PRF [10]. However, Qin et al. showed that TGF-β1 had a slow release for 13 days [11]. In a contrasting study, the levels of growth factors released (except bFGF) did not differ significantly among PRP, PRF, and CGF [12].

Growth factors act on target tissues and regulate a variety of cellular events including cell migration, proliferation, and differentiation. Borsani et al. have ascertained that CGF addition enhanced cell proliferation of fibroblasts, endothelial cells, and osteoblasts which are involved in angiogenesis, tissue remodelling and regeneration [13].

There are two case reports in the literature which describe the utilization of CGF in periapical surgery. In the first, CGF was not prepared with the special centrifuge [14]. In the second, CGF was used along with the sticky bone and Mphi laser [15]. Even though both the cases had unfavourable prognostic factors, the follow-up has affirmed the encouraging effect of CGF which has shortened the healing time of extensive periapical lesions to 6 months. This finding corroborates with the outcome of the case reports by Sohn which described two cases of sinus augmentation in which CGF alone was used as a substitute for bone graft and the results established that healing was reduced to half the average healing period without bone graft placement [16]. The benefits of CGF are that it is autologous, can be easily prepared, and cost-effective than bone grafts and membranes in extensive periapical lesions. Taking into account the above benefits, CGF can be earmarked as an ingenious biomaterial for bone regeneration.

4. Conclusion

Considering the encouraging result of these case reports, concentrated growth factors could be recommended as an alternative to bone grafts and membranes in extensive periapical lesions to enhance bone regeneration and to decrease the healing time. However, this case series is an initiative for application of CGF in endodontic surgery. The utilization of CGF in endodontics can be extended to revascularization procedures and endo-perio lesions also. However, the major limitation is that according to the CEBM level of evidence, the case reports have the lowest level of evidence. A well-designed randomized clinical trial is recommended to comprehend the long-term risks and benefits of using CGF in regenerative endodontics.

Acknowledgments

We thank Dr. Sri Prakash for CGF preparation and Dr. Susila for helping during manuscript preparation.

References

[1] Y.-L. Ng, V. Mann, S. Rahbaran, J. Lewsey, and K. Gulabivala, "Outcome of primary root canal treatment: systematic review of the literature–part 1. Effects of study characteristics on probability of success," *International Endodontic Journal*, vol. 40, no. 12, pp. 921–939, 2007.

[2] W. H. Archer, *Oral and Maxillofacial Surgery*, WB Saunders Company, 1975.

[3] L. M. Lin, D. Ricucci, and T. von Arx, "Guided tissue regeneration in endodontic surgery: principle, efficacy, and complications," in *Complications in Endodontic Surgery*, Springer, 2014.

[4] M. Del Fabbro, V. Ceresoli, A. Lolato, and S. Taschieri, "Effect of platelet concentrate on quality of life after periradicular surgery: a randomized clinical study," *Journal of Endodontia*, vol. 38, no. 6, pp. 733–739, 2012.

[5] T. Kawase and T. Tanaka, "An updated proposal for terminology and classification of platelet-rich fibrin," *Regenerative Therapy*, vol. 7, pp. 80-81, 2017.

[6] N. Meschi, A. B. Castro, K. Vandamme, M. Quirynen, and P. Lambrechts, "The impact of autologous platelet concentrates on endodontic healing: a systematic review," *Platelets*, vol. 27, no. 7, pp. 613–633, 2016.

[7] the CARE Group, J. J. Gagnier, G. Kienle et al., "The CARE guidelines: consensus-based clinical case reporting guideline development," *Journal of Medical Case Reports*, vol. 7, no. 1, p. 223, 2013.

[8] C. Estrela, M. R. Bueno, B. C. Azevedo, J. R. Azevedo, and J. D. Pécora, "A new periapical index based on cone beam computed tomography," *Journal of Endodontia*, vol. 34, no. 11, pp. 1325–1331, 2008.

[9] M. Serrano-Giménez, A. Sanchez-Torres, and C. Gay-Escoda, "Prognostic factors on periapical surgery: a systematic review," *Medicina Oral Patología Oral y Cirugia Bucal*, vol. 20, no. 6, pp. e715–e722, 2015.

[10] H. C. Park, S. G. Kim, J. S. Oh et al., "Early bone formation at a femur defect using CGF and PRF grafts in adult dogs: a comparative study," *Implant Dentistry*, vol. 25, no. 3, pp. 387–393, 2016.

[11] J. Qin, L. Wang, L. Zheng et al., "Concentrated growth factor promotes Schwann cell migration partly through the integrin $\beta 1$-mediated activation of the focal adhesion kinase pathway," *International Journal of Molecular Medicine*, vol. 37, no. 5, pp. 1363–1370, 2016.

[12] L. F. Rodella, G. Favero, R. Boninsegna et al., "Growth factors, CD34 positive cells, and fibrin network analysis in concentrated growth factors fraction," *Microscopy Research and Technique*, vol. 74, no. 8, pp. 772–777, 2011.

[13] E. Borsani, V. Bonazza, B. Buffoli et al., "Biological characterization and in vitro effects of human concentrated growth factor preparation: an innovative approach to tissue regeneration," *Biology and Medicine*, vol. 7, no. 5, p. 726, 2015.

[14] S. Mirković, T. Đurđević-Mirković, and T. Puškar, "Application of concentrated growth factors in reconstruction of bone defects after removal of large jaw cysts: the two cases report," *Vojnosanitetski Pregled*, vol. 72, no. 4, pp. 368–371, 2015.

[15] N. Doan, L. Nguyen-Pham, C. Liang, and Q. T. Duong, "A review on the application of concentrated growth factors and MPhi laser to regenerate oral defects in the oral and maxillofacial region and a two cases report," *International Journal of Oral and Maxillofacial Surgery*, vol. 46, Supplement 1, pp. 203-204, 2017.

[16] D. S. Sohn, *The Use of Concentrated Growth Factors as Alternative to Bone Substitutes for Sinus Augmentation*, Dental Inc., 2009.

14

Guided Periodontal Surgery: Association of Digital Workflow and Piezosurgery for the Correction of a Gummy Smile

Tatiana Miranda Deliberador, Suyany Gabriely Weiss, Alexandre Teixeira Domingues Neto, Isabela Zago Zetola, Maria Eduarda Santana Prix, Darlan Rigo Júnior, Heloysa Hoffman Martins, and Carmen Lucia Mueller Storrer

School of Health Sciences, Positivo University, 5300 Professor Pedro Viriato Parigot de Souza Street, Campo Comprido, Curitiba, PR, Brazil 81280-330

Correspondence should be addressed to Tatiana Miranda Deliberador; tdeliberador@gmail.com

Academic Editor: Giuseppe Alessandro Scardina

Digital flow has become a part of currently practiced dentistry. Virtual planning ensures predictable aesthetic and functional rehabilitation, painless postoperative recovery, and better communication with patients, thus meeting their expectations. The purpose of this case report is to demonstrate the digital planning for the correction of a gummy smile with a personalized preparation using a piezoelectric surgical guide (PerioGuide) for gingival contouring and flapless osteotomy. The guide was designed using Nemo Studio software, based on the patient's facial aesthetic analysis, through photos, videos, and facial scanning. These images were aligned with the scan and placed over the cone beam computed gingival tomography for prediction of results, based not only on the distance from the cementoenamel junction to the bone crest but also on the best gingival margin contour according to virtual aesthetic planning. Digital planning, combined with the use of a piezoelectric device, allows for a flapless guided surgical technique for gingival contouring and osteotomy. As a result, the surgical procedure is safer, faster, and more predictable with better postoperative outcomes.

1. Introduction

A perfect smile is dictated by a balance between three parameters: teeth, gum, and lips. Excessive gingival display while smiling is a concern for many patients, affecting both esthetics and psychosocial behavior [1]. Excessive gingival display, also described as "gummy smile" (GS), has been observed in 7% of men and 14% of women in the age group 20–30 years [2].

GS has several etiologies, such as vertical maxillary excess, anterior dentoalveolar extrusion, altered passive eruption, lip length and activity, and over compensatory eruption, among others, and although there are distinct causes, it is often the result of a multifactorial effect [3–5]. An accurate differential diagnosis is crucial for proper therapeutic application, as the treatment of a gummy smile includes facial surgery, periodontal surgery, laser, and botulinum toxin injection. More recently, digital workflow and flapless surgery (piezosurgery), among others [1, 6, 7], have been associated with treatment planning.

Given the growing demand for aesthetics and less invasive techniques, the digital workflow concept allows better communication with patients, offers the clinician a diagnostic tool to make the most appropriate therapeutic choice, and enables accurate treatment planning with predictable results [8]. Digital treatment planning is based on diagnostic methods such as cone beam computed tomography for the analysis of hard and soft tissues. When the buccal mucosa and the tongue are retracted from the gingival tissues, the images produced allow visualization of the facial and lingual mucosa, determination of the size of the gingival unit (gingival phenotype), and assessment of the ideal relationship between hard and soft tissues for surgical planning of gummy smile correction. The ability to determine the need

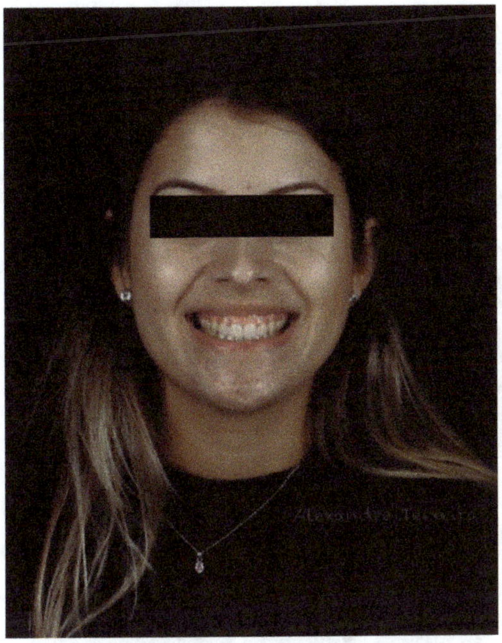

FIGURE 1: Initial smile.

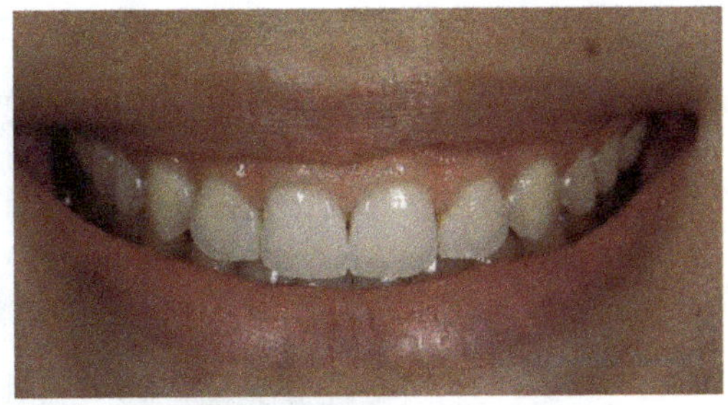

FIGURE 2: Initial smile, approximate view.

for osteoplasty increases the accuracy and predictability of the surgical procedure [6, 9]. Moreover, facial scanning may also be used to evaluate digital photographs and intraoral scanning within the digital workflow. With the facial scan information integrated with data, obtained from intra- and extraoral scanners, the treatment design is more likely to reflect the aesthetic demands imposed by the patient [10]. Moreover, piezoelectric bone surgery overcomes the limitations of traditional instrumentation in oral bone surgery, allowing greater intraoperative control and safe cutting [11].

The purpose of this study is to report a clinical case of guided periodontal surgery for the treatment of a gummy smile using digital planning and piezosurgery.

2. Case Presentation

A 19-year-old woman (M.K.S.) with leukoderma sought clinical service dissatisfied with the aesthetics of her smile due to excessive gingival exposure (Figures 1 and 2). Clinical examination revealed short maxillary anterior teeth with excess gingival tissue. Periodontal examination revealed probing depths 2–3 mm with adequate levels of periodontal health (no plaque, bleeding, or periodontal pockets). After clinical and periodontal examination, previous photographs, intraoral scans, and facial scans were obtained. Tooth-gingival computed tomography was requested, and the patient signed a consent form.

2.1. Digital Planning. Digital treatment planning begins with an analysis of digital photographs, intraoral scanning (STL) images (3Shape, Copenhague K, Dinamarca), facial scanning (OBJ) (Done 3D, Ribeirão Preto, São Paulo), and tomography images, performed to delimit all dental faces, in addition to soft and hard tissues. Three-dimensional images are loaded in the NEMOTEC program (Nemotec, Madrid, Spain) in which the STL model is aligned with the patient's initial photos. Lines are drawn to mark the symmetry of the face and tooth-gingival proportion in the face-guided intraoral planning. The interpupillary line which establishes the horizontal plane should be parallel to the incisal line and the gingival margin contour. The midline of the face is determined by tracing the glabella, nose, filter, and chin to enable an analysis of facial symmetry. If any deviation is noted, a previous treatment (orthodontics, orthognathic surgery, and prosthetic) may be indicated. The incisal line is a horizontal tracing over the lower lip that facilitates the initial evaluation between the facial lines with the smile. The smile zenith curve is to be demarcated: the canine should be 0.5 to 1 mm higher than the central incisors and the lateral incisors 0.5 to 1 mm lower than the central incisors. The position of the interdental papillae must be beyond the interproximal contact point, closing the interdental space, to promote an aesthetically balanced smile. Finally, the aesthetic aspect ratio, height × width, of the latter elements is verified. The size of the central incisors is based on the ideal proportion to provide a pleasant aesthetic smile, between 9.5 mm and 11 mm (Kurbad et al., 2013).

Based on the face-guided intraoral planning analysis, digital wax-up was prepared (Figure 3). A correlation was made between the facial shape and the shape of the teeth (square, ovoid, or triangular). Above all, one should always plan a smile that fits the patient's desire, physical appearance, and personality, providing an aesthetic and functional result. After the digital teeth wax-up was completed, the facial scan was juxtaposed with the initial photos of the case (3D Planning) to ensure that the newly acquired positions would be harmonious for the patient's face.

The digital wax-up was printed on acrylic resin (Printed-Mockup BDS, Curitiba, Brazil) for patient approval. It was then fixed in the mouth with the aid of flow A1 composite resin (Yller, Pelotas, Brazil). Next, new photographs and videos of the patient's case with the mockup were taken.

2.2. Periodontal Profile Analysis. 3D digital planning was performed with the Nemo Studio program (Nemotec, Madrid, Spain). Through this feature, it was possible to estimate the ideal amount of gingival tissue to be removed in each dental element to achieve a more aesthetic gingival contour. The measurement obtained through digital planning was superimposed on the images acquired in the dental gingival tomography to observe the relationship between biological distances and define the best surgical approach.

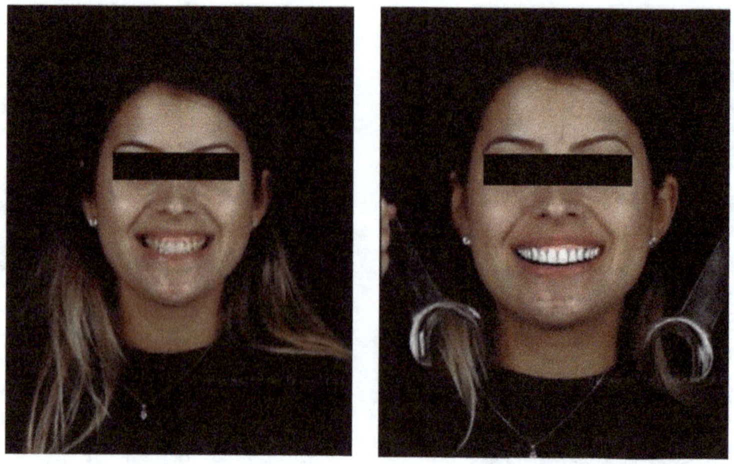

(a) (b)

FIGURE 3: (a) Initial smile. (b) Digital waxing.

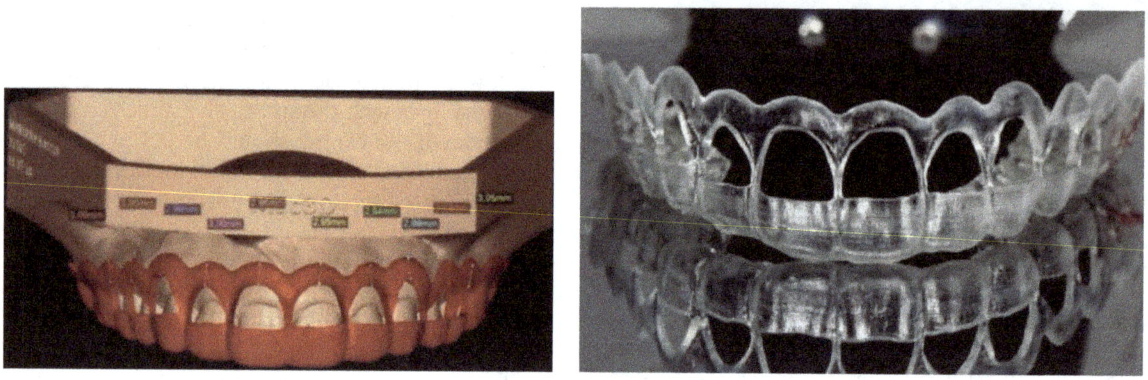

(a) (b)

FIGURE 4: (a) Periodontal analysis and digital planning of the guide. (b) Printed surgical guide.

In the Nemo Studio program, the tomography contrast change (threshold) is made for better visualization of hard tissues. STL overlap with DICOM (cone beam tomography) is performed to delimit the amount of soft and hard tissue that will be removed. The accuracy of the surgical guide is increased through this alignment as tomography facilitates visualization of the distance from the cementoenamel junction to the bone crest and from the gingival margin to the cementoenamel junction in millimeters. Moreover, clinical and radiographic examination revealed a diagnosis of altered passive eruption.

2.3. Periodontal Surgical Guide. The surgical guide was designed in the same software, according to the waxing of the new gingival margin position, and printed on resin (PerioGuide) (Figures 4(a) and 4(b)), with 1 mm thickness. The superior contour of the guide denoted a measurement of 3.0 mm above the new position of the gingival margin defined by the aesthetic waxing, aiming to reestablish biological distances (Figure 5). In the "windows" of the guide, a cut was made for the design of the new regular concave arch gingival margin. The purpose of this cutout was to establish the exact limit for gingival tissue incision, avoid excessive tissue removal, and establish the ideal contour determined by the treatment plan.

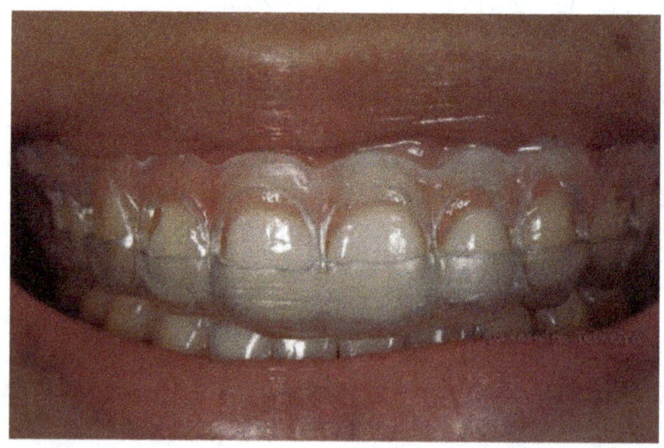

FIGURE 5: Surgical guide in the mouth. The superior contour of the guide denoted a measurement of 3.0 mm above the new position of the gingival margin defined by the aesthetic waxing.

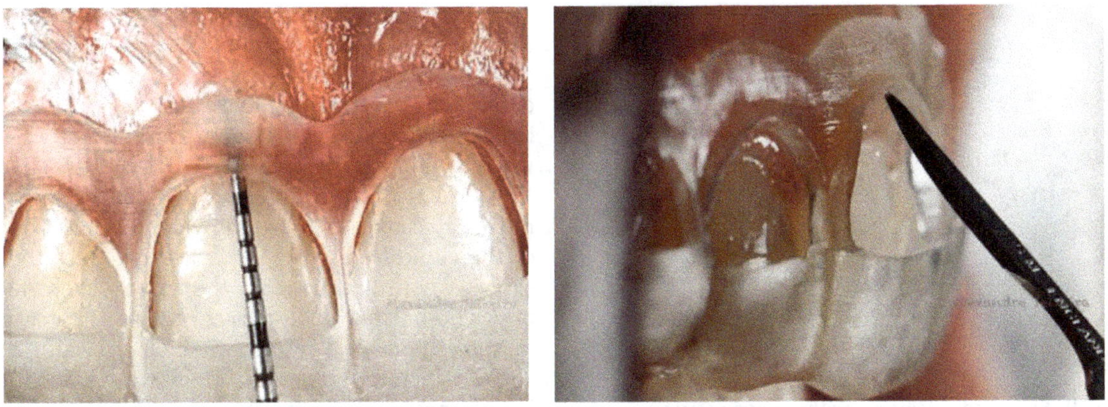

(a) (b)

FIGURE 6: (a) CEJ was located. (b) Primary internal bevel incision.

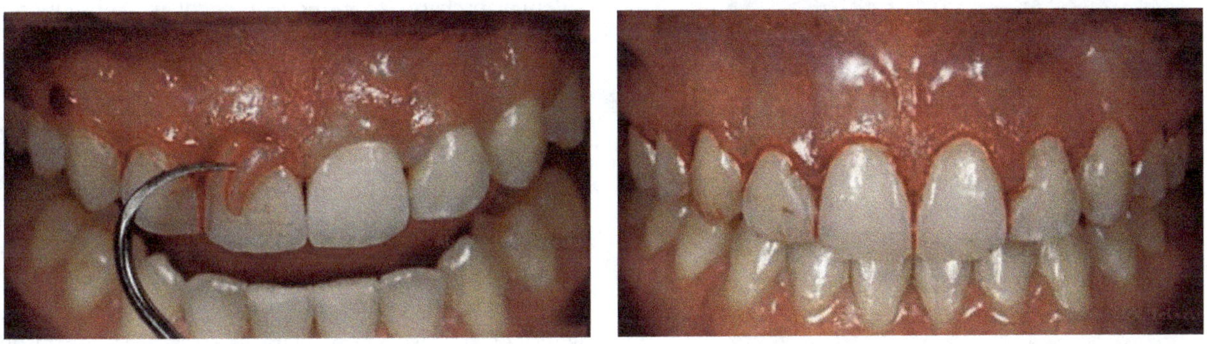

(a) (b)

FIGURE 7: (a) Gingival collar removal. (b) Gingival collar removed.

2.4. Surgery. In the surgical stage, firstly, extraoral asepsis was performed with a 10% povidone-iodine (PVPI) solution and the patient was asked to rinse the mouth with 0.12% chlorhexidine digluconate for one minute. Subsequently, infiltrative local anesthesia with 4% articaine (Nova DFL, Industry and Commerce S.A, Rio de Janeiro, Brazil) was administered at the bottom of the maxillary vestibule. Using a millimeter probe (Hu-Friedy, Chicago, USA), the CEJ was located and compared with the delimitation of the surgical guide positioned in the mouth (Figures 6(a)). The primary internal bevel incision was performed with a 15C blade (Figure 6(b)) (Swann-Morton, England), followed by intrasulcular incisions for collar removal (Figures 7(a) and 7(b)).

Gingival tunneling was performed with the aid of a tunneling instrument, and tunneled osteotomy (tunneling) was performed with a piezoelectric device with a specific insert for this purpose. The frequency of the piezoelectric device is regulated for bone, and not for cementum and dentin, thus preventing damage to the tooth root and crown. Also, a slight inclination of the insert is made so that it touches the bone (Figure 8). Its tips measuring 3 mm were inserted into the gingival sulcus to reestablish biologic width (Figure 9). The patient was medicated for pain and edema control with paracetamol 750 mg and ibuprofen 600 mg every 8 hours for 3 days.

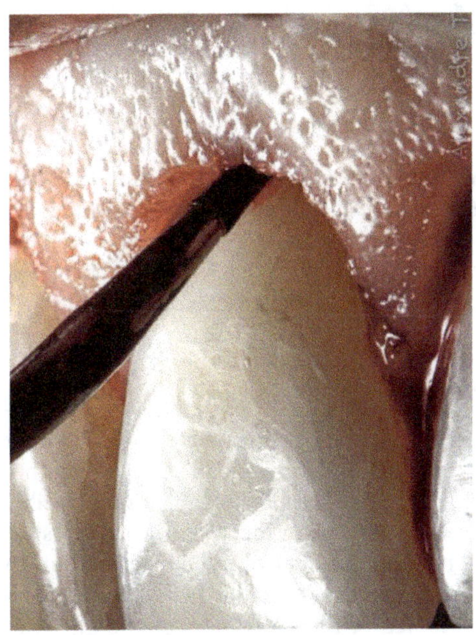

FIGURE 8: Specific insertion for tunneled osteotomy with the piezoelectric device, where the cut is only at the tip to avoid damage to the tooth root.

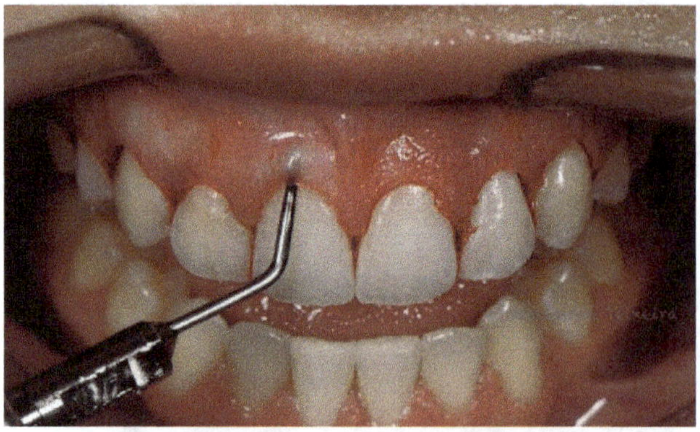

FIGURE 9: Tunneled osteotomy with a piezoelectric.

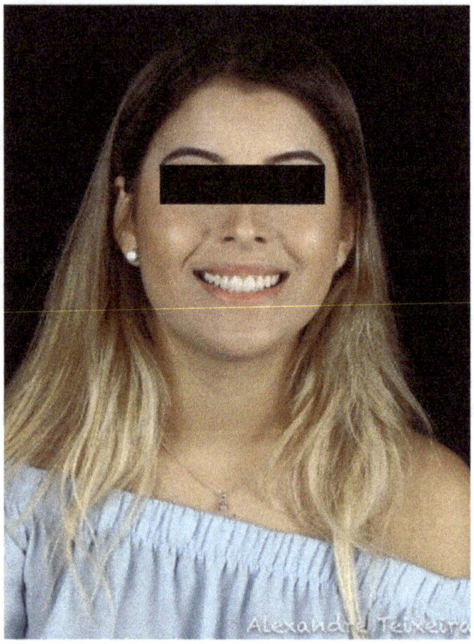

FIGURE 10: 60 days after surgery.

In the immediate postoperative period, the patient presented better gingival contour and was completely satisfied with the treatment at the 60-day evaluation (Figure 10). Whitening was performed after 90 days of surgery, and class III resins were subsequently corrected to harmonize the smile.

3. Discussion

This case report reinforces the interrelationship of periodontics and aesthetic dentistry, considering that both require a multidisciplinary treatment plan in gummy smile patients. Preapproved reverse planning with the diagnostic mockup increased patient confidence. The preview of the result helped in aesthetic and functional evaluation. In the search for smile aesthetics, the correction of the gingival contour before rehabilitation is crucial to obtain better results, and a differential diagnosis is needed to proceed with the specific treatment plan for each etiology [3]. In this case, digital planning supported the obtained results.

Altered passive eruption (APE) is a condition in which the gingiva does not migrate to its final position in the apical direction. In the present case report, clinical examination and dental gingival tomography revealed that APE was the etiological factor. However, a gum exposure of less than 3 mm when smiling is considered acceptable. In an ideal smile, 1 mm to 2 mm of the gum is exposed when the upper lip moves apically [3]. For gummy smile correction, the length of the clinical crown is increased to reduce the amount of exposed gum and increase the crown height to follow the upper lip line [13]. Most cases require osteoplasty to reduce marginal bone and restore the biologic width, as described above. When the gingival margin is too close to the CEJ, there is not enough space for the establishment of the biological space [14], leading to a greater likelihood of gingival growth recurrence after gingival contouring surgery [15]. Therefore, studies have demonstrated a gingivectomy technique initiated by an internal bevel incision and followed by an intrasulcular incision to remove the collar. Subsequently, the flap is raised to the mucogingival line for osteotomy and osteoplasty to reestablish the biologic width [12, 15–19]. Digital treatment planning enables the clinician to plan the amount of osteotomy needed on each tooth to maintain the biologic width.

Silva et al. [23] described a "flapless" approach with gingival sulcus osteotomy using microchisels in the treatment of a gummy smile with altered passive eruption. The results are aesthetically favorable and predictable in patients with thin or intermediate gingival biotypes and a keratinized gingival width of at least 3 mm. Flapless surgery is contraindicated in patients with a thick gingival phenotype because a precise and well-designed osteotomy is needed to obtain a better adaptation of the soft tissues in the cervical region and harmonize the papillae [20]. In our case, the thick periodontal biotype was conducive to the flapless technique. However, piezoelectric surgery was used instead of chisels for osteotomy. The benefits of this method include better soft tissue healing, reduced surgical time, no suture, and less postoperative discomfort. Due to the characteristics of the piezosurgery, also known as piezoelectric bone surgery, the osteotomy technique has become more predictable. The microvibrations allow a precise cut of only mineralized structures without damaging soft tissues, even in case of accidental contact. It also provides a bloodless site and decreases undesirable inflammatory responses such as edema and pain [21, 22]. Moreover, it is important to note that we used a piezoelectric with a specific periodontal tip with a 3 mm marking that guided the clinician to a more accurate and safer osteotomy.

Periodontics walks in a digital stream. Technology resources such as dental gingival computed tomography, facial scanning, surgical guides, stereolithography, and the piezoelectric technique have enriched treatment planning and surgery, from the initial clinical examination to the outcome. Clinical probing has been the standard method to localize the CEJ [17]. However, three-dimensional computed tomography with the use of labial and lingual retractors for image acquisition merged with the STF file (generated through intraoral scanning) in specific software was a less invasive method. This provided visualization of the periodontal structures and their relationship to the hard and soft tissues. Besides, it provides measurements of the relationship of the gingival margin to the bone crest, the bone crest to the CEJ, and the CEJ to the gingival margin, buccal and lingual gingival thickness, bone density, and total biologic width [14].

Reverse planning is a concept in dentistry that allows the clinician to visualize the outcome before initiating treatment. In this case, the patient was extremely pleased when the digital wax-up was presented to her. Through the innovations of digital workflow, it has become possible to refine this technique and use it in periodontics with specific software. Before starting the treatment, patients can see themselves using digital wax-ups (3D Planning, BDS) based on measurements and proportions obtained after aesthetic-facial and intrabuccal analysis. Subsequently, the clinician can use the "Printed-Mockup" (digital waxing, printed on resin) to describe the severity of the case and the desired corrections to the patients. They can discuss the prognosis together and reach a consensus to proceed with the ideal treatment plan. We noticed that the patient was deeply moved when the guide was placed in her mouth, which contributed positively to successful treatment.

4. Conclusion

We can conclude that guided periodontal surgery for the treatment of a gummy smile using piezoelectric digital planning favors postoperative results, making treatment more predictable and consistent with patient expectations. The procedure is faster, more accurate, and safer.

References

[1] A. Diaspro, M. Cavallini, P. Piersini, and G. Sito, "Gummy smile treatment: proposal for a novel corrective technique and a review of the literature," *Aesthet Surg J*, vol. 38, no. 12, pp. 1330–1338, 2018.

[2] A. H. L. Tjan, G. D. Miller, and J. G. P. The, "Some esthetic factors in a smile," *The Journal of Prosthetic Dentistry*, vol. 51, no. 1, pp. 24–28, 1984.

[3] D. A. Garber and M. A. Salama, "The aesthetic smile: diagnosis and treatment," *Periodontology 2000*, vol. 11, no. 1, pp. 18–28, 1996.

[4] J. W. Robbins, "Differential diagnosis and treatment of excess gingival display," *Practical Periodontics and Aesthetic Dentistry*, vol. 11, no. 2, pp. 265–72; quiz 273, 1999.

[5] A. Ramesh, R. Vellayappan, S. Ravi, and K. Gurumoorthy, "Esthetic lip repositioning: a cosmetic approach for correction of gummy smile - a case series," *Journal of Indian Society of Periodontology*, vol. 23, no. 3, pp. 290–294, 2019.

[6] M. B. Dutra, D. E. Ritter, A. Borgatto, C. D.'. A. Derech, and R. Rocha, "Influência da exposição gengival na estética do sorriso," *Dental Press Journal of Orthodontics*, vol. 16, no. 5, pp. 111–118, 2011.

[7] E. Sucupira and A. Abramovitz, "A simplified method for smile enhancement: botulinum toxin injection for gummy smile," *Plastic and Reconstructive Surgery*, vol. 130, no. 3, pp. 726–728, 2012.

[8] G. Cervino, L. Fiorillo, A. V. Arzukanyan, G. Spagnuolo, and M. Cicciu, "Dental restorative digital workflow: digital smile design from aesthetic to function," *Dental Journal*, vol. 7, no. 2, p. 30, 2019.

[9] L. G. Farkas, W. Bryson, and J. Klotz, "Is photogrammetry of the face reliable?," *Plastic and Reconstructive Surgery*, vol. 66, no. 3, pp. 346–355, 1980.

[10] B. Hassan, M. Greven, and D. Wismeijer, "Integrating 3D facial scanning in a digital workflow to CAD/CAM design and fabricate complete dentures for immediate total mouth rehabilitation," *The Journal of Advanced Prosthodontics*, vol. 9, no. 5, pp. 381–386, 2017.

[11] M. Thomas, U. Akula, K. K. Ealla, and N. Gajjada, "Piezosurgery: a boon for modern periodontics," *Journal of International Society of Preventive and Community Dentistry*, vol. 7, no. 1, pp. 1–7, 2017.

[12] F. Cairo, F. Graziani, L. Franchi, E. Defraia, and G. P. Pini Prato, "Periodontal Plastic Surgery to Improve Aesthetics in Patients with Altered Passive Eruption/Gummy Smile: A Case Series Study," *International Journal of Dentistry*, vol. 2012, Article ID 837658, 6 pages, 2012.

[13] S. Ting-Shu and S. Jian, "Intraoral digital impression technique: a review," *Journal of Prosthodontics*, vol. 24, no. 4, pp. 313–321, 2015.

[14] A. W. Gargiulo, F. M. Wentz, and B. Orban, "Dimensions and relations of the dentogingival junction in humans," *Journal of Periodontology*, vol. 32, no. 3, pp. 261–267, 1961.

[15] B. Paolicci, M. Calamita, C. Coachman, G. Galip, A. Shayder, and P. Hallawell, "Visagism: the art of dental composition," *Quintessence of Dental Technology*, pp. 1–14, 2012.

[16] F. Alpiste-Illueca, "Altered passive eruption (APE):A little-known clinical situation," *Medicina Oral Patología Oral y Cirugia Bucal*, vol. 16, no. 1, pp. e100–e104, 2011.

[17] J. G. Coslet, R. Vanarsdall, and A. Weisgold, "Diagnosis and classification of delayed passive eruption of the dentogingival junction in the adult," *The Alpha Omegan*, vol. 70, no. 3, pp. 24–28, 1977.

[18] F. M. Lima dos Santos, M. Serra, F. Cabral et al., "Odontologia digital: transformando sorrisos utilizando a tecnologia CAD/-CAM," *Journal of Clinical Dentistry and Research*, vol. 14, no. 2, pp. 109–117, 2017.

[19] E. R. Watanabe, M. Gabrielli, E. R. Vieira Filho, and O. Freitas, "Utilização do motor piezoelétrico em cirurgia buco maxili facial," *Revista de Odontologia da UNESP*, vol. 42, 2013.

[20] J. C. Joly, P. F. M. Carvalho, and R. C. Silva, *Reconstrução Tecidual Estética - Procedimentos Plás-ticos e Regenerativos Periodontais e Peri-implantares*, Artes Médicas, São Paulo, 2009.

[21] R. Pontoriero and G. Carnevale, "Surgical crown lengthening: a 12-month clinical wound healing study," *Journal of Periodontology*, vol. 72, no. 7, pp. 841–848, 2001.

[22] T. Vercellotti, "Technological characteristics and clinical indications of piezoelectric bone surgery," *Minerva Stomatologica*, vol. 53, no. 5, pp. 207–214, 2004.

[23] P. F. M. De Carvalho, R. C. Silva, and J. C. Joly, "Aesthetic crown lengthening: a flapless, new approach," *Revista da Associação Paulista de Cirurgiões Dentistas*, vol. 1, pp. 26–33, 2010.

15

Tongue Osseous Choristoma in an 11-Year-Old Female: A Case Report and Literature Review Focusing on Pediatric Cases

Satomi Arimoto,[1] **Manabu Shigeoka**,[2] **and Masaya Akashi**[1]

[1]*Division of Oral and Maxillofacial Surgery, Department of Surgery Related, Kobe University Graduate School of Medicine, Kobe, Japan*
[2]*Division of Pathology, Department of Pathology, Kobe University Graduate School of Medicine, Kobe, Japan*

Correspondence should be addressed to Manabu Shigeoka; shigeokamanabu@gmail.com

Academic Editor: Eugenio Maiorano

Osseous choristoma is an uncommon benign lesion characterized by the presence of ectopic mature bone within soft tissue. In most cases, these lesions occur on the dorsum of the tongue in patients in their third and fourth decades of life. This article describes a case of lingual osseous choristoma in a pediatric patient. An eleven-year-old girl with a lingual mass was referred to our hospital from a dental clinic. Total excisional biopsy and histological examination were performed, and osseous choristoma was diagnosed. The postoperative course was uneventful with no signs of recurrence during the 12 months after surgery. Moreover, a literature review focusing on pediatric cases with lingual osseous choristoma was performed to know the etiology, clinicopathological characteristics, and course of treatment of the lesion.

1. Introduction

Choristoma is defined as a tumor-like lesion that is composed of normal tissue in an abnormal location. In 1971, Krolls et al. proposed the term "osseous choristoma" for soft tissue osteoma in the head and neck region [1], and this term has been widely used since. Osseous choristoma is a rare benign lesion characterized by the presence of ectopic mature bone within soft tissue and is more often composed of bone and cartilage [2]. Lingual osseous choristoma is a rather rare entity with less than 100 reported cases in the literature [3]. The pathogenesis of these lesions has remained unexplained [4]. Most cases of intraoral osseous choristoma occur in the tongue (especially its dorsal surface) [2]. Most patients with lingual osseous choristoma are women in their third or fourth decade of life [2]. These lesions are considered self-limiting in their growth. On oral examination, they frequently appear as painless, pedunculated nodules on the tongue that are firm on palpation [5]. Lingual masses can include osseous choristoma or other lesions such as fibroma, papilloma, pyogenic granulomas, squamous cell carcinomas, or hemangiomas [6]. Even though some patients may be asymptomatic, a wide array of symptoms, including gagging, dysphagia, foreign body sensation, throat irritation, discomfort, and pain, have been reported [7]. Physical examination and diagnostic imaging may assist in identifying the mass; however, a definitive diagnosis requires histologic examination. The microscopic features of osseous choristoma include a well-circumscribed mass of viable lamellar bone with haversian canals, a well-developed mass of mature viable cartilage, or a mixture of bone and cartilage surrounded by dense fibrous connective tissue with thin stratified squamous epithelium. Only a few pediatric patients with lingual osseous choristoma have been reported so far [4]. On the other hand, no previous reports of lingual osseous choristoma have highlighted the features of pediatric patients. This report is aimed at presenting another case of lingual osseous choristoma in a pediatric patient and at reviewing the relevant literature focusing on pediatric cases. A thorough literature search was carried out on PubMed and Google Scholar using search terms like "osseous choristoma," "soft tissue osteoma," and "lingual" or "tongue."

2. Case Presentation

An 11-year-old Japanese girl told her dentist about a mass in her tongue and was referred to our hospital. She had noticed an asymptomatic nodule at the dorsum of the tongue. However, the fear of being diagnosed with a malignant condition prevented her from consulting a doctor, at least for a while. She had been aware of its existence for 2–3 years before her first visit. She was diagnosed with pneumonia at the age of one year but had no other remarkable medical history. She was not on any long-term medications. Her clinical examination revealed a pedunculated mass covered with normal mucosa in the tongue's posterior portion (Figure 1). The lesion was approximately 7 mm in diameter. Although the lesion was asymptomatic and clinically diagnosed as a benign soft tissue tumor, the patient and her parents were concerned about the possibility of malignancy. A total excisional biopsy was thus performed under general anesthesia. Our patient's lesion was composed of mature bone tissue surrounded by fibrous stroma and lined by normal squamous epithelium. This lesion was regarded as ectopic bone tissue localized far away from the maxilla-mandibular bone, and the histological diagnosis of osseous choristoma was made microscopically (Figure 2). Since the pathological specimen's preparation required the resected sample's decalcification, the final diagnosis could not be determined until ~30 days postsurgery, when the histological diagnosis was revealed as osseous choristoma. This waiting period was difficult for the patient and her family. Twelve months postoperatively, no symptoms of recurrence have been observed.

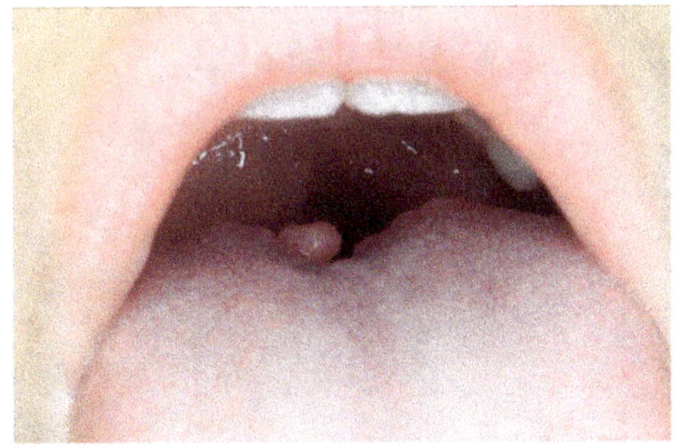

Figure 1: Intraoral clinical findings of the 11-year-old female patient. A mass approx. 7 mm in dia. was observed on the posterior dorsum of the tongue. This lesion with no symptoms was diagnosed clinically as a fibroma.

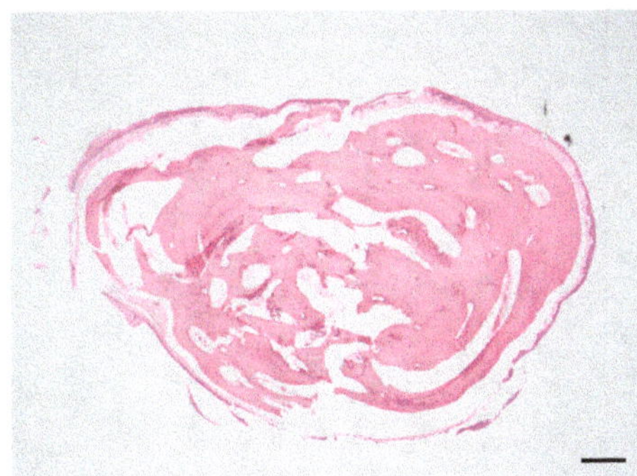

(a)

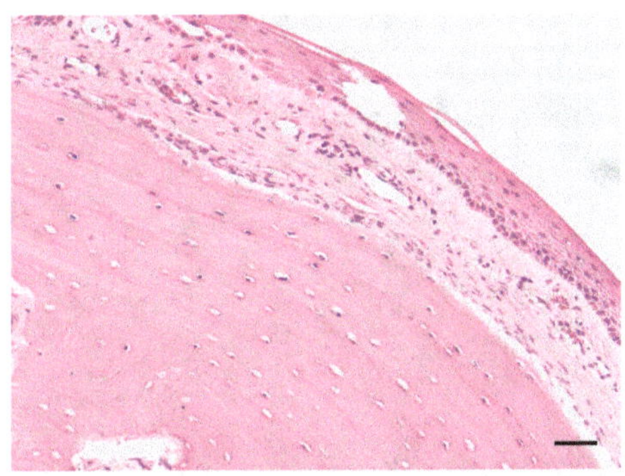

(b)

Figure 2: Histological findings. (a) Low-power image. A nodule consisting of matured bone surrounded by normal fibrous tissue was observed. Squamous epithelium that covered them is seen. Few inflammatory cells infiltrated into the lesion. Scale bar: 500 μm. (b) High-power image. Several osteocytes are observed in the matured bone. The squamous epithelium has no atypia. Scale bar: 50 μm.

3. Discussion

Lingual osseous choristoma is rare among pediatric patients. In this manuscript, we present another pediatric case of lingual osseous choristoma and review the relevant literature.

In Japan, most children attend pediatric clinics until the age of ~12 years. Thus, we focused on patients below the age of 13 years with osseous choristoma in our literature search. To our knowledge, in the literature, 62 cases have been described on patients above the age of 13 years (Table 1) [1, 3, 6, 8–45]. On the other hand, 16 cases have been described in children below the age of 13 years (Table 2) [1, 2, 4, 6, 31, 44, 46–55]. On the other hand, only one pediatric case with intraoral nonlingual osseous choristoma was found [34]. We could not detect the crucial differences in clinicopathological features between pediatric cases and the others.

We summarized the characteristics of the 17 cases with pediatric lingual osseous choristoma including our case in Table 2. Most pediatric patients with lingual osseous choristoma are females (4 males, 13 females). Although these findings are consistent with previous reports [4, 54], we could not identify the reason for the sexual predisposition. The patients' ages ranged from 5 years to 11 years (mean 9.3 years, median 10 years using Excel function). It has been demonstrated that most of the lesions develop as symptomless 3–50 mm masses located in the tongue's posterior third in the area of circumvallate papillae or close to the foramen caecum [4, 54]. The findings reported in our manuscript are in line with previous reports. It has been reported that dysphagia, a gapping sensation, pain, vomiting reflex, and nausea are the most frequent symptoms of this condition [4]. Five patients had a history of these symptoms (29.4%). Moreover, a systematic review reported a correlation

TABLE 1: Reports of cases of intraoral osseous choristomas of the tongue on >13-year-old patients.

Year	Author	Pathogenesis	Age (y)	Sex	Location on tongue	Size	Symptom	Duration	Course of discovered events	Diagnostic imaging	Preoperative diagnosis	Local recurrence	Follow-up	Reference number
1950	Breckenridge and Lukens	Developmental malformation theory	23	F	Right anterior 2/3	1 cmØ	None	Un.	Un.	None	Fibroma	Un.	Un.	8
1956	Peimer et al.	Developmental malformation theory	27	F	Left anterior 2/3	0.7 × 0.6 × 0.3 cm	Gagging, foreign body sensation	5 months	Un.	None	Fibroma	Un.	Un.	9
1967	Cataldo et al.	Developmental malformation theory	39	F	Posterior tongue	1 cmØ	None	4 months	Physical examination	None	Un.	Un.	Un.	10
1968	Jahnke and Daly	Not trauma, developmental malformation theory	22	F	Posterior to CP	1.3 × 0.8 × 0.7 cm	Lump	13 years	Asymptomatic	None	Un.	Un.	Un.	11
1968	Begel et al.	Developmental malformation theory	22	F	Area of CP	1 × 0.5 cm	Dysphagia	2 years	Slowly getting bigger	None	Fibroma	Un.	Un.	12
1968	Kaye	Un.	26	F	Base of the tongue	1 × 1 cm	Lump	Childwood	Slowly getting bigger	Un.	Un.	Un.	Un.	13
1971	Krolls et al.	Un.	22	F	Anterior to CP	0.75 cmØ	None	2 years	Un.	None	Papilloma	Un.	Un.	1
1971	Krolls et al.	Un.	23	M	Area of CP	0.5 × 0.5 × 0.5 cm	Un.	Un.	Un.	None	Hyperplast papilla	Un.	Un.	1
1971	Krolls et al.	Un.	23	M	Area of FC	Un.	Un.	Un.	Un.	None	Papilloma	Un.	Un.	1
1971	Krolls et al.	Un.	25	F	Posterior tongue	0.5 cmØ	Un.	4 months	Un.	None	Fibroma	Un.	Un.	1
1971	Krolls et al.	Un.	39	M	Area of CP	0.6 × 0.6 cm	None	Un.	Un.	None	Hyperplast papilla	Un.	Un.	1
1971	Krolls et al.	Un.	73	M	Posterior tongue	Un.	Gagging	Several years	Un.	None	Papilloma	Un.	Un.	1
1971	Goldberg et al.	Un.	65	M	Lateral border	1 cmØ	None	Un.	Un.	Un.	Un.	Un.	Un.	14
1975	McClendon	Un.	15	F	Area of FC	1.4 × 0.6 × 0.5 cm	Lump	None	Physical examination	Thyroid scan: failed to show ectopic thyroid tissue, a thyroid scintigram: normal	Lingual thyroid	Un.	Un.	15
1975	McClendon	Un.	20	M	Posterior tongue	0.7 cmØ	None	None	Physical examination	None	Un.	Un.	Un.	15
1976	Engel and Cherrick	Developmental malformation theory	31	M	Mid third right border	2 cmØ	Lump	3 years	Oral cavity examination	Dental X-P	Un.	No	2 years	16
1979	Sugita et al.	Un.	29	F	Area of FC	0.8 × 0.8 × 0.5 cm	None	12 months	Slowly getting bigger	Dental X-P	Un.	No	6 months	17

Table 1: Continued.

Year	Author	Pathogenesis	Age (y)	Sex	Location on tongue	Size	Symptom	Duration	Course of discovered events	Diagnostic imaging	Preoperative diagnosis	Local recurrence	Follow-up	Reference number
1981	Ohno et al.	Un.	44	M	Posterior to FC	0.4 × 0.8 × 0.5 cm	Un.	6 years	Slowly getting bigger	Dental X-P	Benign tumor	Un.	Un.	18
1981	Sato et al.	Un.	14	F	Anterior to CP	0.4 cmØ	Lump	4 years	Slowly getting bigger	None	Un.	Un.	Un.	19
1982	Esguep et al.	Developmental malformation theory	63	F	Right border	0.5 cmØ	Lump	Un.	Un.	Un.	Un.	Un.	Un.	20
1983	Wasserstein et al.	Developmental malformation theory	50	F	Mid third	1.5 × 0.75 cm	Lump	3 months	Oral cavity examination	None	Un.	Un.	Un.	21
1984	Main	The posterior tongue: embryological development The anterior tongue: trauma or inflammation	54	F	Posterior to FC	1.5 cmØ	Lump	Childwood	Un.	None	Un.	No	1 month	22
1984	Sheridan	Un.	20	F	Anterior to CP	1 cmØ	Lump	From birth	Un.	None	Un.	Un.	Un.	23
1984	Shimono et al.	Not trauma, developmental malformation theory	37	F	Area of FC	1.5 × 1.5 × 0.7 cm	Lump	8 years	Un.	None	Lingual thyroid	Un.	Un.	24
1984	Shimono et al.	Not trauma, developmental malformation theory	47	F	Posterior tongue	1 cmØ	Lump	12 months	Slowly getting bigger	Dental X-P	Benign tumor	Un.	Un.	24
1985	Weitzner	Developmental malformation theory	25	F	Posterior tongue	0.8 × 0.4 × 0.4 cm	Lump	None	Physical examination	None	Cyst	No	6 weeks	25
1985	Weitzner	Developmental malformation theory	27	F	Posterior tongue	0.8 × 0.7 × 0.3 cm	Lump	None	Physical examination	None	Benign tumor	No	7 weeks	25
1985	Weitzner	Developmental malformation theory	52	F	Mid third	1 × 0.6 × 0.5 cm	None	None	Physical examination	None	Benign tumor	No	2 months	25
1987	Markaki et al.	Un.	25	F	Posterior to FC	0.8 × 0.4 × 0.3 cm	Lump	5 months	Asymptomatic	The thyroid gland was normal to palpation	Un.	Un.	Un.	26
1987	Tohill et al.	Un.	26	F	Right anterior 2/3	0.9 × 0.9 × 0.5 cm	None	None	Oral cavity examination	None	Fibroma	Un.	Un.	27
1987	Tohill et al.	Un.	31	F	Anterior to CP	1 × 0.8 × 0.7 cm	None	Un.	Examination	None	Lingual thyroid, fibroma, salivary gland neoplasm	Un.	Un.	27
1987	Tohill et al.	Un.	68	M	Left posterior 1/3	0.7 × 0.5 × 0.3 cm	None	2 years	Oral cavity examination	None	Papilloma	Un.	Un.	27
1987	Van Der Wal and van der Waal	Developmental malformation theory	61	F	Anterior to CP	2 cmØ	None	15 years	Slowly getting bigger	None	Un.	No	2.5 years	28

Table 1: Continued.

Year	Author	Pathogenesis	Age (y)	Sex	Location on tongue	Size	Symptom	Duration	Course of discovered events	Diagnostic imaging	Preoperative diagnosis	Local recurrence	Follow-up	Reference number
1988	Cannon and Niparko	Un.	51	F	Posterior tongue	Un.	Lump	20 years	Un.	Un.	Un.	Un.	Un.	29
1989	Bernard et al.	Un.	21	F	Area of FC	2 cmØ	Lump	12 years	Physical examination	CT: densely ossified mass	Un.	No	Un.	30
1993	Ishikawa et al.	Developmental malformation theory	53	F	Area of FC	0.8 cmØ	Foreign body sensation	3 days	Foreign body sensation	None	Benign tumor	No	Un.	31
1996	Wei Cheong et al.	Developmental malformation theory	23	F	Posterior to FC	1.5 cmØ	Un.	13 years	Slowly getting bigger	The thyroid gland was normal to palpation	Lingual thyroid, fibroma	No	12 months	32
1996	Manganaro	Un.	27	M	Posterior tongue	1.0 × 0.5 cm	Gagging	Un.	Slowly getting bigger	None	Un.	Un.	Un.	33
1996	Manganaro	Un.	44	M	Posterior tongue	0.7 × 0.6 cm	Gagging	Several months	Slowly getting bigger	None	Un.	Un.	Un.	33
1998	Lin et al.	Not trauma, the posterior tongue: developmental malformation, other site: trauma	21	F	Posterior tongue	1.2 cmØ	Lump	5 years	Asymptomatic	None	Fibroma	No	4 years	34
1998	Supiyaphun et al.	Un.	19	F	Area of FC	1.1 × 0.7 × 0.7 cm	None	11 years	Un.	None	Un.	No	Un.	6
1998	Supiyaphun et al.	Un.	21	F	Area of FC	1.5 × 1.3 × 0.8 cm	Lump	5 years	Un.	None	Un.	No	Un.	6
1998	Supiyaphun et al.	Un.	22	M	Area of FC	0.9 × 0.8 × 0.6 cm	None	Un.	Examination	None	Un.	No	Un.	6
1998	Supiyaphun et al.	Un.	25	F	Area of FC	0.7 × 0.5 × 0.4 cm	Lump	12 months	Un.	None	Un.	No	Un.	6
1998	Supiyaphun et al.	Un.	27	F	Area of FC	1.2 × 0.9 × 0.6 cm	None	Un.	Examination	None	Un.	No	Un.	6
1998	Supiyaphun et al.	Un.	28	F	Area of FC	1 × 0.8 × 0.6 cm	Throat irritation	4 years	Un.	None	Un.	No	Un.	6
1998	Supiyaphun et al.	Un.	35	F	Area of FC	0.7 × 0.5 × 0.5 cm	None	Un.	Examination	None	Un.	No	Un.	6
1998	Vered et al.	Un.	27	M	Posterior to CP	1 × 0.5 cm	Pain, gagging	None	Slowly getting bigger	None	Un.	Un.	Un.	35
1998	Vered et al.	Un.	44	M	Posterior to CP	0.7 × 0.6 cm	Gagging, nausea, dysphagia	Several months	Un.	None	Un.	Un.	Un.	35
2007	Benamer and Elmangoush	Un.	14	F	Midline posterior 1/3	1 cmØ	Gagging	More than ten years	Painless but slowly getting bigger	None	Un.	Un.	Un.	36
2007	Demirseren and Aydin	Not trauma	28	M	Anterior 2/3	2 × 1.5 × 1 cm	Gagging	4 years	Slowly getting bigger	None	Pyogenic granuloma	No	48 months	37

Table 1: Continued.

Year	Author	Pathogenesis	Age (y)	Sex	Location on tongue	Size	Symptom	Duration	Course of discovered events	Diagnostic imaging	Preoperative diagnosis	Local recurrence	Follow-up	Reference number
2008	Andressakis et al.	Local trauma from dentures	72	M	Area of CP	1.5 × 1.0 cm	Pain, dysphagia	Several years	Asymptomatic	None	Un.	Un.	Un.	38
2009	Naik et al.	Not trauma	25	F	Posterior tongue	1.2 × 1.1 × 0.5 cm	Lump	5 years	Slowly getting bigger	Un.	Un.	Un.	Un.	39
2011	Liu et al.	Not trauma	17	M	Area of FC	0.5 × 0.5 cm	Lump	Several years	Asymptomatic	None	Un.	No	Un.	40
2016	Adhikari et al.	Not trauma	15	F	Area of FC	0.5cmØ	Throat irritation	12 months	Painless but gradually swelling	None	Fibroma	No	5 months	41
2016	Adhikari et al.	Not trauma	21	F	Area of FC	0.5 mØ	Pain	Un.	Oral cavity examination	None	Un.	No	48 months	41
2016	Turan et al.	Un.	41	F	Posterior tongue	1 × 0.5 cm	Throat irritation	6 months	Examination	Ultrasonographic evaluation: normal thyroid gland	Lingual thyroid, mucocele, lingual thyroglossal duct cyst	No	4 months	42
2017	Heinz et al.	Not trauma	21	F	Base of the tongue	0.5 cmØ	Lump	Un.	Asymptomatic	Fiberoptic examination	Un.	No	3 months	43
2020	Sun et al.	Un.	23	M	Base of the tongue	0.8 × 0.7 × 0.5 cm	Lump	Un.	Un.	None	Benign tumor	Un.	Un.	3
2020	Sun et al.	Un.	27	M	Base of the tongue	0.8 × 0.5 × 0.5 cm	Lump	3 months	Un.	None	Benign tumor	Un.	Un.	3
2020	Leigh et al.	Developmental malformation theory	37	F	Base of the tongue	0.7 × 0.4 × 0.3 cm	Gagging	3 months	Physical examination	Ultrasonographic evaluation: normal thyroid gland	Un.	No	26 months	44
2020	Hemmi et al.	Not trauma	89	M	Base of the tongue	1 cmØ	Cough	Un.	Prolonged cough	Cervical spine CT: well-defined, rounded, high-density mass	Un.	No	15 months	45

CP: circumvallate papillae; FC: foramen caecum; M: male; F: female; CT: computed tomography; Un.: unknown.

TABLE 2: Reports of cases of intraoral osseous choristomas of the tongue on <13-year-old patients.

Year	Author	Age (y)	Sex	Location on tongue	Size	Symptom	Duration	Pathogenesis	Course of discovered events	Diagnostic imaging	Preoperative diagnosis	Local recurrence	Follow-up	Reference number
1964	Church	11	F	Area of FC	0.5 cmØ	Dysphagia	Un.	Un.	Slowly getting bigger	None	Un.	Un.	Un.	46
1971	Krolls et al.	9	F	Area of FC	Un.	Gagging	2.5 years	Un.	Un.	None	Fibroma	Un.	Un.	1
1971	Krolls et al.	11	F	Posterior tongue	2 cmØ	Un.	12 months	Un.	Un.	None	Papilloma	Un.	Un.	1
1977	Busuttil	8	F	Area of CP	Pea-sized	Lump	9 months	Un.	Slowly getting bigger	None	Un.	Un.	Un.	47
1986	Cabbabe et al.	5	F	Base of the tongue	0.6 × 0.5 × 0.3 cm	Lump	2 years	Not trauma, developmental malformation theory	Asymptomatic	None	Fibroma	Un.	Un.	48
1992	Maqbool et al.	8	F	Right vallecula	5 × 4 cm	Dysphagia, distress	Un.	Not trauma, developmental malformation theory	Un.	Un.	Un.	Un.	Un.	49
1993	Ishikawa et al.	5	F	Anterior to CP	0.3 → 0.8 cmØ	Lump	1-month follow-up: 16 months	Developmental malformation theory	Asymptomatic	None	Fibroma	No	Un.	31
1993	Lutcavage and Fulbright	11	F	Area of FC	1 cmØ	Lump	12 months	Enclavement of mesenchymal cells	Slowly getting bigger	A thyroid scintigram: normal	Un.	Un.	Un.	50
1998	Supiyaphun et al.	9	F	Area of FC	0.7 × 0.6 × 0.5 cm	None	Un.	Un.	Examination	None	Un.	No	Un.	6
2001	Horn et al.	11	F	Posterior tongue	Un.	Lump	Un.	Un.	Un.	Un.	Un.	Un.	Un.	51
2014	Gorini et al.	10	F	Area of FC	1 cmØ	Lump	Since the first months of life	Developmental malformation theory	Asymptomatic	Thyroid scan: failed to show ectopic thyroid tissue	Un.	No	12 months	4
2014	Yamamoto et al.	11	M	Posterior to CP	0.8 × 0.6 cm	Dysphagia	5 years	Developmental malformation theory	Slowly getting bigger	MRI: T1 and T2WI (fat saturation): oval no-signal area	Papilla fibroma	No	12 months	52
2015		11	M		1.1 × 0.9 × 0.8 cm		Un.	Un.	Examination		Un.	Un.	Un.	53

Table 2: Continued.

Year	Author	Age (y)	Sex	Location on tongue	Size	Symptom	Duration	Pathogenesis	Course of discovered events	Diagnostic imaging	Preoperative diagnosis	Local recurrence	Follow-up	Reference number
	Stanford et al.			Base of the tongue		Throat irritation				Thyroid uptake scan: normal CT: densely calcified lesion				
2016	Davidson et al.	11	M	Base of the tongue	Un.	Foreign body sensation	Un.	Un.	Slowly getting bigger	Thyroid scan: failed to show ectopic thyroid tissue CT: a calcified ovoid mass	Un.	Un.	Un.	2
2018	Yoshimura et al.	7	F	Posterior tongue	0.5 cmØ → 0.6 cmØ	None	Un.	Ectopic bone formation by secretion of BMPs	Slowly getting bigger	T1- and T2-weighted images: low-signal intensity Dermoscopy dental X-P: radiopaque trabeculated mass	Benign tumor	No	36 months	54
2018	Macêdo et al.	9	M	Posterior 1/3	2.3 × 2.0 × 0.8 cm	Symptomatic	3 months	Developmental malformation theory associated with adenoidectomy	Oral cavity examination	CT: pseudotumor	Un.	No	2.5 years	55
2021	Present case	11	F	Posterior tongue	0.7 cmØ	Lump	2–3 years	Developmental malformation theory	Oral cavity examination	None	Papilloma	No	12 months	

CP: circumvallate papillae; FC: foramen caecum; M: male; F: female; CT: computed tomography; MRI: magnetic resonance imaging; Un.: unknown.

between these symptoms and lesion size [4]; however, another review concluded that there was no correlation between them [6]. Hemmi et al. reported an adult case of lingual osseous choristoma with prolonged cough. They concluded that the cough was due to gastroesophageal reflux disease. Regarding the correlation in pediatric cases, we could not conclude from only 5 cases (29.4%). To resolve this discordance, it is necessary to recruit more cases [45]. The follow-up period ranged from one year to three years. No evidence of spontaneous loss or malignant transformation has been reported. No case of pediatric lingual osseous choristoma showed any sign of recurrence [7], while only two recurrent nonpediatric cases of the buccal mucosa lesion were reported [56, 57]. Long et al. reported that the recurrent lesion could have arisen as a result of the surgical trauma caused by the removal of the original lesion; however, this theory could not explain the occurrence of the original lesion because the patient denied any history of trauma [56]. Besides, according to Dalkiz et al., lesions do not recur once excised and the recurrent lesion might have been caused by a new fibrotic region that underwent ossification an uncalcified lesion that subsequently ossified [57]. Although the mechanisms of recurrence remain uncertain, cases of extralingual lesions should have a longer follow-up period. Our patient's clinical findings were consistent with previous reports. Taking into account the fact that our patient was referred from a private dental clinic, not only head and neck clinicians but also dentists should be familiar with the clinical features of this disease.

The pathogenesis of osseous choristoma is not yet known, a "developmental malformation hypothesis" and a "chronic trauma-associated reactive hypothesis" were proposed [4, 16, 41, 54, 58]. The involvement of systemic diseases has not been reported. With respect to the former, the lesion arises at the line of fusion of the first and third brachial arches between the anterior two-thirds and posterior one-third of the tongue [41]. Additionally, some researchers indicated that the lingual thyroid remnant ossification is associated with developmental malformation theory due to it occurring at the posterior tongue near the foramen cecum [12, 30]. However, no thyroid tissue was observed in the current case. With respect to the latter, on the other hand, the osseous lesion on the tongue appeared due to a reactive or posttraumatic center of ossification [41]. There were no previous cases that support the reactive hypothesis. In the current case, there was no evidence of irritational factors. Moreover, our patient's microscopic findings showed no reactive epithelial change, including acanthosis and cell atypia, and little inflammatory cell infiltration and fibrosis were observed. From these clinicopathological features, the "developmental malformation hypothesis" seems likely to apply in this case.

Finally, it cannot be overlooked that the 30-day waiting period until the histological diagnosis of the patient's lesion was stressful for the patient and her family. Although the reason for the long waiting time was the need to decalcify the bone tissue, the psychological care we provided was insufficient. It was speculated that the information provided by imaging modalities can help reduce patients' anxiety.

Diagnostic imaging was conducted in five pediatric cases. Given that no attending surgeons considered the possibility of an osseous choristoma, we did not conduct any imaging examination in this case. An earlier study reported computed tomography (CT) images are useful for the radiological diagnosis of lingual osseous choristoma [45]. Also, Yoshimura et al. reported the usefulness of not only radiographic examination for the surgical specimen. Additionally, they proposed developing a miniaturized, flexible dermoscopy that enabled the detailed examination of the whole oral cavity [54]. However, it is difficult for children to follow instructions when undergoing a CT scan, which often leads to motion artifacts [45]. It is also important to consider the effect of radiation exposure in pediatric patients. Furthermore, a case that occurred in the choroid was diagnosed using ultrasonography [59]; however, there are no reports of ultrasonography being used to diagnose lingual osseous choristoma as it might be difficult to use ultrasonography on the base of the tongue. Therefore, radiographic examination of the surgical specimen might be the most useful tool in the diagnosis of lingual osseous choristoma in pediatric patients.

In conclusion, we presented a pediatric case of lingual osseous choristoma and conducted a review of the literature to identify the characteristics of pediatric cases of the lesion.

Authors' Contributions

S.A. was responsible for the manuscript drafting, literature search, and collection of clinical records. M.S. was responsible for the histological evaluation and the revision of the manuscript. M.A. supervised the work. All authors reviewed and accepted the final version of the manuscript.

Acknowledgments

We thank Prof. Tomoo Ito for the valuable discussions and histopathological suggestions and all technicians of the Division of Diagnostic Pathology, Department of Pathology, Kobe University, for the excellent technical assistance.

References

[1] S. O. Krolls, J. R. Jacoway, and W. N. Alexander, "Osseous choristomas (osteomas) of intraoral soft tissues," *Oral Surgery, Oral Medicine, and Oral Pathology*, vol. 32, no. 4, pp. 588–595, 1971.

[2] S. Davidson, M. Steiner, and M. Nowicki, "Lingual osseous choristoma," *The Journal of Pediatrics*, vol. 168, pp. 247–247.e1, 2016.

[3] H. A. Sun, W. T. Lee, and H. J. Hsu, "Lingual osteoma-a case report and literature review," *Ear, Nose, & Throat Journal*, no. -article 145561320977469, 2020.

[4] E. Gorini, M. Mullace, L. Migliorini, and E. Mevio, "Osseous choristoma of the tongue: a review of etiopathogenesis," *Case Reports in Otolaryngology*, vol. 2014, Article ID 373104, 5 pages, 2014.

[5] J. E. Bouquot and M. S. H. Nikai, "Lesions of oral cavity," in *Diagnostic surgical pathology of the head and neck*, D. Gnepp, Ed., Saunders Elsevier, Amstedam, 2nd ed edition, 2009.

[6] P. Supiyaphun, P. Sampatanakul, V. Kerekhanjanarong, P. Chawakitchareon, and V. Sastarasadhit, "Lingual osseous choristoma: a study of eight cases and review of the literature," *Ear, Nose, & Throat Journal*, vol. 77, no. 4, pp. 316–325, 1998.

[7] Z. J. Shareef, S. J. Shareef, C. C. Kerndt, A. Aughenbaugh, and A. Di Ponio, "Lingual osseous choristoma: a systematic review of lesion presentation, histology, and morphology," *Spartan Medical Research Journal*, vol. 5, no. 2, p. 17543, 2020.

[8] R. L. Breckenridge and R. M. Lukens, "Osteoma of the tongue," *Archives of Otolaryngology*, vol. 52, no. 1, pp. 19–24, 1950.

[9] D. H. Dreizin, Y. Masugi, and R. Peimer, "Osteoma of the tongue," *A.M.A. Archives of Otolaryngology*, vol. 64, no. 2, pp. 148–150, 1956.

[10] E. Cataldo, G. Shklar, and I. Meyer, "Osteoma of the tongue," *Archives of Otolaryngology*, vol. 85, no. 2, pp. 202–206, 1967.

[11] V. Jahnke and J. F. Daly, "Osteoma of the tongue," *The Journal of Laryngology and Otology*, vol. 82, no. 3, pp. 273–275, 1968.

[12] H. Begel, H. Wilson, G. Stratigos, and R. F. Zambito, "Osteoma of the tongue: report of case," *Journal of Oral Surgery*, vol. 26, no. 10, pp. 662–664, 1968.

[13] W. H. Kaye, "Osteoma of the tongue," *The Journal of Laryngology and Otology*, vol. 82, no. 3, pp. 269–271, 1968.

[14] A. F. Goldberg, D. F. Skuble, and R. J. Latronica, "Osteoma of the tongue: report of case," *Journal of Oral Surgery*, vol. 28, no. 6, p. 457, 1970.

[15] E. H. McClendon, "Lingual osseous choristoma: Report of two cases," *Oral Surgery, Oral Medicine, and Oral Pathology*, vol. 39, no. 1, pp. 39–44, 1975.

[16] P. Engel and H. M. Cherrick, "Extraosseous osteomas of the tongue," *Journal of Oral Medicine*, vol. 31, no. 4, pp. 99–103, 1976.

[17] H. Sugita, E. Yamamoto, H. Sunakawa, T. Matsubara, I. Furuta, and G. I. Kohama, "Lingual osseous choristoma: report of a case," *Japanese Journal of Oral and Maxillofacial Surgery*, vol. 25, no. 6, pp. 1417–1421, 1979.

[18] T. Ohno, H. Y. E. Morii, A. Takahashi et al., "Osseous choristoma situated on the dorusum of the root of the tongue: report of a case," *Japanese Journal of Oral and Maxillofacial Surgery*, vol. 27, no. 8, pp. 1106–1109, 1981.

[19] Y. Sato, S. O. N. Aria, I. Toguchi, T. Fukuda, Y. Ueda, and T. Yoshimoto, "Osseous Choristoma of the tongue: report of a case," *Japanese Journal of Oral and Maxillofacial Surgery*, vol. 27, no. 1, pp. 93–95, 1981.

[20] A. Esguep, E. Espinoza, and G. Diaz, "Lingual osteoma," *Journal of Oral Medicine*, vol. 37, no. 1, pp. 27–29, 1982.

[21] M. H. Wasserstein, M. SunderRaj, R. Jain, G. Yamane, and A. P. Chaudhry, "Lingual osseous choristoma," *Journal of Oral Medicine*, vol. 38, no. 3, pp. 87–89, 1983.

[22] D. M. Main, "Osseous polyp of the tongue: osteoma or choristoma?," *British Dental Journal*, vol. 156, no. 8, pp. 285-286, 1984.

[23] S. M. Sheridan, "Osseous choristoma: A report of two gases," *The British Journal of Oral & Maxillofacial Surgery*, vol. 22, no. 2, pp. 99–102, 1984.

[24] M. Shimono, T. Tsuji, Y. Iguchi et al., "Lingual osseous choristoma: Report of 2 cases," *International Journal of Oral Surgery*, vol. 13, no. 4, pp. 355–359, 1984.

[25] S. Weitzner, "Osseous choristoma of the tongue," *Southern Medical Journal*, vol. 79, no. 1, pp. 69-70, 1986.

[26] S. Markaki, J. Gearty, and P. Markakis, "Osteoma of the tongue," *The British Journal of Oral & Maxillofacial Surgery*, vol. 25, no. 1, pp. 79–82, 1987.

[27] M. J. Tohill, J. G. Green, and D. M. Cohen, "Intraoral osseous and cartilaginous choristomas: report of three cases and review of the literature," *Oral Surgery, Oral Medicine, and Oral Pathology*, vol. 63, no. 4, pp. 506–510, 1987.

[28] N. van der Wal and I. van der Waal, "Osteoma or chondroma of the tongue; a clinical and postmortem study," *International Journal of Oral and Maxillofacial Surgery*, vol. 16, no. 6, pp. 713–717, 1987.

[29] S. C. Cannon and J. K. Niparko, "Pathologic quiz case 1. Lingual osteoma," *Archives of Otolaryngology – Head & Neck Surgery*, vol. 114, no. 1, pp. 92–94, 1988.

[30] P. J. Bernard, J. M. A. Shugar, R. Mitnick, P. M. Som, and R. Meyer, "Lingual osteoma," *Archives of Otolaryngology – Head & Neck Surgery*, vol. 115, no. 8, pp. 989-990, 1989.

[31] M. Ishikawa, T. Mizukoshi, K. I. Notani, T. Iizuka, A. Amemiya, and H. Fukuda, "Osseous choristoma of the tongue: Report of two cases," *Oral Surgery, Oral Medicine, and Oral Pathology*, vol. 76, no. 5, pp. 561–563, 1993.

[32] N. Wei Cheong, L. C. Boon, and P. Shanmahasuntharam, "Osseous choristoma of the tongue," *The Journal of Nihon University School of Dentistry*, vol. 38, no. 1, pp. 49–51, 1996.

[33] A. M. Manganaro, "Lingual osseous choristoma," *General Dentistry*, vol. 44, no. 5, pp. 430-431, 1996.

[34] C. C. Lin, C. H. Chen, Y. K. Chen, Y. H. Shen, and L. M. Lin, "Osseous choristoma of oral cavity–report of two cases and review of the literature," *The Kaohsiung Journal of Medical Sciences*, vol. 14, no. 11, pp. 727–733, 1998.

[35] M. Vered, J. P. Lustig, and A. Buchner, "Lingual osteoma: a debatable entity," *Journal of Oral and Maxillofacial Surgery*, vol. 56, no. 1, pp. 9–13, 1998.

[36] M. H. Benamer and A. M. Elmangoush, "Lingual osseous choristoma case report and review of literature," *Libyan Journal of Medicine*, vol. 2, no. 1, pp. 46–48, 2007.

[37] M. E. Demirseren and N. E. Aydin, "A lingual osteoid mass originating from hyaline cartilage," *Journal of Cranio-Maxillo-Facial Surgery*, vol. 35, no. 2, pp. 132–134, 2007.

[38] D. D. Andressakis, A. G. Pavlakis, E. Chrysomali, and A. Rapidis, "Infected lingual osseous choristoma. Report of a case and review of the literature," *Medicina Oral, Patología Oral y Cirugía Bucal*, vol. 13, no. 10, pp. E627–E632, 2008.

[39] V. R. Naik, W. A. Wan Faiziah, and M. Y. Musa, "Choristoma of the base of the tongue," *Indian Journal of Pathology & Microbiology*, vol. 52, no. 1, pp. 86-87, 2009.

[40] J. Y. Liu and K. K. Tan, "Lingual osteoma: case report and literature review," *Singapore Medical Journal*, vol. 52, no. 10, pp. e198–e200, 2011.

[41] B. R. Adhikari, J. Sato, T. Morikawa et al., "Osseous choristoma of the tongue: two case reports," *Journal of Medical Case Reports*, vol. 10, no. 1, p. 59, 2016.

[42] S. Turan, M. Ö. Pınarbaşlı, M. Açıkalın, E. Kaya, and E. Özüdoğru, "Lingual osseous choristoma," *Turkish Archives of Otorhinolaryngology*, vol. 54, no. 2, pp. 86–88, 2016.

[43] M. J. Heinz, S. M. Peters, S. M. Caruana, and A. J. Yoon, "Lingual osseous choristoma of the tongue base: unusual presentation of a rare entity," *Case Reports in Otolaryngology*, vol. 2017, Article ID 3234086, 3 pages, 2017.

[44] N. Leigh, R. Anteby, T. Awan, and C. Sinclair, "Lingual osseous choristoma causing odynophagia in a young female," *Ear, Nose, & Throat Journal*, no. article 145561320968928, 2020.

[45] T. Hemmi, J. Suzuki, S. Sato et al., "A case of an incidentally removed lingual osseous choristoma," *Case Reports in Otolaryngology*, vol. 2020, Article ID 3498915, 4 pages, 2020.

[46] L. E. Church, "Osteoma of the tongue: Report of a case," *Oral Surgery, Oral Medicine, and Oral Pathology*, vol. 17, no. 6, pp. 768–770, 1964.

[47] A. Busuttil, "An osteoma of the tongue," *The Journal of Laryngology and Otology*, vol. 91, no. 3, pp. 259–261, 1977.

[48] E. B. Cabbabe, C. Sotelo-Avila, S. T. Moloney, and M. V. Makhlouf, "Osseous choristoma of the tongue," *Annals of Plastic Surgery*, vol. 16, no. 2, pp. 150–152, 1986.

[49] M. Maqbool, R. Ahmad, and R. Ahmad, "Osteoma of the tongue: a rare cause of upper airway obstruction," *Indian Pediatrics*, vol. 29, no. 11, pp. 1429–1431, 1992.

[50] G. J. Lutcavage and D. K. Fulbright, "Osteoma of the tongue," *Journal of Oral and Maxillofacial Surgery*, vol. 51, no. 6, pp. 697–699, 1993.

[51] C. Horn, H. M. Thaker, D. A. Tampakopoulou, L. M. D. Serres, J. L. Keller, and J. Haddad Jr., "Tongue lesions in the pediatric population," *Otolaryngology and Head and Neck Surgery*, vol. 124, no. 2, pp. 164–169, 2001.

[52] M. Yamamoto, M. Migita, S. Ogane et al., "Osseous choristoma in child with strong vomiting reflex," *The Bulletin of Tokyo Dental College*, vol. 55, no. 4, pp. 207–215, 2014.

[53] J. K. Stanford 2nd, J. C. Spencer, and J. M. Reed, "Case presentation and images of a lingual osseous choristoma in a pediatric patient," *American Journal of Otolaryngology*, vol. 36, no. 6, pp. 753-754, 2015.

[54] H. Yoshimura, S. Ohba, Y. Imamura, and K. Sano, "Osseous choristoma of the tongue: a case report with dermoscopic study," *Molecular and Clinical Oncology*, vol. 8, no. 2, pp. 242–245, 2018.

[55] M. B. Macêdo, S. E. M. Borges, P. . S. Macêdo, and P. . T. M. Borges, "Lingual osteoma as a fortuitous finding on a boy with post-adenoidectomy inflammatory pseudotumor," *Oral and Maxillofacial Surgery Cases*, vol. 4, no. 3, pp. 115–117, 2018.

[56] D. E. Long and A. W. Koutnik, "Recurrent intraoral osseous choristoma: Report of a case," *Oral Surgery, Oral Medicine, and Oral Pathology*, vol. 72, no. 3, pp. 337–339, 1991.

[57] M. Dalkiz, R. H. Yurdakul, E. Pakdemirli, and B. Beydemir, "Recurrent osseous choristoma of the masseter muscle: case report," *Journal of Oral and Maxillofacial Surgery*, vol. 59, no. 7, pp. 836–839, 2001.

[58] A. C. Veni, K. Ashokan, and K. C. Sekar, "Osseous choriostoma of the upper lip," *Iranian Journal of Otorhinolaryngology*, vol. 32, no. 111, pp. 259–262, 2020.

[59] L. Joffe, J. A. Shields, and J. R. Fitzgerald, "Osseous choristoma of the choroid," *Archives of Ophthalmology*, vol. 96, no. 10, pp. 1809–1812, 1978.

16

Periodontal Regenerative Treatment of Intrabony Defects Associated with Palatal Grooves: A Report of Two Cases

Stefano Corbella,[1,2,3] **Alice Alberti**,[1,2] **Beatrice Zotti**,[1,2] **and Luca Francetti**[1,2]

[1]*Department of Biomedical, Surgical and Dental Sciences, Università degli Studi di Milano, Milan, Italy*
[2]*IRCCS Istituto Ortopedico Galeazzi, Milan, Italy*
[3]*Institute of Dentistry, I.M. Sechenov First Moscow State Medical University, Moscow, Russia*

Correspondence should be addressed to Alice Alberti; alice.alberti3@gmail.com

Academic Editor: Jiiang H. Jeng

A palatal radicular groove (PRG) is a morphological deformity, occurring during tooth development. It is usually located on the palatal aspect of maxillary incisors and frequently associated with periodontal or endodontic-periodontal lesions. Some treatment options were described for such lesions, including primary endodontic treatment and periodontal surgery and extraction with intentional replantation after removal of a PRG and endodontic treatment. The present paper reported two cases of PRG-associated deep intrabony defects, successfully treated with periodontal surgery with enamel matrix derivative (EMD) application and mechanical removal of PRGs, avoiding endodontic treatment or retreatment. The complexity of the diagnostic process was also discussed.

1. Introduction

In scientific literature, palatal radicular grooves (PRGs) were first described by Lee and coworkers in 1968 [1], who discussed its clinical characteristics and potential etiology [1]. A PRG is usually described as a kind of morphological deformity, occurring during tooth development as a failed attempt to form a new root [2], usually located on the palatal aspect of permanent maxillary lateral incisors [3, 4]. From the anatomical point of view, PRGs are heterogeneous, generally extending from the central fossa of the incisor, over the cingulum and down apically, on the root surface [4, 5]. In some cases, the presence of one PRG was considered as an important adverse prognostic factor, because of the frequently associated wide endodontic-periodontal lesions [6]. Even though a recent classification scheme for tooth, root, and canal anomalies was recently proposed [7], the most common classification for a PRG was proposed by Gu [8], who described three different types on the basis of its anatomical extension.

Considering that, in the past, many terms were used to describe this particular kind of deformity (such as palate-gingival groove, development of radicular anatomy, distolingual groove, palatal-radicular groove, and radicular groove [5]), PRG incidence was described, with this limitation, to range between 2.8% and 18% [5, 9–11] and one study on a cohort of Taiwanese people found PRGs in more than 40% of the subjects [12].

With regard to the clinical features, the presence of a PRG provides an ideal pathway for oral bacteria to reach deep periodontal tissues, since it can be difficultly cleaned by standard oral hygiene maneuvers. The apical migration of bacteria could lead to the formation of intrabony pockets, which are located in correspondence of the PRG and are usually deep and narrow [10, 13, 14]. In some cases, probably due to rapid progression of the infection, the lesion could reach the apical tissues, thus causing pulp necrosis and consequently an endodontic-periodontal lesion of periodontal origin [2, 9, 11, 15, 16]. In some cases, the diagnosis could

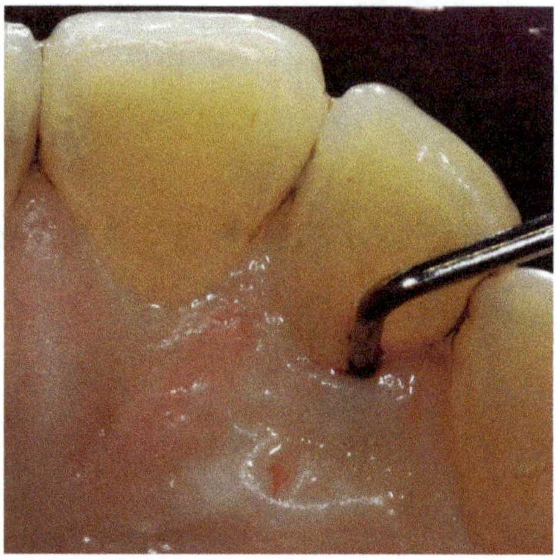

FIGURE 1: Clinical examination revealed the presence of a 13 mm deep periodontal pocket associated with an enamel alteration on the palatal side of 1.2.

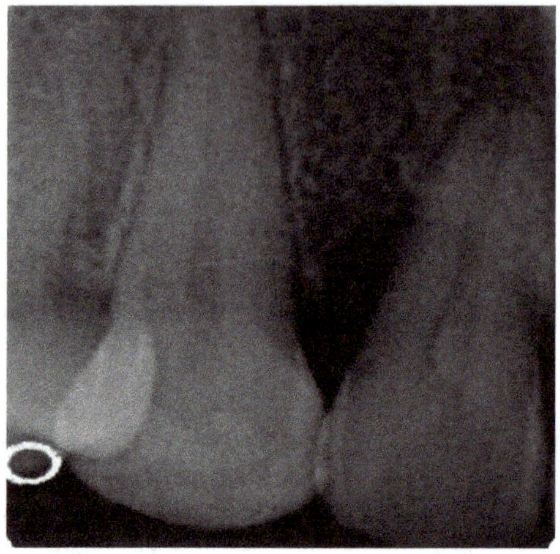

FIGURE 2: An angular bone defect was also visible through intraoral radiographic examination.

be complicated by the presence of the sinus tract usually on the vestibular mucosa, in correspondence of the affected tooth [4].

The treatment options for endodontic-periodontal lesions related to the presence of a PRG include primary endodontic treatment [4] usually associated with periodontal surgery that was limited in the site of the defect [5, 9, 15]. Other authors described the extraction of the affected tooth when a complete loss of the periodontal support occurred [4] or extraction and intentional replantation after removal of a PRG and extraoral endodontic treatment [11]. Ideally, a timely diagnosis could prevent the pulpal involvement, thus allowing successful treatment of the defect through a merely periodontal approach.

The aim of this paper was to present two case reports of PRG-associated deep intrabony defects treated with periodontal surgery and enamel matrix derivative (EMD) application, avoiding endodontic treatment or retreatment.

2. Case Presentation

Both subjects were treated following the principles of the Helsinki Declaration [17]. The operator (SC) informed the patients about the treatment alternatives and about the planned intervention, and both patients signed a written informed consent form before performing the treatment procedures.

2.1. Case Report 1. One female patient, aged 49 at the time of the first visit, without any systemic disease (ASA-1 following the classification proposed by the American Society of Anesthesiologists) presented referring an episode of acute abscess in the region of 1.1, 1.2, and 1.3 that was treated with systemic administration of Amoxicillin 875 mg+Clavulanate 125 mg twice a day for six days.

The clinical examination revealed the presence of one isolated periodontal pocket (measuring 13 mm) in correspondence of the palatal aspect of 1.2, in the presence of one enamel alteration (PRG) (Figure 1). Mild pain was associated with percussion of 1.2, and the element was vital, without any caries. Full-mouth clinical evaluation excluded the presence of generalized periodontitis. Adjacent sites did not show the presence of any pathological periodontal pocket, with probing depth less than 4 mm in all sites. Radiographic examination showed a deep intrabony defect distal to 1.2 (Figure 2).

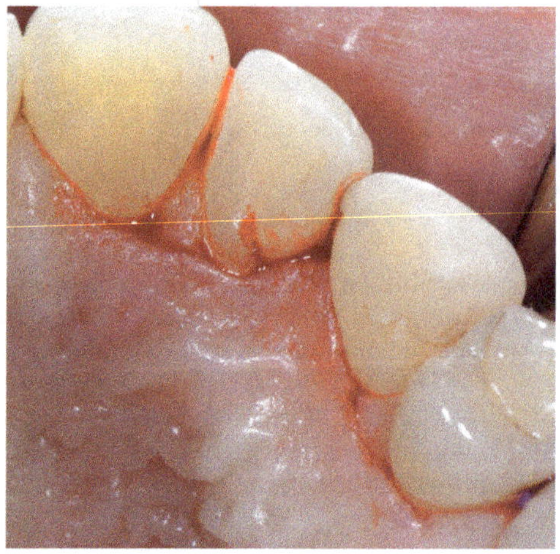

FIGURE 3: A horizontal incision on the palatal aspect was performed, preserving the interdental papilla.

Differential diagnosis reasonably excluded the presence of a vertical root fracture (VRF) since the tooth was vital and no history of trauma was reported. The treatment option was to elevate a palatal flap to allow the debridement of the pocket, to remove physically the etiologic factor (the PRG) maintaining tooth vitality, and to stimulate periodontal regeneration by using enamel matrix derivative (EMD).

After local anesthesia on the vestibular and palatal side with Articaine 4%+epinephrine 1 : 100.000, a horizontal incision was performed on the palatal aspect preserving interdental papilla between 1.1 and 1.2 and between 1.3 and 1.4 (Figure 3). The papilla between 1.2 and 1.3 was separated from the vestibular portion and reflected in order to directly visualize the PRG and the defect (Figure 4). After

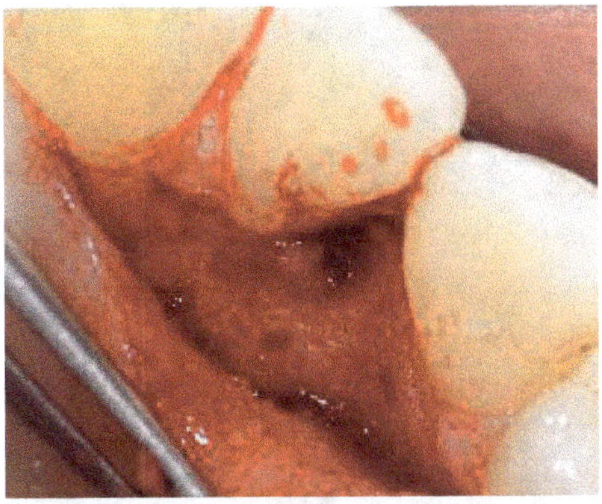

FIGURE 4: The reflection of the flap, including the papilla between 1.2 and 1.3, allowed a direct visualization of the intrabony defect and the radicular groove.

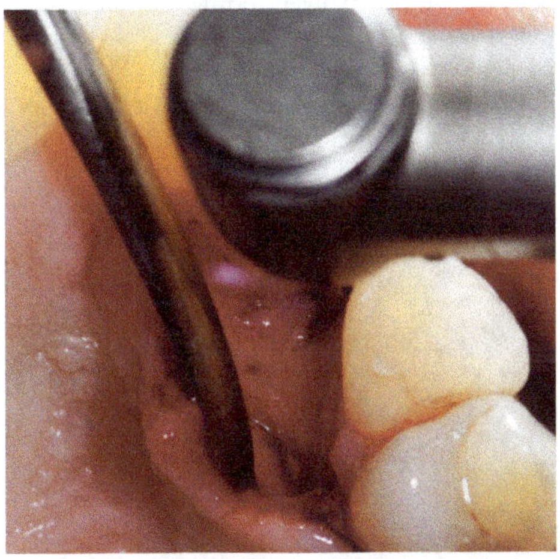

FIGURE 5: Granulation tissue was removed from the intrabony defect.

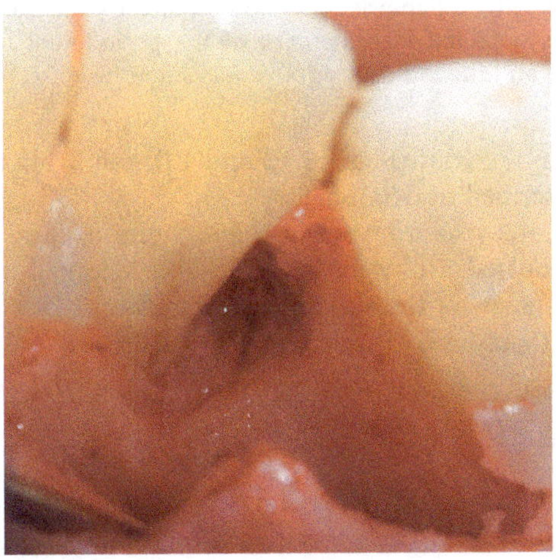

FIGURE 6: Using a diamond bur with copious irrigation of sterile saline solution, the enamel alteration was removed.

the debridement of the defect, by removing the granulation tissue, the PRG was smoothed by the use of a diamond bur under abundant irrigation of sterile saline solution (Figures 5 and 6). Following the instructions provided by

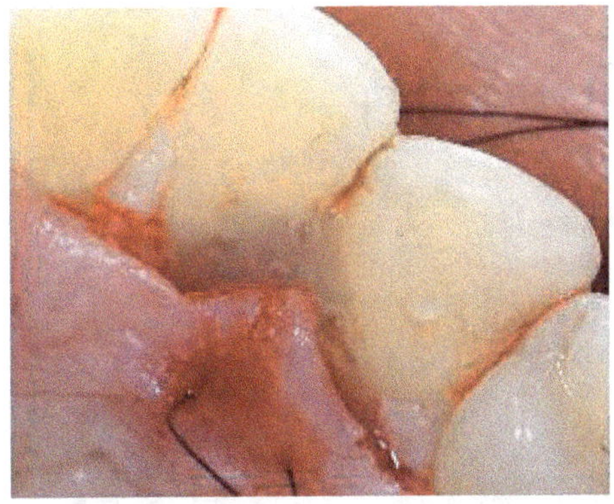

FIGURE 7: The bone substitute was placed in the osseous defect after it had been conditioned through a 24% EDTA gel and irrigated with abundant sterile saline solution.

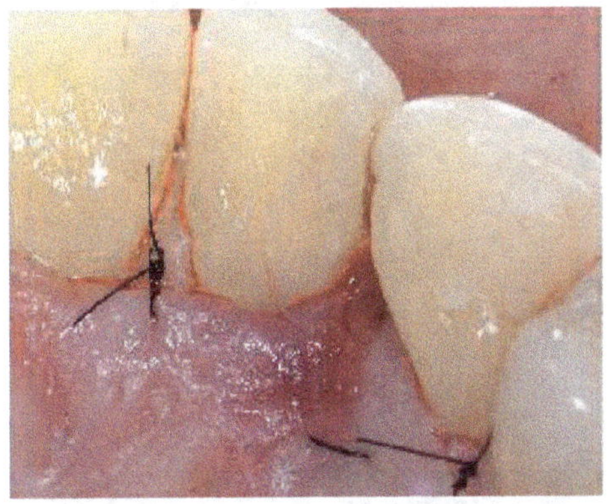

FIGURE 8: Single 5/0 and 6/0 sutures were placed.

the manufacturer, tooth surface was conditioned for two minutes with 24% EDTA gel (Straumann® PrefGel®, Straumann AG, Basel, Switzerland) and, after its removal through copious irrigation with sterile saline solution, EMD (Straumann® Emdogain®, Straumann AG, Basel, Switzerland) was placed in the defect (Figure 7). The flap was then sutured with single 5/0 and 6/0 sutures (ETHILON®, Ethicon Inc., Johnson & Johnson, Piscataway, NJ, United States) (Figure 8). The patient was advised to avoid any trauma or traction in the region of surgery and not to consume hard food during the first five days. Ibuprofen 400 mg was prescribed twice a day for three days for inflammation control and pain relief. Healing completed without any adverse event.

Clinical and radiographic examination 12 months after surgical intervention revealed a complete healing with bone regeneration in the site of the defect (Figures 9 and 10).

2.2. Case Report 2. One female patient, aged 36 at the time of the first visit, without any systemic disease (ASA-1 following the classification proposed by the American Society of Anesthesiologists) presented referring mild pain sensation while touching with the tongue the palatal-gingival margin of 1.2.

The clinical examination revealed the presence of one deep narrow isolated periodontal pocket (PD = 10 mm) in correspondence of the palatal aspect of 1.2, in the presence of bleeding on probing, no plaque accumulation, and one

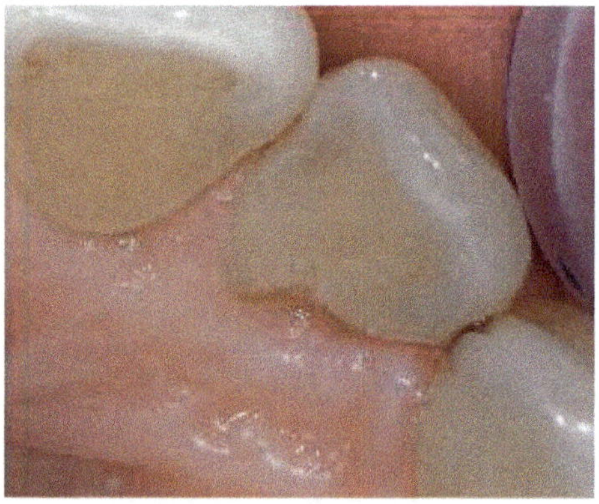

FIGURE 9: Clinical examination after 12 months.

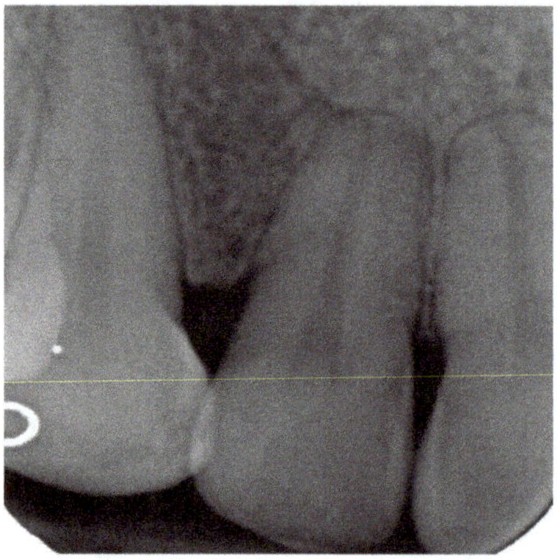

FIGURE 10: Radiographic examination after 12 months.

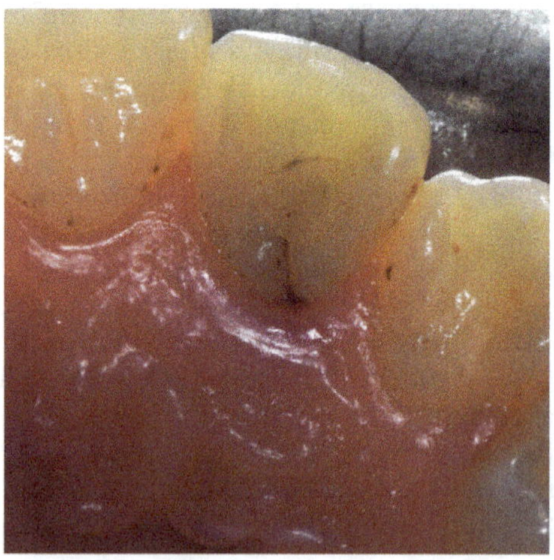

FIGURE 11: Clinical examination: a 10 mm periodontal pocket is associated with 1.2 in correspondence of a palatal groove.

PRG (Figure 11). Full-mouth clinical evaluation excluded the presence of periodontitis. Radiographic examination showed no evidence of one visible intrabony defect (Figure 12). The tooth was endodontically treated and did not show signs and symptoms of a lesion of endodontic origin.

The treatment was by a regenerative approach, using EMD, on the palatal aspect, removing mechanically the

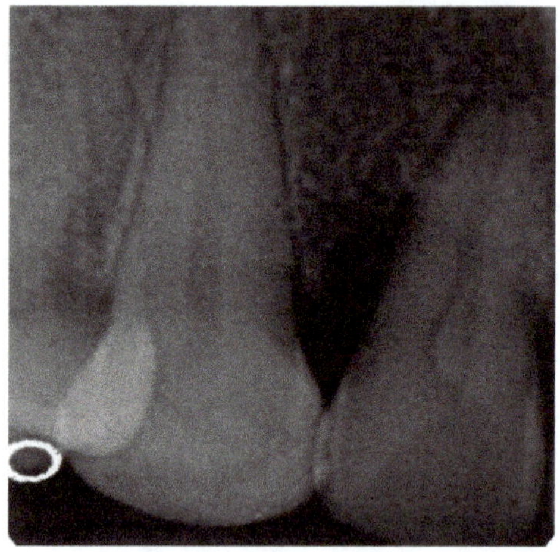

FIGURE 12: Radiographic examination: no bone resorption is visible in correspondence of the involved tooth.

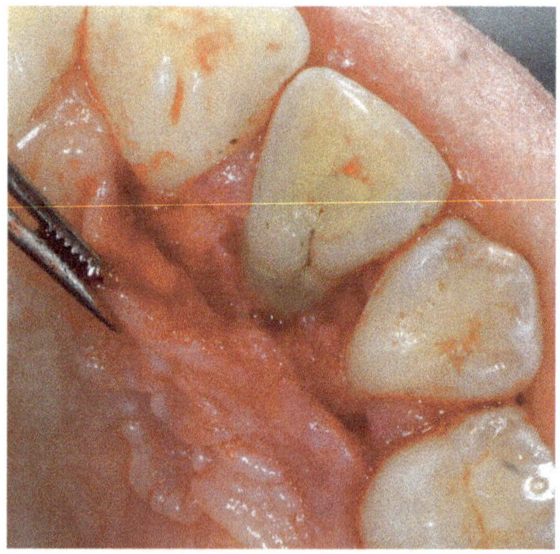

FIGURE 13: After a flap was reflected and direct visualization of the defect was obtained, debridement of the periodontal lesion was performed and the radicular groove was smoothed.

PRG from the root (Figures 13 and 14), following the technique described in detail before.

After one year from surgical intervention, clinical examination showed a physiological probing depth (less than 4 mm) in the site of the surgery and the absence of symptoms (Figures 15 and 16).

3. Discussion

The described case reports showed the clinical and radiographic success of one treatment option for PRG-related intrabony lesions. The periodontal regenerative treatment resulted in the resolution of the cases, maintaining tooth vitality when present and avoiding the recurrence of symptoms.

The presented results should be considered with caution, in particular when evaluating external validity, since they are derived on just two cases not included in one clinical trial. Even considering this important limitation, some considerations could be made on the basis of the outcomes obtained.

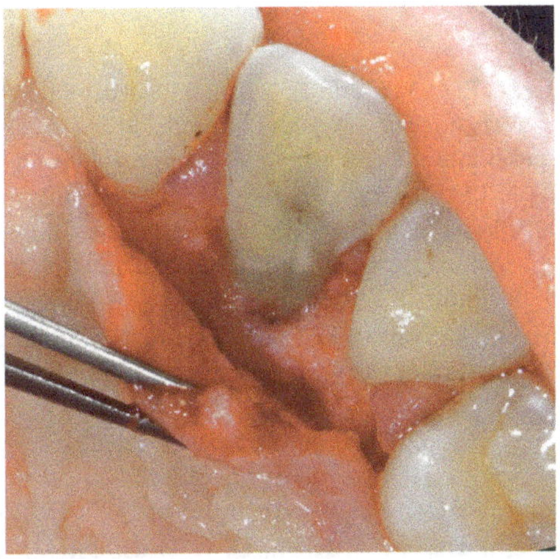

Figure 14: The radicular groove was smoothed using a diamond bur.

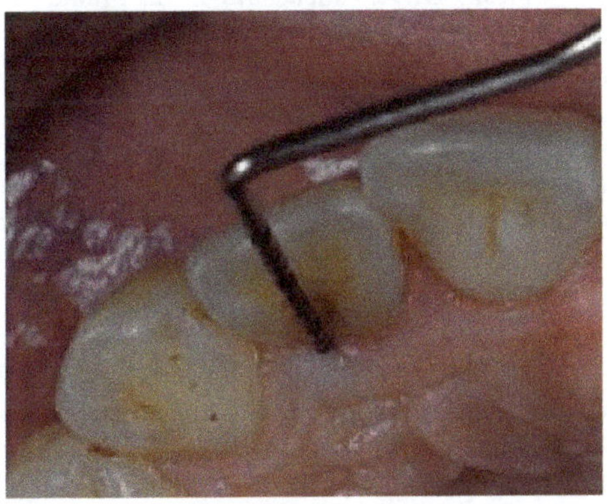

Figure 15: Clinical examination after 12 months.

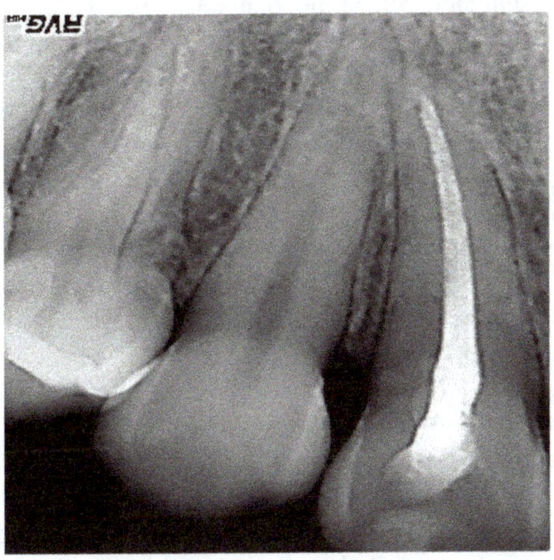

Figure 16: Radiographic examination after 12 months.

The first issue to be discussed is about the diagnostic procedure that led to the diagnosis of PRG-related intrabony defect.

Both patients referred some nonspecific symptoms that could be related to various conditions of periodontal or endodontic origin. In order to identify the etiologic factor, an accurate clinical examination was performed, revealing no caries, no restorations, and the presence of a deep and narrow periodontal pocket on the lingual aspect of the tooth.

Purely periodontal lesions could be obviously related to the presence of periodontal disease. In the presented cases, a full-mouth examination excluded the presence of periodontitis. For this reason, we considered other factors which can be related to localized periodontal lesions, with or without acute abscess. Those include endodontic periapical or lateral lesions of the involved or of an adjacent tooth which find a drainage route through the periodontal ligament and the gingival sulcus [18], vertical root fractures with or without pulpal involvement, local plaque retention factors, such as the presence of inadequate restorations [19], developmental anomalies such as gemination, fused roots, and radicular grooves [1], and other rare conditions, such as ectopic gingival sebaceous glands [20]. All these options should be considered and tested.

Even though no caries was visible, no previous restoration was present, and no dental trauma was reported by the patients, the hypothesis of a purely endodontic lesion was not excluded since it can also result, for example, from longitudinal tooth fractures such as split tooth or VRF, which cannot be easily detected [21]. Thus, tooth vitality was tested and a radiographic examination was performed; in both cases involved, the presence of a fracture was excluded.

Vertical root fractures are usually related to dental trauma and excessive occlusal forces, and they are referred to as “acute” and “chronic” or “fatigue fractures,” respectively [22]. They usually occur in restored endodontically treated teeth with or without endodontic posts, even though they can be encountered in vital and nonendodontically treated teeth [23–25]. The diagnosis of VRFs can be challenging, since signs and symptoms are not specific, including pain with lateral percussion or while chewing, gingival swelling, sinus tract, and periodontal defect. Only the presence of two deep and narrow periodontal pockets on the buccal and lingual sides of the tooth can be considered a pathognomonic sign of VRF. Its radiographical features are also heterogeneous, varying from vertical bone resorption to radiographic thickening of the periodontal ligament and to the typical “halo” effect, a combined periapical and perilateral radiolucency [22, 26]. Surgical exploration, consisting of direct visualization after lifting a full-thickness flap, can confirm VRF diagnosis. In the reported cases, no characteristic sign of VRF was found and no previous endodontic treatment or large restoration was present; on the other side, PRGs typically occur in maxillary lateral incisors [3, 4].

Once the diagnosis of a PRG is confirmed (through direct visualization in the presented cases), some authors proposed a classification of such deformity, distinguishing three types of grooves on the basis of their depth evaluated before intervention by Cone-Beam Computed Tomography (CBCT) [4]. Other classifications were proposed on the basis of groove characteristics as evaluated after tooth extraction [8].

With regard to the treatment options, a combined approach (both from the endodontic side and the periodontal side) was widely described and proposed when the bony defect caused the loss of tooth vitality [5, 9, 11, 15, 16]. Schwartz and coworkers in 2006 described a combined endoperiodontal treatment that was complicated by the complex root canal anatomy [5]. Other authors proposed the extraction, endodontic treatment, and sealing of the groove using composite resin or glass ionomer cement and subsequent replantation of the affected teeth [11, 27]. Al-Hezaimi and coworkers associated intentional extraction and replantation with EMD application to treat residual bone defect [28]. Cho and coworkers published in 2017 the description of three cases treated with a combined endoperiodontal approach with odontoplasty in order to remove/flatten, after endodontic treatment, the groove from root surface [16].

Some studies reported the results of EMD application alone for the treatment of periodontal defects associated with a PRG, in teeth with preserved pulp vitality [29, 30], even though the techniques described were different from the one adopted for the described case reports. However, the use of such biomaterial found a wide justification in previously published scientific papers on the regenerative treatment of deep and narrow periodontal defects, mainly self-contained [31].

Many reviews described the mechanisms of action of EMD in the stimulation of a number of cells (fibroblast and epithelial cells of the gingiva and of the periodontium) involved in the regenerative process, by influencing cell attachment, spreading, proliferation, and, finally, bone remodeling [32–34].

With regard to the clinical applications of EMD, since the first paper published by Heijl in 1997, the results of a number of studies confirmed the efficacy of EMD (even when used alone) in the treatment of deep intrabony defects [35, 36].

The multicentric study by Tonetti and coworkers, published in 2002, compared open flap debridement and EMD application alone in the treatment of intrabony defects [35]. The authors found that the use of EMD resulted in a mean PD reduction of 3.9 ± 1.7 mm and CAL gain of 3.1 ± 1.5 mm 12 months after surgery. These results were similar to those obtained in other studies comparing the same treatment options [36, 37]. Our case reports confirmed that EMD alone could be successfully used for the treatment of PRG-related periodontal defects, when an adequate primary closure was obtained.

In conclusion, the two case reports described a technique that resulted in clinical and radiographic resolution of PRG-related periodontal defect by a periodontal regenerative approach with the application of EMD, furthermore preventing loss of tooth vitality (Case 1). Well-designed randomized controlled clinical trials with an adequate sample size are needed in order to establish which treatment procedure would lead to better results. However, even considering the limitations of the present study, we can speculate that a timing and early diagnosis of PRG-related defect can modify importantly the prognosis of the affected teeth.

Consent

Informed consent was obtained from all individual participants included in the study.

References

[1] K. W. Lee, E. C. Lee, and K. Y. Poon, "Palato-gingival grooves in maxillary incisors. A possible predisposing factor to localised periodontal disease," *British Dental Journal*, vol. 124, no. 1, pp. 14–18, 1968.

[2] M. D. Peikoff and J. R. Trott, "An endodontic failure caused by an unusual anatomical anomaly," *Journal of Endodontia*, vol. 3, no. 9, pp. 356–359, 1977.

[3] V. S. Lara, A. Consolaro, and R. S. Bruce, "Macroscopic and microscopic analysis of the palato-gingival groove," *Journal of Endodontia*, vol. 26, no. 6, pp. 345–350, 2000.

[4] X. Tan, L. Zhang, W. Zhou et al., "Palatal radicular groove morphology of the maxillary incisors: a case series report," *Journal of Endodontia*, vol. 43, no. 5, pp. 827–833, 2017.

[5] S. A. Schwartz, M. A. Koch, D. E. Deas, and C. A. Powell, "Combined endodontic-periodontic treatment of a palatal groove: a case report," *Journal of Endodontia*, vol. 32, no. 6, pp. 573–578, 2006.

[6] J. H. S. Simon, D. H. Glick, and A. L. Frank, "Predictable endodontic and periodontic failures as a result of radicular anomalies," *Oral Surgery, Oral Medicine, and Oral Pathology*, vol. 31, no. 6, pp. 823–826, 1971.

[7] H. M. A. Ahmed and P. M. H. Dummer, "A new system for classifying tooth, root and canal anomalies," *International Endodontic Journal*, vol. 51, no. 4, pp. 389–404, 2018.

[8] Y. C. Gu, "A micro-computed tomographic analysis of maxillary lateral incisors with radicular grooves," *Journal of Endodontia*, vol. 37, no. 6, pp. 789–792, 2011.

[9] K. Attam, R. Tiwary, S. Talwar, and A. K. Lamba, "Palatogingival groove: endodontic-periodontal management—case report," *Journal of Endodontia*, vol. 36, no. 10, pp. 1717–1720, 2010.

[10] F. G. Everett and G. M. Kramer, "The disto-lingual groove in the maxillary lateral incisor; a periodontal hazard," *Journal of Periodontology*, vol. 43, no. 6, pp. 352–361, 1972.

[11] I. Garrido, F. Abella, R. Ordinola-Zapata, F. Duran-Sindreu, and M. Roig, "Combined endodontic therapy and intentional replantation for the treatment of palatogingival groove," *Journal of Endodontia*, vol. 42, no. 2, pp. 324–328, 2016.

[12] G. L. Hou and C. C. Tsai, "Relationship between palato-radicular grooves and localized periodontitis," *Journal of Clinical Periodontology*, vol. 20, no. 9, pp. 678–682, 1993.

[13] R. T. Walker, "The disto-palatal groove in maxillary incisors; a predisposing factor in periodontal disease," *Journal of the Royal Naval Medical Service*, vol. 62, no. 1, pp. 30–32, 1976.

[14] J. A. Withers, M. A. Brunsvold, W. J. Killoy, and A. J. Rahe, "The relationship of palato-gingival grooves to localized periodontal disease," *Journal of Periodontology*, vol. 52, no. 1, pp. 41–44, 1981.

[15] P. Castelo-Baz, I. Ramos-Barbosa, B. Martin-Biedma, A. B. Dablanca-Blanco, P. Varela-Patino, and J. Blanco-Carrion, "Combined endodontic-periodontal treatment of a palatogingival groove," *Journal of Endodontia*, vol. 41, no. 11, pp. 1918–1922, 2015.

[16] Y. D. Cho, J. E. Lee, Y. Chung et al., "Collaborative management of combined periodontal-endodontic lesions with a palatogingival groove: a case series," *Journal of Endodontia*, vol. 43, no. 2, pp. 332–337, 2017.

[17] World Medical Association, "World Medical Association Declaration of Helsinki: ethical principles for medical research

involving human subjects," *JAMA*, vol. 310, no. 20, pp. 2191–2194, 2013.

[18] G. W. Harrington, D. R. Steiner, and W. F. Ammons, "The periodontal-endodontic controversy," *Periodontology 2000*, vol. 30, no. 1, pp. 123–130, 2002.

[19] M. Halperin-Sternfeld, M. Saminsky, E. E. Machtei, and J. Horwitz, "The association between dental proximal restorations and periodontal disease: a retrospective 10-18 years longitudinal study," *Quintessence International*, vol. 47, no. 3, pp. 249–259, 2016.

[20] R. E. Cohen, A. Aguirre, A. J. Drinnan, M. E. Neiders, and A. J. Mastroianni, "Ectopic gingival sebaceous glands presenting as localized periodontitis," *Journal of Periodontology*, vol. 61, no. 1, pp. 58–60, 1990.

[21] L. H. Berman and S. Kuttler, "Fracture necrosis: diagnosis, prognosis assessment, and treatment recommendations," *Journal of Endodontia*, vol. 36, no. 3, pp. 442–446, 2010.

[22] I. Tsesis, E. Rosen, A. Tamse, S. Taschieri, and A. Kfir, "Diagnosis of vertical root fractures in endodontically treated teeth based on clinical and radiographic indices: a systematic review," *Journal of Endodontia*, vol. 36, no. 9, pp. 1455–1458, 2010.

[23] C. P. Chan, C. P. Lin, S. C. Tseng, and J. H. Jeng, "Vertical root fracture in endodontically versus nonendodontically treated teeth: a survey of 315 cases in Chinese patients," *Oral Surgery, Oral Medicine, Oral Pathology, Oral Radiology, and Endodontics*, vol. 87, no. 4, pp. 504–507, 1999.

[24] S. F. Yang, E. M. Rivera, and R. E. Walton, "Vertical root fracture in nonendodontically treated teeth," *Journal of Endodontia*, vol. 21, no. 6, pp. 337–339, 1995.

[25] C. J. Yeh, "Fatigue root fracture: a spontaneous root fracture in non-endodontically treated teeth," *British Dental Journal*, vol. 182, no. 7, pp. 261–266, 1997.

[26] S. Cohen, L. Blanco, and L. Berman, "Vertical root fractures: clinical and radiographic diagnosis," *The Journal of the American Dental Association*, vol. 134, no. 4, pp. 434–441, 2003.

[27] J. Forero-Lopez, L. Gamboa-Martinez, L. Pico-Porras, and J. L. Nino-Barrera, "Surgical management with intentional replantation on a tooth with palato-radicular groove," *Restorative Dentistry & Endodontics*, vol. 40, no. 2, pp. 166–171, 2015.

[28] K. Al-Hezaimi, J. Naghshbandi, J. H. S. Simon, and I. Rotstein, "Successful treatment of a radicular groove by intentional replantation and Emdogain therapy: four years follow-up," *Oral Surgery, Oral Medicine, Oral Pathology, Oral Radiology, and Endodontics*, vol. 107, no. 3, pp. e82–e85, 2009.

[29] M. P. Rethman, "Treatment of a palatal-gingival groove using enamel matrix derivative," *Compendium of Continuing Education in Dentistry*, vol. 22, no. 9, pp. 792–797, 2001.

[30] G. Zucchelli, M. Mele, and L. Checchi, "The papilla amplification flap for the treatment of a localized periodontal defect associated with a palatal groove," *Journal of Periodontology*, vol. 77, no. 10, pp. 1788–1796, 2006.

[31] R. J. Miron, M. Dard, and M. Weinreb, "Enamel matrix derivative, inflammation and soft tissue wound healing," *Journal of Periodontal Research*, vol. 50, no. 5, pp. 555–569, 2015.

[32] D. D. Bosshardt, "Biological mediators and periodontal regeneration: a review of enamel matrix proteins at the cellular and molecular levels," *Journal of Clinical Periodontology*, vol. 35, 8 Suppl, pp. 87–105, 2008.

[33] R. J. Miron, L. Wei, S. Yang, O. M. Caluseru, A. Sculean, and Y. Zhang, "Effect of enamel matrix derivative on periodontal wound healing and regeneration in an osteoporotic model," *Journal of Periodontology*, vol. 85, no. 11, pp. 1603–1611, 2014.

[34] M. Zeichner-David, "Is there more to enamel matrix proteins than biomineralization?," *Matrix Biology*, vol. 20, no. 5-6, pp. 307–316, 2001.

[35] M. S. Tonetti, N. P. Lang, P. Cortellini et al., "Enamel matrix proteins in the regenerative therapy of deep intrabony defects," *Journal of Clinical Periodontology*, vol. 29, no. 4, pp. 317–325, 2002.

[36] L. Francetti, M. Del Fabbro, M. Basso, T. Testori, and R. Weinstein, "Enamel matrix proteins in the treatment of intra-bony defects. A prospective 24-month clinical trial," *Journal of Clinical Periodontology*, vol. 31, no. 1, pp. 52–59, 2004.

[37] D. Chambrone, I. M. Pasin, L. Chambrone, C. M. Pannuti, M. C. Conde, and L. A. Lima, "Treatment of infrabony defects with or without enamel matrix proteins: a 24-month follow-up randomized pilot study," *Quintessence International*, vol. 41, no. 2, pp. 125–134, 2010.

17

Biodentine™ Partial Pulpotomy of a Young Permanent Molar with Signs and Symptoms Indicative of Irreversible Pulpitis and Periapical Lesion: A Case Report of a Five-Year Follow-Up

W. Chinadet,[1] T. Sutharaphan,[2] and P. Chompu-inwai[1]

[1]Division of Pediatric Dentistry, Department of Orthodontics and Pediatric Dentistry, School of Dentistry, Chiang Mai University, Thailand
[2]Phrae Hospital, Phrae, Thailand

Correspondence should be addressed to P. Chompu-inwai; papimonin@hotmail.com

Academic Editor: Eugenio Maiorano

The purpose of this paper was to report the five-year success of Biodentine™ partial pulpotomy in a young permanent molar, with signs and symptoms indicative of irreversible pulpitis and periapical lesion, in a nine-year-old girl. Preoperative clinical examination revealed a large carious lesion of the left mandibular permanent first molar. The patient reported pain on percussion. The tooth responded positively to the electric pulp test and had lingering pain after cold testing. A periapical radiograph showed a deep carious lesion and periapical lesion. Based on the clinical and radiographical examination, the tooth had signs and symptoms indicative of irreversible pulpitis and periapical lesion. During caries removal, pulp exposure occurred, and 2-3 mm in depth of pulp tissue at the exposure site was removed. Haemorrhage was controlled within four minutes with 2.5% sodium hypochlorite-moistened cotton pellets. Biodentine™ was then applied as both a pulp dressing and a temporary restoration. At the following visit, composite resin was placed over the Biodentine™ as a final restoration. During a five-year follow-up, the tooth was asymptomatic, had positive responses to sensibility tests, and had no discolouration. Follow-up radiographs showed a dentine bridge and periapical healing.

1. Introduction

Partial pulpotomy, one form of vital pulp therapy, has traditionally been indicated only in a cariously or traumatically exposed vital tooth with a clinical diagnosis of normal pulp or reversible pulpitis [1]. When a tooth has signs and symptoms indicative of irreversible pulpitis and periapical lesion, root canal treatment has traditionally been recommended [1]. However, root canal treatment is an expensive, complicated, and time-consuming procedure. Recently, the success of vital pulp therapy in challenging cases has been demonstrated [2].

Mineral trioxide aggregate (MTA) has been recommended as the gold standard for vital pulp therapy; however, it has some disadvantages, such as long setting time, poor handling properties, high cost, and the potential for tooth discolouration [3]. Biodentine™ (Septodont, Saint-Maur-des-Fossés, France), one of the new-generation, bioactive endodontic cements, has been claimed to have improved properties over MTA.

Biodentine™ presents high biocompatibility with human dental pulp cells [4]. The pulp tissue in contact with Biodentine™ does not show an irreversible inflammatory response [5]. Previous studies have reported that Biodentine™ has high antibacterial effects and antifungal activity [6, 7]. It has a shorter setting time than MTA, as the result of calcium chloride in the liquid component of Biodentine™ [8]. The easy manipulation of Biodentine™ is the result of hydrosoluble polymer in the liquid component, which is based on polycarboxylate, a component that induces flocculation and increases flowability at low water/cement ratios [9]. Biodentine™ has higher flexural strength [10], compressive strength [11], and modulus of elasticity than does MTA [12]. Consequently, Biodentine™ can be used simultaneously as a pulp

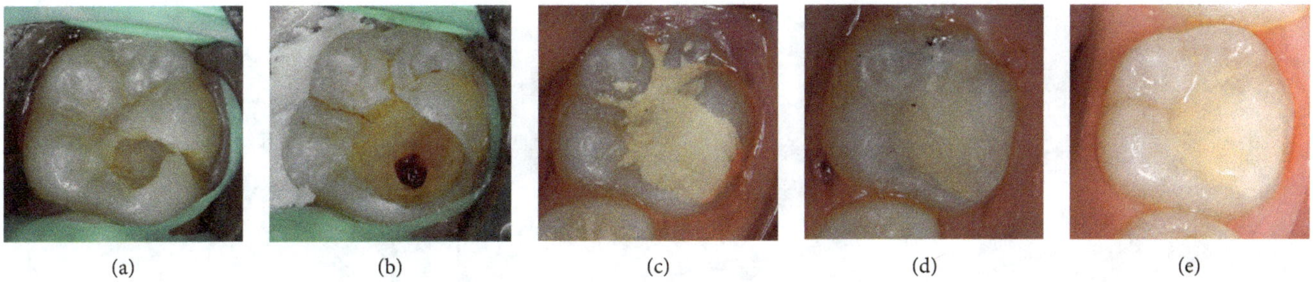

FIGURE 1: Intraoral photographs: (a) initial clinical appearance, (b) after pulp tissue removal and haemorrhage was controlled, (c) Biodentine™ was placed as a temporary filling, (d) restored with composite resin, and (e) colour stability of the tooth after a five-year follow-up.

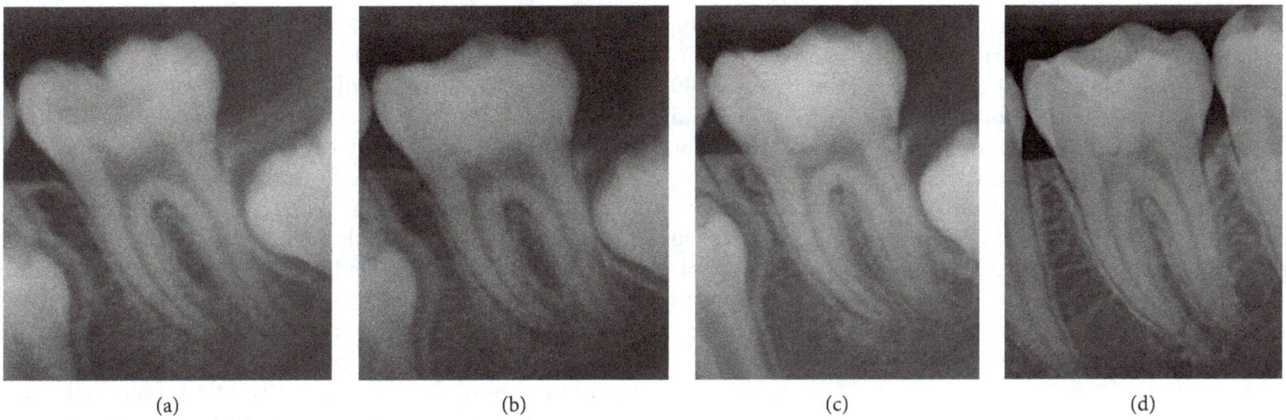

FIGURE 2: Periapical radiographs recorded (a) before treatment, (b) immediately after treatment, (c) six months postoperative, and (d) five years postoperative, showing dentine bridge and improvement of the periapical area.

dressing as well as a base material. Moreover, bismuth oxide in MTA is replaced with zirconium oxide in Biodentine™, thus resulting in better colour stability [13].

The purpose of this paper was to report the long-term success of partial pulpotomy using Biodentine™ in a young permanent molar, with signs and symptoms indicative of irreversible pulpitis and periapical lesion.

2. Case Report

A nine-year-old healthy Thai girl presented to the Pediatric Dentistry Clinic, Faculty of Dentistry, Chiang Mai University, because of pain in the lower left quadrant upon eating and upon drinking cold liquids. Clinical examination revealed a large carious lesion involving the occlusal and buccal surfaces of the left mandibular permanent first molar (Figure 1(a)). The patient reported pain on percussion. The tooth responded positively to the electric pulp test (EPT; Kerr Vitality Scanner; SybronEndo, Glendora, CA, USA) and had lingering pain for more than 10 seconds after cold testing (Green Endo-Ice®, Coltene Whaledent, Cuyahoga Falls, OH, USA). A periapical radiograph showed a deep carious lesion in close proximity to the pulp and periapical lesion, including loss of lamina dura, widened periodontal ligament space, and condensing osteitis (Figure 2(a)). Based on the clinical and radiographical examination, the tooth had signs and symptoms indicative of irreversible pulpitis and periapical lesion. The options of treatment, root canal treatment or vital pulp therapy, with their risks and benefits were explained to the patient and her legal guardian. Both preferred vital pulp therapy and signed assent and informed consent forms, respectively.

A local anaesthetic was administered, and a rubber dam was placed. During caries removal, there was a carious pulp exposure, approximately 2.5 mm in diameter. The exposed pulp appeared vital, judged by its appearance, bright red colour, and bleeding overflowing from the exposure site. Then, approximately 2-3 mm in depth of pulp tissue at the exposure site was removed with a sterilized long-shank, high-speed, round carbide bur and irrigated with 2.5% sodium hypochlorite (NaOCl). The bleeding was controlled with 2.5% NaOCl-moistened cotton pellets within four minutes (Figure 1(b)). Biodentine™ was mixed according to the manufacturer's instructions and then applied to the exposed site and surrounding dentine as a pulp dressing as well as a temporary restorative material. Biodentine™ was allowed to initially set for 12 minutes (Figure 1(c)). A periapical radiograph was recorded immediately after treatment (Figure 2(b)).

Two days later, the patient returned for a definitive restoration. The outer layer of Biodentine™ was removed leaving 2 mm of space for final restoration with resin composite. A two-step total-etch adhesive (Scotchbond™ etchant and Adper™ Single Bond; 3M ESPE, St. Paul, MN, USA) was applied, according to the manufacturer's

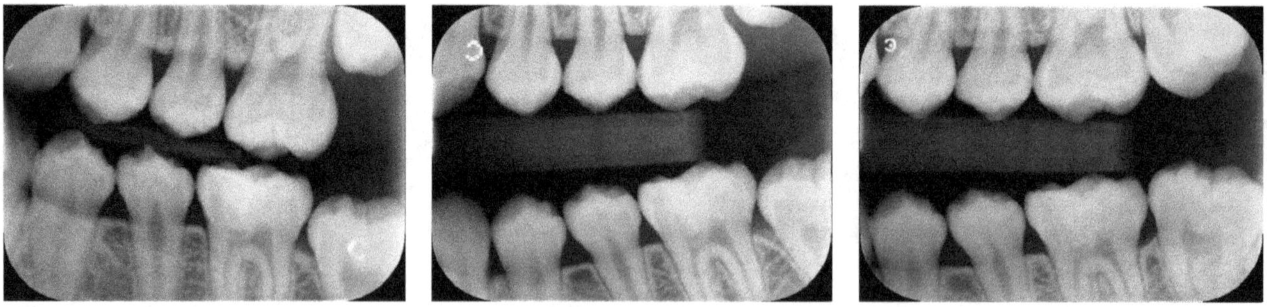
(a) (b) (c)

FIGURE 3: Bitewing radiographs recorded (a) three years postoperative, (b) four years postoperative, and (c) five years postoperative, showing dentine bridge in the left mandibular permanent first molar.

instructions, over the Biodentine™ and the surrounding dentine wall. Finally, the cavity was filled with resin composite (Filtek™ Z350 XT; 3M ESPE) and light cured for 40 seconds for each surface, followed by the finishing and polishing procedures (Figure 1(d)). The treated tooth was followed up every six months, for five years. The tooth had positive responses to EPT and cold testing. The colour stability of the tooth was noted (Figure 1(e)). The follow-up periapical radiographs showed a dentine bridge and periapical healing (Figures 2(c) and 2(d)). Bitewing radiographs at different follow-up periods showed a dentine bridge underneath the Biodentine™ layer (Figure 3).

3. Discussion

Although contrary to the traditional recommendation [1], partial pulpotomy was performed successfully in this case with signs and symptoms indicative of irreversible pulpitis and periapical lesion. Clinical diagnosis of the pulp status has traditionally been used as the main criterion for choosing treatment; however, the correlation between clinical and histological pulpal status varies from weak to high [14, 15]. Moreover, a periapical lesion in teeth with vital pulp in young patients may be the result of the process of immunological response to an irritating factor invading from the corona, diffusing through the radicular pulp tissue [16]. Information derived from preoperative clinical and radiographic examination should not be the sole criterion used to determine treatment, and direct evaluation of the pulp can also aid in the evaluation of pulp vitality.

When there is a pulp exposure, the appearance of the pulp tissue, the colour of the bleeding, and haemorrhage control at the exposure site are also clinical criteria commonly used to judge the vitality of the pulp. In this case report, the exposed pulp appeared vital, judged by its resilient texture, bright red colour, and bleeding overflowing from the exposure site. After pulp amputation, the bleeding was controlled within four minutes, indicating that the remaining pulp tissue was healthy and thus could be preserved. Some authors agree that pulpal bleeding can be used as a clinical indicator of pulpal inflammation [16, 17]; however, there is no consensus regarding the specific time required to control bleeding. On the other hand, Mutluay et al. [18] suggested that the evaluation of pulpal bleeding is subjective and may not reflect the actual pulpal status. Methods aiding in correct diagnosis of the pulp status should be further studied.

Moreover, there is still controversy regarding the type of irrigating solution and haemostatic agent most suitable for vital pulp therapy. NaOCl has been one of the most commonly used disinfectants for root canal treatment for many years; consequently, clinicians have arbitrarily adopted the use of NaOCl for vital pulp therapy [17, 19, 20]. NaOCl readily controls bleeding, while at the same time disinfects the cavity [19]. One point five per cent to 6% NaOCl appears to be the most effective and inexpensive haemostatic agent for direct pulp capping procedures [20, 21] because these concentrations do not negatively affect pulp cell recruitment, cytodifferentiation, or reparative dentin deposition when used against pulp tissue [22]. Moreover, NaOCl has been recommended as a diagnostic tool to assess inflammation of pulpal tissue; when haemorrhage is controlled within ten minutes, the prognosis can be favorable [23].

Similar to our case report, previous studies have reported successful outcomes of vital pulp therapy, using bioactive endodontic cement, in teeth diagnosed with irreversible pulpitis and periapical lesion [17, 24]. The advancement of bioactive endodontic cements may play a role in the success of challenging cases. The follow-up radiographs of the presented case show a dentine bridge underneath the Biodentine™ layer. The odontogenic effect of Biodentine™ involves the creation of a suitable environment for healing, including the release of calcium ions, production of calcium hydroxide, and formation of an apatite-like layer between the contact surface of dentine and the material [3, 4]. Moreover, Biodentine™ has been shown to stimulate the release of bioactive molecules, such as transforming growth factor-β1 (TGF-β1), nerve growth factor (NGF), and glial cell line-derived growth factor (GDNF) in dentine, contributing to the induction of tertiary dentinogenesis [25]. De Rossi et al. evaluated the pulpal and periapical responses of dogs' teeth after pulpotomy with Biodentine™ and MTA and demonstrated that Biodentine™ allows for mineralized tissue bridge formation after pulpotomy in all specimens with similar morphology and integrity to those formed with use of MTA [26].

Compared to MTA, Biodentine™ has a shorter setting time, better physical and mechanical properties, and easier handling [27]. The sealing ability of Biodentine™ has been shown to be equal to or better than that of MTA [28], thus allowing it to be used as a temporary restorative material. Moreover, as shown in this case report, Biodentine™ does not cause discolouration of the treated tooth because it contains zirconium dioxide, instead of bismuth oxide, the radiopacifier that causes tooth discolouration when MTA is used [29].

In conclusion, Biodentine™ might be a suitable biomaterial in partial pulpotomy of young permanent molars, with signs and symptoms indicative of irreversible pulpitis and periapical lesion. However, further clinical studies with longer follow-up periods and larger sample sizes are recommended.

Acknowledgments

The authors wish to thank Dr. M. Kevin O Carroll, Professor Emeritus of the School of Dentistry, University of Mississippi, and Faculty Consultant with the Faculty of Dentistry, Chiang Mai University, Thailand, for his assistance in the preparation of the manuscript.

References

[1] American Academy of Pediatric Dentistry, "Guideline on pulp therapy for primary and immature permanent teeth," *Pediatric Dentistry*, vol. 38, no. 6, pp. 280–288, 2016.

[2] S. Asgary, M. J. Eghbal, M. Fazlyab, A. A. Baghban, and J. Ghoddusi, "Five-year results of vital pulp therapy in permanent molars with irreversible pulpitis: a non-inferiority multicenter randomized clinical trial," *Clinical Oral Investigations*, vol. 19, no. 2, pp. 335–341, 2015.

[3] M. Parirokh, M. Torabinejad, and P. M. H. Dummer, "Mineral trioxide aggregate and other bioactive endodontic cements: an updated overview - part I: vital pulp therapy," *International Endodontic Journal*, vol. 51, no. 2, pp. 177–205, 2018.

[4] M. O. Daltoé, F. W. G. Paula-Silva, L. H. Faccioli, P. M. Gatón-Hernández, A. de Rossi, and L. A. Bezerra Silva, "Expression of mineralization markers during pulp response to Biodentine and mineral trioxide aggregate," *Journal of Endodontics*, vol. 42, no. 4, pp. 596–603, 2016.

[5] C. Tziafa, E. Koliniotou-Koumpia, S. Papadimitriou, and D. Tziafas, "Dentinogenic responses after direct pulp capping of miniature swine teeth with Biodentine," *Journal of Endodontics*, vol. 40, no. 12, pp. 1967–1971, 2014.

[6] V. Bhavana, K. P. Chaitanya, P. Gandi, J. Patil, B. Dola, and R. B. Redd, "Evaluation of antibacterial and antifungal activity of new calcium-based cement (Biodentine) compared to MTA and glass ionomer cement," *Journal of Conservative Dentistry*, vol. 18, no. 1, pp. 44–46, 2015.

[7] M. S. Chopra and M. N. Gulve, "Evaluation of the antibacterial and antifungal activity of three retrograde filling materials: an in vitro study," *International Journal of Contemporary Medical Research*, vol. 3, no. 8, pp. 2286–2288, 2016.

[8] E. A. Bortoluzzi, N. J. Broon, C. M. Bramante, W. T. Felippe, M. Tanomaru Filho, and R. M. Esberard, "The influence of calcium chloride on the setting time, solubility, disintegration, and pH of mineral trioxide aggregate and white Portland cement with a radiopacifier," *Journal of Endodontics*, vol. 35, no. 4, pp. 550–554, 2009.

[9] J. Camilleri, "Mineral trioxide aggregate: present and future developments," *Endodontic Topics*, vol. 32, no. 1, pp. 31–46, 2015.

[10] M. Kaur, H. Singh, J. S. Dhillon, M. Batra, and M. Saini, "MTA versus Biodentine: review of literature with a comparative analysis," *Journal of Clinical and Diagnostic Research*, vol. 11, no. 8, pp. ZG1–ZG5, 2017.

[11] M. Torabinejad, M. Parirokh, and P. M. H. Dummer, "Mineral trioxide aggregate and other bioactive endodontic cements: an updated overview-part II: other clinical applications and complications," *International Endodontic Journal*, vol. 51, no. 3, pp. 284–317, 2018.

[12] W. N. Ha, T. M. Nicholson, B. Kahler, and L. J. Walsh, "Rheological characterization as an alternative method to indentation for determining the setting time of restorative and endodontic cements," *Materials*, vol. 10, no. 12, article 1451, 2017.

[13] S. Rajasekharan, L. C. Martens, R. G. E. C. Cauwels, R. P. Anthonappa, and R. M. H. Verbeeck, "Biodentine™ material characteristics and clinical applications: a 3 year literature review and update," *European Archives of Paediatric Dentistry*, vol. 19, no. 1, pp. 1–22, 2018.

[14] A. Garfunkel, J. Sela, and M. Ulmansky, "Dental pulp pathosis. Clinicopathologic correlations based on 109 cases," *Oral Surgery, Oral Medicine, Oral Pathology*, vol. 35, no. 1, pp. 110–117, 1973.

[15] D. Ricucci, S. Loghin, and J. F. Siqueira Jr., "Correlation between clinical and histologic pulp diagnoses," *Journal of Endodontics*, vol. 40, no. 12, pp. 1932–1939, 2014.

[16] M. Tsukiboshi, D. Ricucci, and J. F. Siqueira Jr., "Mandibular premolars with immature roots and apical periodontitis lesions treated with pulpotomy: report of 3 cases," *Journal of Endodontics*, vol. 43, no. 9, pp. S65–S74, 2017.

[17] N. Parinyaprom, A. Nirunsittirat, P. Chuveera et al., "Outcomes of direct pulp capping by using either ProRoot Mineral Trioxide Aggregate or Biodentine in permanent teeth with carious pulp exposure in 6- to 18-year-old patients: a randomized controlled trial," *Journal of Endodontics*, vol. 44, no. 3, pp. 341–348, 2018.

[18] M. Mutluay, V. Arikan, S. Sari, and U. Kisa, "Does achievement of hemostasis after pulp exposure provide an accurate assessment of pulp inflammation?," *Pediatric Dentistry*, vol. 40, no. 1, pp. 37–42, 2018.

[19] G. Bogen, J. S. Kim, and L. K. Bakland, "Direct pulp capping with mineral trioxide aggregate: an observational study," *Journal of the American Dental Association*, vol. 139, no. 3, pp. 305–315, 2008.

[20] T. Matsuo, T. Nakanishi, H. Shimizu, and S. Ebisu, "A clinical study of direct pulp capping applied to carious-exposed pulps," *Journal of Endodontics*, vol. 22, no. 10, pp. 551–556, 1996.

[21] D. E. Witherspoon, "Vital pulp therapy with new materials: new directions and treatment perspectives—permanent teeth," *Journal of Endodontics*, vol. 34, no. 7, pp. S25–S28, 2008.

[22] T. Demir and Z. C. Cehreli, "Clinical and radiographic evaluation of adhesive pulp capping in primary molars following hemostasis with 1.25% sodium hypochlorite: 2-year results," *American Journal of Dentistry*, vol. 20, no. 3, pp. 182–188, 2007.

[23] G. Bogen and N. P. Chandler, "Pulp preservation in immature permanent teeth," *Endodontic Topics*, vol. 23, no. 1, pp. 131–152, 2012.

[24] S. Asgary and M. J. Eghbal, "Treatment outcomes of pulpotomy in permanent molars with irreversible pulpitis using biomaterials: a multi-center randomized controlled trial," *Acta Odontologica Scandinavica*, vol. 71, no. 1, pp. 130–136, 2013.

[25] W. L. O. da Rosa, E. Piva, and A. F. da Silva, "Disclosing the physiology of pulp tissue for vital pulp therapy," *International Endodontic Journal*, vol. 51, no. 8, pp. 829–846, 2018.

[26] A. de Rossi, L. A. B. Silva, P. Gatón-Hernández et al., "Comparison of pulpal responses to pulpotomy and pulp capping with Biodentine and mineral trioxide aggregate in dogs," *Journal of Endodontics*, vol. 40, no. 9, pp. 1362–1369, 2014.

[27] S. Rajasekharan, L. C. Martens, R. G. E. C. Cauwels, and R. M. H. Verbeeck, "Biodentine material characteristics and clinical applications: a review of the literature," *European Archives of Paediatric Dentistry*, vol. 15, no. 3, pp. 147–158, 2014.

[28] H. M. El-Khodary, D. J. Farsi, N. M. Farsi, and A. Z. Zidan, "Sealing ability of four calcium containing cements used for repairing furcal perforations in primary molars: an in vitro study," *The Journal of Contemporary Dental Practice*, vol. 16, no. 9, pp. 733–739, 2015.

[29] L. J. Marconyak Jr., T. C. Kirkpatrick, H. W. Roberts et al., "A comparison of coronal tooth discoloration elicited by various endodontic reparative materials," *Journal of Endodontics*, vol. 42, no. 3, pp. 470–473, 2016.

18

Efficacy of the Combination of rhBMP-2 with Bone Marrow Aspirate Concentrate in Mandibular Defect Reconstruction after a Pindborg Tumor Resection

Kamel Alraei,[1] **Jameel Sharqawi**,[2] **Somaya Harcher**,[3] **and Ibrahim Ghita**[4]

[1]*Department of Oral and Maxillofacial Surgery, Al-Noor Specialist Hospital, Makkah, Saudi Arabia*
[2]*Department of Oral and Maxillofacial Surgery, Royal Commission Hospital, Jubail, Saudi Arabia*
[3]*General Dentist, Saudi Arabia*
[4]*Department of Hematology, Al-Noor Specialist Hospital, Makkah, Saudi Arabia*

Correspondence should be addressed to Kamel Alraei; drkamel2@yahoo.com

Academic Editor: Daniel Torres-Lagares

Recombinant human bone morphogenetic protein-2 (rhBMP-2) is an osteoinductive growth factor used in oral and maxillofacial surgery. It offers a feasible alternative for various regenerative procedures, including reconstruction of mandibular defects. In this study, we report a case of a large Pindborg tumor involving the left mandible. The treatment consisted of surgical resection, followed by off-label use of rhBMP-2 in addition to bone marrow aspirate concentrate, together with an allograft in a titanium mesh. The patient was rehabilitated with dental implants, and a good clinical outcome was achieved. We found no evidence of bone resorption or complications in both clinical and radiographic evaluations during the one-year follow-up period. In conclusion, we have demonstrated the efficacy of using rhBMP-2 combined with bone marrow aspirate concentrate, and an allograft with a titanium mesh, for the reconstruction of long mandibular bone defects. Not only is this combination feasible, but it also has the advantages of lower morbidity and cost.

1. Introduction

The reconstruction of mandibular defects poses a significant challenge in oral and maxillofacial surgery, particularly in cases with bone continuity defects [1]. Mandibular defects can be a result of trauma, benign tumors, or malignancies [2]. For successful reconstruction of mandibular defects, the surgeon must establish mandibular continuity, in addition to restoring the height and width of the bone to allow further dental rehabilitation [3].

Autogenous bone grafts are considered the gold standard for surgical repair of most osseous defects [4, 5]; however, there are major drawbacks to this treatment modality, including donor site morbidity and the limited amount of bone that can be harvested [6, 7]. With recent breakthroughs in tissue engineering, many new graft materials and treatment modalities for the reconstruction of mandibular defects have been developed. One of the alternatives to traditional bone grafting is the use of recombinant human bone morphogenetic protein-2 (rhBMP-2), which is a potent osteoinductive growth factor that attracts mesenchymal stem cells, and stimulates them to proliferate and differentiate into osteoblasts [8, 9]. rhBMP-2 can be used alone or in combination with different types of grafts, such as allografts and autografts. Allografts are osteoconductive materials, which maintain space for bone ingrowth, whereas bone marrow aspirate concentrate (BMAC) increases the supply of stem cells and cytokines, thus increasing the osteogenic potential of the graft [10].

In this study, we sought to evaluate the results of using rhBMP-2 combined with BMAC, and an allograft with a titanium mesh, for the reconstruction of segmental bone defects.

2. Case Presentation

A 27-year-old woman presented to the clinic for evaluation of a persistent swelling on the left side of the mandible

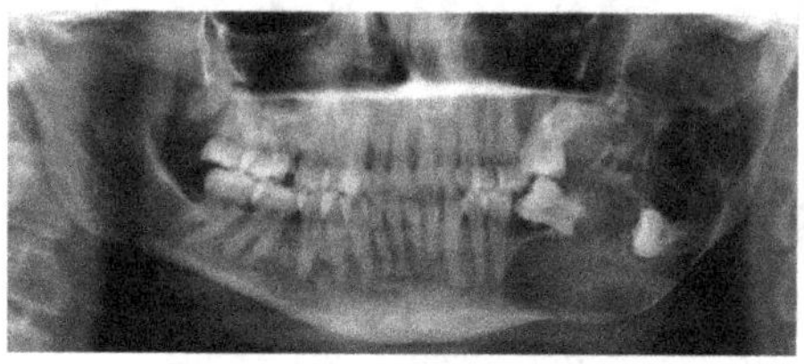
(a)

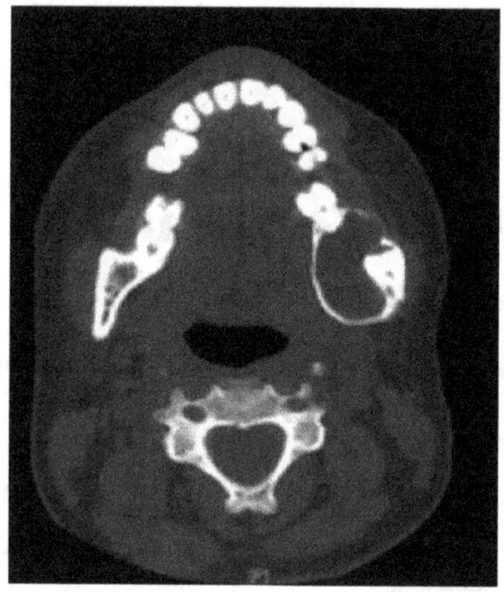
(b)

FIGURE 1: (a) Orthopantomogram showing an impacted 38 with an associated multilocular radiolucent lesion involving the left posterior mandible, which extends from the second premolar to the left condyle. (b) Axial view of a computed tomographic image of the facial bone showing a hypodense lesion in the left posterior mandible, with expansion and thinning of both the buccal and lingual cortices.

causing facial asymmetry. Radiographic imaging showed a multilocular, radiolucent lesion involving the left posterior mandible, extending into the left condyle (Figure 1). We performed a biopsy which revealed a calcifying, cystic, odontogenic tumor (a Pindborg tumor). As this tumor is aggressive, we decided to proceed with a transcutaneous segmental resection under general anesthesia, followed by immediate reconstruction using a 2.7 mm reconstruction plate (Figure 2). The patient's postoperative course was uneventful. After nine months, the patient returned for the reconstruction of the mandibular defect using rhBMP-2 combined with BMAC, and an allograft with a titanium mesh.

Under general anesthesia, we cannulated the patient's posterior left iliac crest; 60 cc of bone marrow was then aspirated and concentrated using density gradient centrifugation. We placed the patient into maxillomandibular fixation and made a transcutaneous submandibular incision at the scar site of the previous incision. After proper dissection, we exposed the entire defect, together with the reconstruction plate, and recontoured the adjacent bony margins. The titanium mesh was then adapted to reconstruct the mandibular contour, while acting as a protective matrix to contain the graft material. We then secured the mesh in place with a wire. We placed a total of 12 mg of rhBMP-2 (Infuse® Bone Graft from Medtronic Sofamor Danek, Inc.; Tennessee, USA) in four absorbable collagen sponges (1.5 mg/ml). Two sponges were placed inside the mesh, and the two other sponges were cut into small pieces and mixed with 16 mm of allogenic cancellous bone (LifeNet Health; Virginia, USA) in combination with BMAC. The graft material was then packed into the osseous defect. An additional allogenic block (measuring 3×1.5 cm) soaked in BMAC was placed in the posterior aspect of the defect, to allow greater dimensional stability (Figure 3). A "watertight" seal closure was performed. The postoperative course was uneventful.

The patient showed radiographic evidence of bone formation three months after the operation; mandibular continuity was regained, as demonstrated both radiographically and clinically (Figure 4(a)). After six months of follow-up, the reconstruction plate was removed as it would have blocked the subsequent placement of implants (Figure 4(b)). Three dental implants were placed under local anesthesia (Figure 4(c)), and prosthetic rehabilitation with implant-supported partial dentures was initiated three months later (Figure 4(d)). After four years of follow-up, a good implant stability and cosmetic outcome was achieved.

3. Discussion

Successful reconstruction of mandibular continuity defects requires the restoration of both vertical and horizontal dimensions of the bone for further functional rehabilitation and implant placement; this step is essential for the creation of an appropriate facial form [11]. In the case of the patient presented herein, we were able to meet these objectives while minimizing morbidity.

Autogenous bone grafts are still considered the gold standard for the reconstruction of osseous defects since they incorporate all the properties necessary for bone regeneration, i.e. osteogenesis, osteoinduction, and osteoconduction. Furthermore, they are histocompatible, meaning that they do not trigger a specific immune response and are not associated with the risk of infection transmission [12, 13]. The most common donor site for obtaining autogenous bone grafts is the iliac crest; the main advantage of this site is the availability of sufficient quantities of bone with the desired quality [12, 14, 15]. Despite all the benefits, the use of autogenous bone grafts is still associated with a high morbidity and a number of potential complications (namely increased overall time of the surgical procedure, risk of hematoma, pelvic instability, sensory disturbances, poor cosmetic appearance,

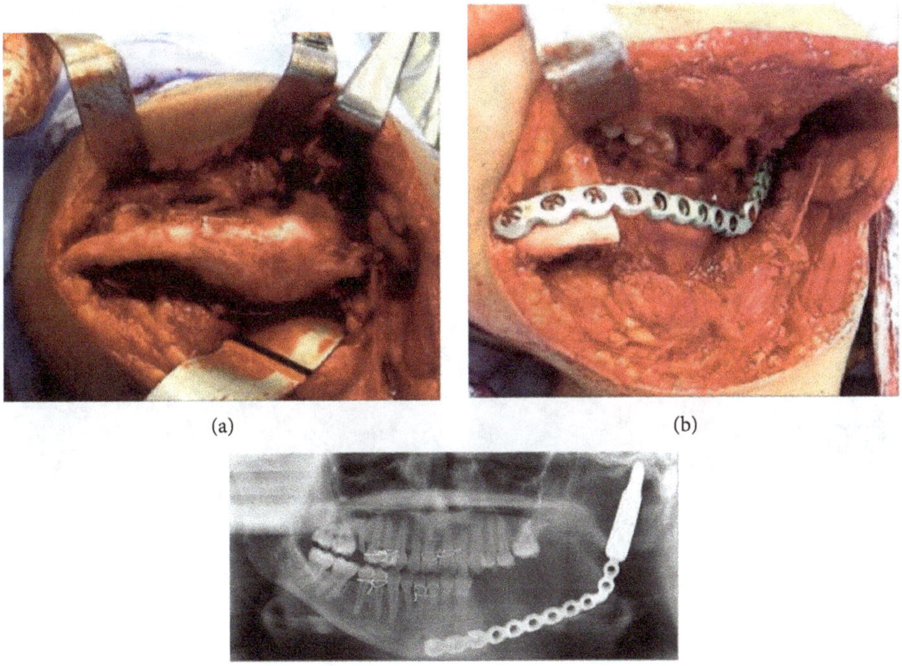

(a) (b) (c)

FIGURE 2: (a) Photograph showing the tumor and the expansion of both the buccal and lingual cortices. (b) Segmental resection of the left mandible stabilized with a 2.7 mm reconstruction plate. (c) Postoperative orthopantomogram.

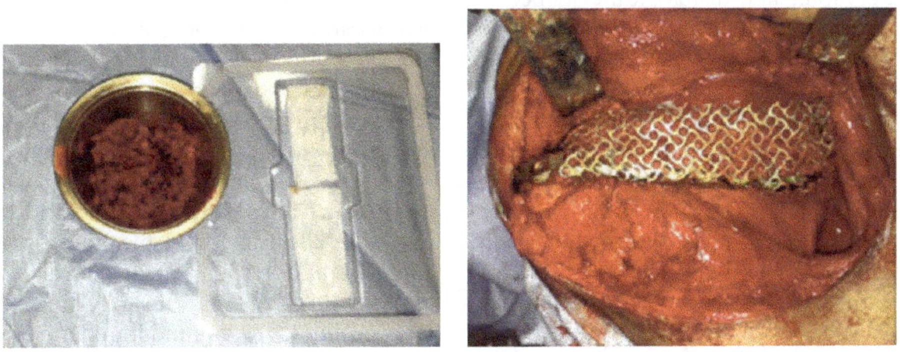

(a) (b)

FIGURE 3: (a) Absorbable collagen sponges (ACS) impregnated with recombinant human bone morphogenetic protein-2 (rhBMP-2) (right side) and allogenic chips soaked in bone marrow aspirate concentrate (BMAC) with small cut pieces of ACS with rhBMP-2 (left side). (b) Photograph showing the entire defect filled with rhBMP-2 combined with demineralized bone allograft and BMAC.

gait disturbance, infections, herniation of abdominal content, and acute or chronic pain). However, the surgical technique also has an important role in determining postoperative complications [16–18]. The use of autogenous bone grafts in mandibular defects provides a reasonable long-term survival and high success rate (up to 70%); however, the chances of a successful outcome are lower if the defect is longer than 6 cm [19, 20].

Allografts are mainly space-occupying, osteoconductive structures with minimal osteoinductive capability, as they are designed to have minimal antigenicity and risk of infection transmission [21, 22]. Several studies have compared different types of allograft materials in procedures such as ridge augmentation, sinus lift, and bone reconstruction in the maxillofacial region. These studies have concluded that allografts provide an acceptable material for grafting, with the main advantage being the saving of surgical time as no additional bone harvest site is required, as in autogenous bone grafts [23–27].

Members of the transforming growth factor beta superfamily have superior osteoinductive capabilities, with rhBMP-2 and rhBMP-7 being the most extensively studied for the treatment of bone defects. Studies have shown that rhBMP-2 can stimulate osteoblastic differentiation of mesenchymal stem cells, resulting in newly formed bone that has the same composition as that of natural bone [28, 29]. Therefore, rhBMP-2 is one of the most promising growth factors for the regeneration of osseous defects. In addition, it also overcomes most of the problems associated with both autogenous and allogenous bone grafts.

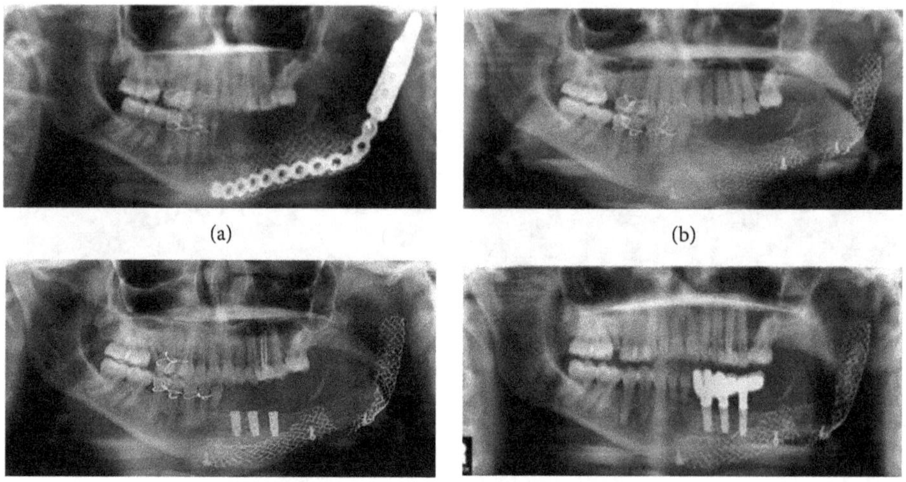

(a) (b) (c) (d)

Figure 4: (a) Orthopantomogram (OPG) at the three-month follow-up. (b) OPG after removing the reconstruction plate. Bone regeneration can be observed on the left mandible. (c) OPG showing implant rehabilitation. (d) OPG showing prosthetic rehabilitation with dental implants and an implant-supported partial denture.

Moghadam et al. reported in 2001 the first application of rhBMP-2 in a human mandibular reconstruction. In this study, the authors demonstrated successful bone formation in a 6 cm long mandibular discontinuity defect after segmental resection, with radiographic and histological evidence of new bone formation [30]. Since then, several reports have mentioned the off-label use of rhBMP-2 in mandibular reconstruction [31–34]. For instance, Sheikh et al. reported in 2015 that a predictable reconstruction of continuity bone defects larger than 6 cm could be achieved with the use of rhBMP-2 (12 mg) and BMAC (10 ml), as an alternative to autogenous bone grafting [35].

Studies in animals and humans have shown that when rhBMP-2 is combined with absorbable collagen sponges, it can induce new bone formation even in defects of critical size [34, 36]. Absorbable collagen sponges are ideal carriers for rhBMP-2, as they strongly bind it and provide a continuous release of the protein into the surrounding milieu over a period of three weeks. Nevertheless, absorbable collagen sponges lack structural stability and have a limited ability to prevent soft tissue compression at the surgical site; this further negatively affects vascular growth in bone [35, 37].

Degidi et al. reported in 2003 that titanium mesh has the necessary stiffness for maintaining the space required for bone regeneration, especially in large mandibular or maxillary defects. Furthermore, it can be adapted and contoured into the desired form [38]. Carter et al. have reported in 2008 that one of the possible factors contributing to graft failure in cases of mandibular defect reconstruction was the lack of a space maintainer [39]. An additional benefit of titanium mesh is that it retains the graft material in position with more stability; this was especially useful, as our patient had previously undergone marginal resection [40]. The titanium mesh was easy to handle, molded around the reconstruction plate, and produced successful outcomes with neither wound dehiscence nor infections.

The rationale behind the use of BMAC is that it contains a considerable number of mesenchymal stem cells, which can differentiate into osteoprogenitor cells [41]. Bone marrow aspirate can be easily harvested by aspirating the iliac bone; the procedure is cost-effective and has low morbidity [42]. The aspirate is then concentrated by centrifugation to increase the ratio of mesenchymal stem cells to growth factors [43].

When bone marrow aspirate is combined with graft material, bone regeneration is enhanced; in some cases, it has been shown to be comparable to the results obtained from using an autograft alone. For instance, Taghavi et al. have shown in 2010 that a combination of bone marrow aspirate with allograft is a viable alternative to autogenous bone grafts [44]. Moreover, Hernigou et al. in 2014 studied approximately 1000 patients who were treated with bone grafts for delayed-union or nonunion fractures, and found that the number of adverse events was significantly lower for the bone marrow aspirate group when compared to the autograft group [45]. Furthermore, Carter et al. reported in 2008 that when rhBMP-2 was combined with bone marrow cells, two out of three cases showed successful regeneration of the mandibular defect, while one case failed to form bone due to chronic infection and lack of space maintenance by the graft [39].

The case described in this study shows that it is possible to perform mandibular reconstruction using rhBMP-2 in combination with BMAC mixed with an allograft; it is logical to combine them all with a titanium mesh to bring about bone neoformation. Even if the use of this combination seems to result in a predictable outcome, further studies are needed to determine the ideal combination of grafting materials that would result in maximal clinical and cost-effectiveness.

Consent

We discussed our treatment plan with the patient, including risks and potential complications. We obtained written informed consent from the patient.

Authors' Contributions

Kamel Alraei conceptualized the study and collected the data. Kamel Alraei and Somaya Harcher contributed to data analysis and the writing of the manuscript. Jameel Shrqawi and Ibrahim Ghita contributed to the drafting and review of the manuscript.

References

[1] C. M. Misch, O. T. Jensen, M. A. Pikos, and J. P. Malmquist, "Vertical bone augmentation using recombinant bone morphogenetic protein, mineralized bone allograft, and titanium mesh: a retrospective cone beam computed tomography study," *The International Journal of Oral & Maxillofacial Implants*, vol. 30, no. 1, pp. 202–207, 2015.

[2] A. S. Herford, "rhBMP-2 as an option for reconstructing mandibular continuity defects," *Journal of Oral and Maxillofacial Surgery*, vol. 67, no. 12, pp. 2679–2684, 2009.

[3] J. M. Lane, A. W. Yasko, E. Tomin et al., "Bone marrow and recombinant human bone morphogenetic protein-2 in osseous repair," *Clinical Orthopaedics and Related Research*, vol. 361, pp. 216–227, 1999.

[4] O. T. Jensen, L. B. Shulman, M. S. Block, and V. J. Iacono, "Report of the sinus consensus conference of 1996," *The International Journal of Oral & Maxillofacial Implants*, vol. 13, Supplement, pp. 11–45, 1998.

[5] R. E. Marx, "Clinical application of bone biology to mandibular and maxillary reconstruction," *Clinics in Plastic Surgery*, vol. 21, no. 3, pp. 377–392, 1994.

[6] Z. H. Baqain, M. Anabtawi, A. A. Karaky, and Z. Malkawi, "Morbidity from anterior iliac crest bone harvesting for secondary alveolar bone grafting: an outcome assessment study," *Journal of Oral and Maxillofacial Surgery*, vol. 67, no. 3, pp. 570–575, 2009.

[7] A. Joshi and G. C. Kostakis, "An investigation of post-operative morbidity following iliac crest graft harvesting," *British Dental Journal*, vol. 196, no. 3, pp. 167–171, 2004.

[8] S. D. Cook, S. L. Salkeld, M. R. Brinker, M. W. Wolfe, and D. C. Rueger, "Use of an osteoinductive biomaterial (rhOP-1) in healing large segmental bone defects," *Journal of Orthopaedic Trauma*, vol. 12, no. 6, pp. 407–412, 1998.

[9] M. F. Sciadini and K. D. Johnson, "Evaluation of recombinant human bone morphogenetic protein-2 as a bone-graft substitute in a canine segmental defect model," *Journal of Orthopaedic Research*, vol. 18, no. 2, pp. 289–302, 2000.

[10] H. Dym and J. Pierse, "Advanced techniques in bone grafting procedures," *Dental Clinics of North America*, vol. 55, no. 3, pp. 453–460, 2011.

[11] C. M. Clokie and G. K. Sándor, "Reconstruction of 10 major mandibular defects using bioimplants containing BMP-7," *Journal of the Canadian Dental Association*, vol. 74, no. 1, pp. 67–72, 2008.

[12] T. W. Bauer and G. F. Muschler, "Bone graft materials: an overview of the basic science," *Clinical Orthopaedics and Related Research*, vol. 371, pp. 10–27, 2000.

[13] V. M. Goldberg and S. Akhavan, "Biology of bone grafts," in *Bone Regeneration and Repair*, J. R. Lieberman and G. E. Friedlaender, Eds., Springer, 2005.

[14] G. Schmidmaier, S. Herrmann, J. Green et al., "Quantitative assessment of growth factors in reaming aspirate, iliac crest, and platelet preparation," *Bone*, vol. 39, no. 5, pp. 1156–1163, 2006.

[15] M. E. Elsalanty and D. G. Genecov, "Bone grafts in craniofacial surgery," *Craniomaxillofacial Trauma & Reconstruction*, vol. 2, no. 3-4, pp. 125–134, 2009.

[16] E. D. Arrington, W. J. Smith, H. G. Chambers, A. L. Bucknell, and N. A. Davino, "Complications of iliac crest bone graft harvesting," *Clinical Orthopaedics and Related Research*, vol. 329, pp. 300–309, 1996.

[17] D. W. Boone, "Complications of iliac crest graft and bone grafting alternatives in foot and ankle surgery," *Foot and Ankle Clinics*, vol. 8, no. 1, pp. 1–14, 2003.

[18] A. Barone, M. Ricci, F. Mangano, and U. Covani, "Morbidity associated with iliac crest harvesting in the treatment of maxillary and mandibular atrophies: a 10-year analysis," *Journal of Oral and Maxillofacial Surgery*, vol. 69, no. 9, pp. 2298–2304, 2011.

[19] R. D. Foster, J. P. Anthony, A. Sharma, and M. A. Pogrel, "Vascularized bone flaps versus nonvascularized bone grafts for mandibular reconstruction: an outcome analysis of primary bony union and endosseous implant success," *Head & Neck*, vol. 21, no. 1, pp. 66–71, 1999.

[20] M. A. Pogrel, S. Podlesh, J. P. Anthony, and J. Alexander, "A comparison of vascularized and nonvascularized bone grafts for reconstruction of mandibular continuity defects," *Journal of Oral and Maxillofacial Surgery*, vol. 55, no. 11, pp. 1200–1206, 1997.

[21] J. M. Wozney, "Bone morphogenetic proteins and their gene expression," in *Cellular and Molecular Biology of Bone*, M. Noda, Ed., Elsevier, 1993.

[22] T. Boyce, J. Edwards, and N. Scarborough, "Allograft bone: the influence of processing on safety and performance," *Orthopedic Clinics of North America*, vol. 30, no. 4, pp. 571–581, 1999.

[23] J. D. Kassolis, P. S. Rosen, and M. A. Reynolds, "Alveolar ridge and sinus augmentation utilizing platelet-rich plasma in combination with freeze-dried bone allograft: case series," *Journal of Periodontology*, vol. 71, no. 10, pp. 1654–1661, 2000.

[24] S. S. Noumbissi, J. L. Lozada, P. J. Boyne et al., "Clinical, histologic, and histomorphometric evaluation of mineralized solvent-dehydrated bone allograft (Puros) in human maxillary sinus grafts," *Journal of Oral Implantology*, vol. 31, no. 4, pp. 171–179, 2005.

[25] J. A. Leonetti and R. Koup, "Localized maxillary ridge augmentation with a block allograft for dental implant placement: case reports," *Implant Dentistry*, vol. 12, no. 3, pp. 217–226, 2003.

[26] J. P. A. van den Bergh, C. M. ten Bruggenkate, G. Krekeler, and D. B. Tuinzing, "Maxillary sinusfloor elevation and grafting with human demineralized freeze dried bone," *Clinical Oral Implants Research*, vol. 11, no. 5, pp. 487–493, 2000.

[27] R. D. Roden Jr., "Principles of bone grafting," *Oral and Maxillofacial Surgery Clinics of North America*, vol. 22, no. 3, pp. 295–300, 2010.

[28] T. A. Einhorn and L. C. Gerstenfeld, "Fracture healing: mechanisms and interventions," *Nature Reviews Rheumatology*, vol. 11, no. 1, pp. 45–54, 2015.

[29] A. Valentin-Opran, J. Wozney, C. Csimma, L. Lilly, and G. E. Riedel, "Clinical evaluation of recombinant human bone

morphogenetic protein-2," *Clinical Orthopaedics and Related Research*, vol. 395, pp. 110–120, 2002.

[30] H. G. Moghadam, M. R. Urist, G. K. B. Sandor, and C. M. L. Clokie, "Successful mandibular reconstruction using a BMP bioimplant," *Journal of Craniofacial Surgery*, vol. 12, no. 2, pp. 119–127, 2001.

[31] R. M. Lustosa, L. C. Iwaki, S. Tolentino Ede, M. Chicarelli da Silva, R. de Oliveira Lazarin, and L. Iwaki Filho, "Mandible reconstruction using rhBMP-2: case report and literature review," *Quintessence International*, vol. 45, no. 10, pp. 869–874, 2014.

[32] M. R. Oliveira, L. F. . O. Gorla, M. A. C. Gabrielli, and V. A. Pereira-Filho, "Off-label use of bone morphogenetic protein 2 in the reconstructions of mandibular continuity defects," *Journal of Craniofacial Surgery*, vol. 28, no. 1, pp. 227–230, 2017.

[33] S. C. Desai, A. Sclaroff, and B. Nussenbaum, "Use of recombinant human bone morphogenetic protein 2 for mandible reconstruction," *JAMA Facial Plastic Surgery*, vol. 15, no. 3, pp. 204–209, 2013.

[34] A. S. Herford and M. Cicciù, "Recombinant human bone morphogenetic protein type 2 jaw reconstruction in patients affected by giant cell tumor," *Journal of Craniofacial Surgery*, vol. 21, no. 6, pp. 1970–1975, 2010.

[35] Z. Sheikh, M. Javaid, N. Hamdan, and R. Hashmi, "Bone regeneration using bone morphogenetic proteins and various biomaterial carriers," *Materials*, vol. 8, no. 4, pp. 1778–1816, 2015.

[36] P. J. Boyne, "Animal studies of application of rhBMP-2 in maxillofacial reconstruction," *Bone*, vol. 19, no. 1, Supplement 1, pp. S83–S92, 1996.

[37] P. J. Boyne, L. C. Lilly, R. E. Marx et al., "De novo bone induction by recombinant human bone morphogenetic protein-2 (rhBMP-2) in maxillary sinus floor augmentation," *Journal of Oral and Maxillofacial Surgery*, vol. 63, no. 12, pp. 1693–1707, 2005.

[38] M. Degidi, A. Scarano, and A. Piattelli, "Regeneration of the alveolar crest using titanium micromesh with autologous bone and a resorbable membrane," *Journal of Oral Implantology*, vol. 29, no. 2, pp. 86–90, 2003.

[39] T. G. Carter, P. S. Brar, A. Tolas, and O. R. Beirne, "Off-label use of recombinant human bone morphogenetic protein-2 (rhBMP-2) for reconstruction of mandibular bone defects in humans," *Journal of Oral and Maxillofacial Surgery*, vol. 66, no. 7, pp. 1417–1425, 2008.

[40] R. M. Lustosa, D. . V. Macedo, L. C. V. Iwaki et al., "Continuity resection of the mandible after ameloblastoma - feasibility of oral rehabilitation with rhBMP-2 associated to bovine xenograft followed by implant installation," *Journal of Cranio-maxillofacial Surgery*, vol. 43, no. 8, pp. 1553–1560, 2015.

[41] J. E. Block, "The role and effectiveness of bone marrow in osseous regeneration," *Medical Hypotheses*, vol. 65, no. 4, pp. 740–747, 2005.

[42] A. L. Gianakos, L. Sun, J. N. Patel, D. M. Adams, and F. A. Liporace, "Clinical application of concentrated bone marrow aspirate in orthopaedics: a systematic review," *World Journal of Orthopedics*, vol. 8, no. 6, pp. 491–506, 2017.

[43] D. R. Martin, N. R. Cox, T. L. Hathcock, G. P. Niemeyer, and H. J. Baker, "Isolation and characterization of multipotential mesenchymal stem cells from feline bone marrow," *Experimental Hematology*, vol. 30, no. 8, pp. 879–886, 2002.

[44] C. E. Taghavi, K. B. Lee, G. Keorochana, S. T. Tzeng, J. H. Yoo, and J. C. Wang, "Bone morphogenetic protein-2 and bone marrow aspirate with allograft as alternatives to autograft in instrumented revision posterolateral lumbar spinal fusion: a minimum two-year follow-up study," *Spine*, vol. 35, no. 11, pp. 1144–1150, 2010.

[45] P. Hernigou, A. Desroches, S. Queinnec et al., "Morbidity of graft harvesting versus bone marrow aspiration in cell regenerative therapy," *International Orthopaedics*, vol. 38, no. 9, pp. 1855–1860, 2014.

19

The Device of Ethylene Vinyl Acetate Sheet for Trismus Caused by Bilateral Mandible Fractures

Yoshiaki Ihara, Yuka Nakamichi, Yuichi Tashimo, Shinji Nozue, Kota Hayashi, Mitsunori Ishiguro, and Koji Takahashi

Division of Oral Rehabilitation Medicine, Department of Special Needs Dentistry, School of Dentistry, Showa University, Tokyo, Japan

Correspondence should be addressed to Yoshiaki Ihara; ikkun@dent.showa-u.ac.jp

Academic Editor: Sreekanth Kumar Mallineni

Trismus is commonly caused by temporomandibular joint disorders and maxillofacial fractures. We report the case of a 62-year-old woman with trismus and difficulty in mastication caused by bilateral mandibular fractures. She had a maximal interincisal opening distance (MID) of 22 mm. Mouth-opening training was administered using a novel dental mouth-training device custom-made using ethylene vinyl acetate sheets and according to the dentition and extent of mouth-opening of the patient. After 2 months of training, the MID increased to 42 mm. With adequate training, this device is effective in treating trismus due to scarring.

1. Introduction

Trismus or restricted mouth-opening is commonly caused by temporomandibular joint (TMJ) disorders, fractures in the maxillofacial region, and treatment of head and neck cancers. The maximal interincisal opening distance (MID), the distance between the upper and lower incisors at maximum opening, is usually measured to assess mouth-opening. Trismus has been previously diagnosed with MID values of 30 mm [1, 2], 35 mm [3, 4], and 40 mm [5, 6]. Traumatic facial fractures often result in malocclusion after treatment due to impaired opening or deviation of the occlusal position. Although manual methods and off-the-shelf mouth-training devices have been used in the past for the treatment of trismus, it is often difficult to achieve sustained therapeutic effects or ensure that the patient can train themselves at home. It was reported that approximately one in four patients does not adhere to the prescribed exercise therapy [7]. We fabricated a novel device for mouth-opening exercises using a dental thermoplastic sheet, which can be fitted according to the individual's dentition and mouth-opening. Herein, we report the application of this device in a patient with trismus following bilateral mandible fractures, which resulted in good therapeutic outcomes.

2. Case Report

A 62-year-old woman complained of trismus and difficulty in mastication following bilateral mandibular fractures. Six months prior, she had lost consciousness in a bus and hit her head when she fell, which resulted in fractures of the jawbone and anterior part of the maxilla, among other injuries. Subsequently, she was immobilized for 3 months. She was referred to our department because of persistent pain and no improvement in mouth-opening despite rehabilitation with a wooden device. She complained of pain in the molar during mouth-opening exercise, which reflected poor adherence to mouth-opening training. She lost her maxillary incisors and used a partial denture. Thus, we measured her MID between incisors of a partial denture and lower incisors. The MID was 22 mm, and she experienced pain on attempting to open the mouth further (Figure 1). Radiography and CT images revealed displacement of the left and right temporomandibular articular heads due to fracture

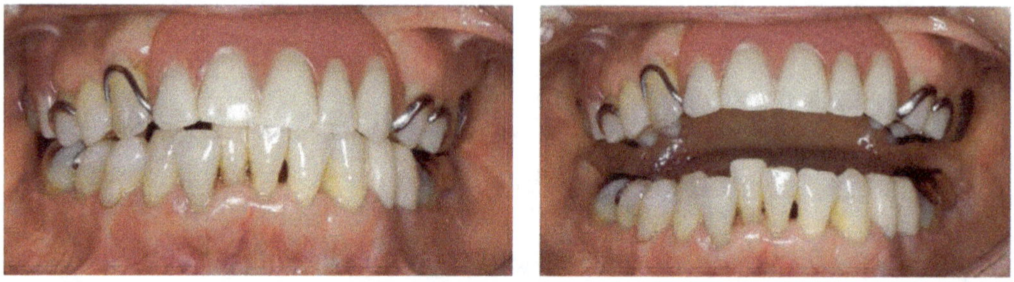

(a) (b)

FIGURE 1: Preoperative views: (a) front view and (b) maximum mandibular opening at preoperation.

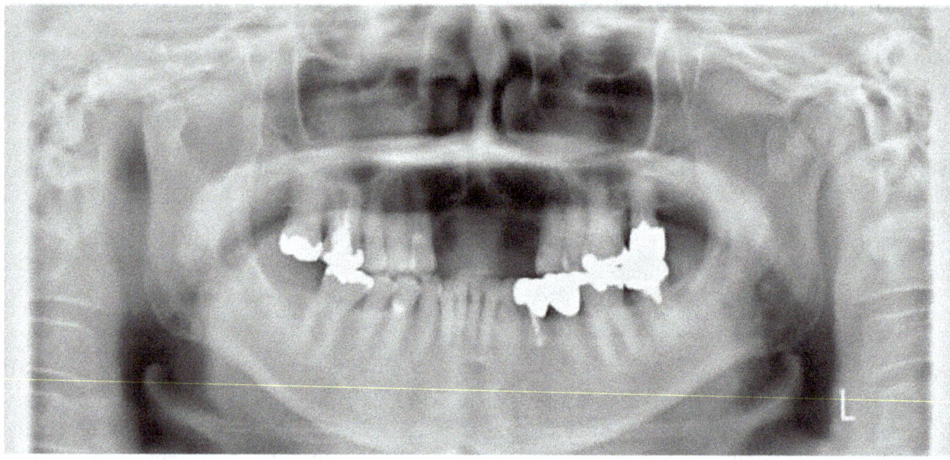

(a)

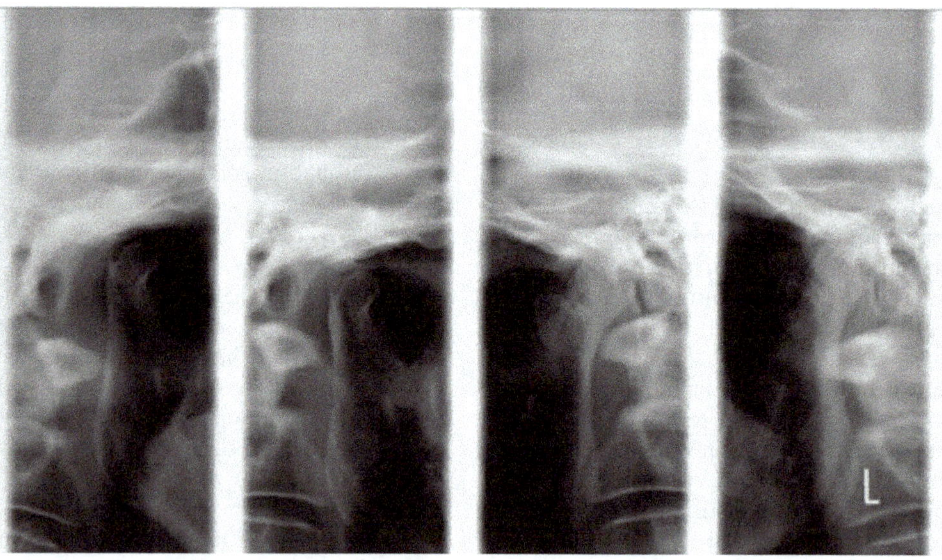

(b)

FIGURE 2: Radiographic findings: (a) panoramic radiograph and (b) lateral projection of the temporomandibular joint.

(Figures 2 and 3). Tooth mobility was noted in the maxillary annular tooth. The General Oral Health Assessment Index (GOHAI) [8] score was 29 points at the first visit. Regarding feeding function, the Fujishima's Food Intake Level Scale [9] value was level 8 (the patient ate three meals, avoiding food that is particularly difficult to swallow).

The patient was treated with intra- and extraoral massaging and a home exercise program to increase the MID using a device made of ethylene vinyl acetate (EVA). A 4 mm thick EVA sheet was cut into 2×6 mm pieces. The surface of the sheets was then softened using a burner, and blocks were created by stacking the sheets (Figure 4). The

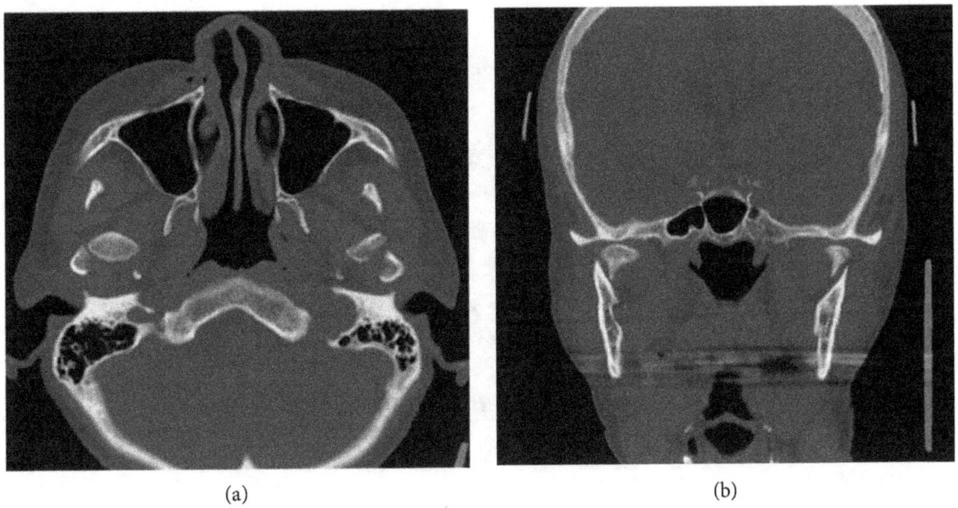

FIGURE 3: CT findings: (a) sagittal reconstruction of CT images and (b) coronal reconstruction of CT images. The bilateral condylar fractures were observed.

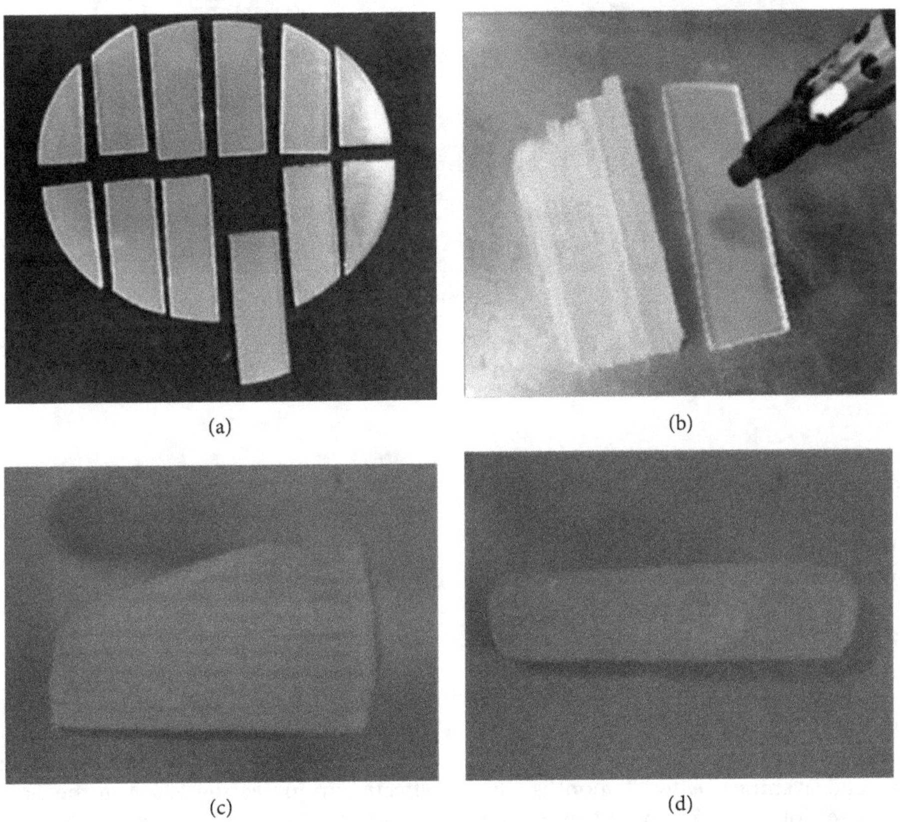

FIGURE 4: Fabrication of the device. (a) A 4 mm thick ethylene vinyl acetate (EVA) sheet was cut into 2 × 6 cm pieces. (b) The surface of the sheets was softened using a burner, and blocks were created. (c) Lateral view of the device. (d) Top view of the device.

thickness of the block was adjusted according to the MID. Furthermore, the device was slanted and inserted from the thin side. The initial thickness of the device was also decided based on the MID. In our patient with MID of 22 mm, the initial thickness of the thin side was 20 mm. The patient received instructions regarding inserting the device, advancing it in the direction of the molar teeth to increase the mouth-opening, and avoiding overloading the teeth and crest (Figure 5). Each training session of 15 minutes was prescribed twice a day whenever possible. Once the device could be easily inserted, the thickness of the device was increased accordingly.

One week after the first visit, the MID improved to 26 mm with training. The thickness of the device was

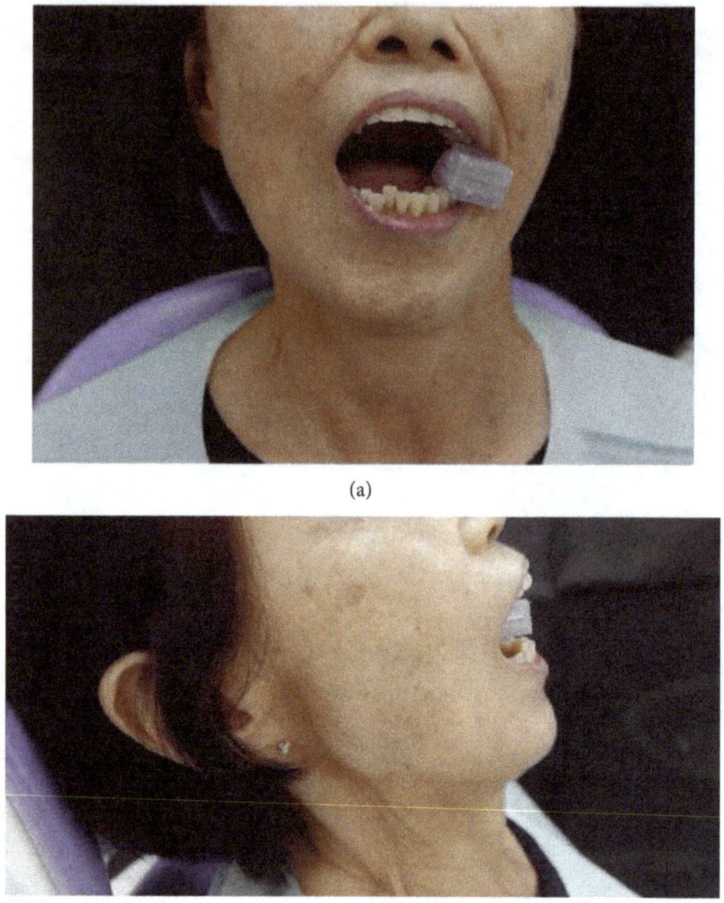

(a)

(b)

FIGURE 5: Mouth-opening training with the device. (a, b) The patient received instructions on how to insert the device and advance it in the direction of the molars.

increased to 24 mm to facilitate further mouth-opening since the patient did not complain of any TMJ, muscular, or teeth-related symptoms. After 2 weeks, the MID improved to 32 mm. Tenderness was observed around the left zygomatic area after training, and she was instructed to massage the surrounding area and prescribed exercise therapy for TMJ after mouth-opening training. The patient complained that the increase in the extent of mouth-opening persisted only for approximately 2 hours after the training. Therefore, the patient was instructed to perform mouth-opening training twice a day (morning and evening). After 2 months, the MID before the training session was 35 mm and improved to 42 mm after training (Table 1 and Figure 6). At this stage, the patient was comfortable and did not experience any issues related to trismus in her daily life. Therefore, it was decided to retain the device thickness at the same level to maintain the improvement in mouth-opening. After 12 months, the MID before training was 41 mm. Oral-related quality of life was assessed using GOHAI score, which improved to 34 after 3 months and 40 after 12 months (Table 1). Regarding feeding function, the Fujishima's Food Intake Level Scale value improved to level 10 (normal; there is no dietary restriction, and the patient ingests three meals orally) after 2 months of training and was sustained after 12 months of training (Table 1).

3. Discussion

The purpose of this case report was to highlight the use of an EVA device in mouth-opening exercises. The low-load and prolonged-stretch properties of EVA have been reported to be effective in treating the range of motion (ROM) in some pathologies [10]. In this case, a device made of EVA was effective in increasing ROM in the TMJ.

In the present case, more than 6 months had passed since the bilateral mandibular fractures were sustained before the initial visit to our department, which would have resulted in advanced scarring and restricted mouth-opening. It is reported that the mechanism of scar formation in muscle tissues after trauma involves proliferation of mesenchymal tissue due to necrosis, contusions, and hemorrhage caused by trauma [11]. In this case, scarring of the TMJ and the lip area was observed at the initial visit, which might have caused trismus and difficulty in sealing the lips.

Mouth-opening training using a device is effective for trismus caused by scarring [11]. In a previous study [12],

Table 1: Measurements before and after mouth-opening training.

	Initial visit	After 2 months	After 12 months
Maximal interincisal opening distance	22 mm	35 mm	41 mm
General Oral Health Assessment Index	29	34	40
Fujishima's Food Intake Level Scale	8	10	10

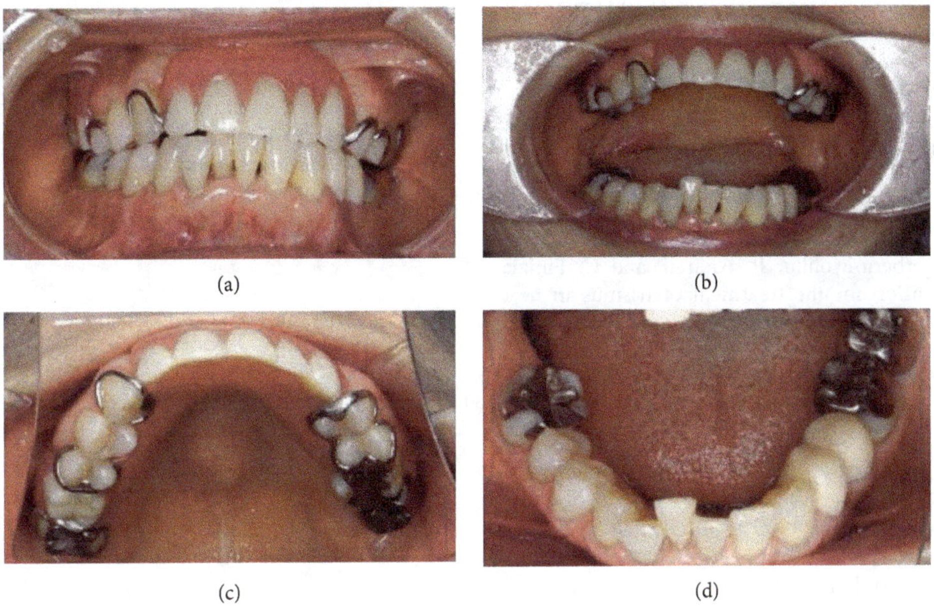

Figure 6: Postoperative views: (a) front view, (b) maximum mandibular opening at postoperation, (c) occlusal view of maxilla, and (d) occlusal view of mandible.

TheraBite® (Atos Medical AB; Hörby, Sweden), a wooden mouth-opening device, was used for such training, which was inserted into the patient's dentition and loaded to force mouth-opening. Some studies have reported that mouth-opening training should be implemented for at least 3 months to be effective [13, 14]. In this case, the patient achieved sufficient mouth-opening (42 mm) after 2 months of training, which suggests that the device used in our case is probably more effective than previously reported training devices, such as wooden devices.

The main difference between the older devices and the present device is the training methodology. Previously, devices were used for a shorter duration of training, lasting only few minutes [15]. In contrast, the device in this study was applied for as long as 15 minutes and demonstrated quicker results. In the field of physical therapy, sustained stretching exercises are often used to prevent restriction of ROM in joints [16]. Mouth-opening training uses continuous stretching movements around the TMJ. It is reported that 30 minutes of sustained extension is most effective for sustained stretching exercises [16]. In this case, we initially instructed the patient to use the device for 30 minutes daily. However, it was difficult for the patient to perform 30 consecutive minutes of training. Therefore, we instructed the patient to use it for 15 minutes twice a day. To obtain more effective outcomes, further studies are needed to examine the ideal duration of training.

EVA sheets are commonly used in devices such as mouth guards to prevent trauma during sports. Therefore, such sheets might have little effect on the patient's teeth during mouth-opening training. In this case, the patient's adherence for training with a wooden device was low. However, her adherence improved for training with the current device. One of the possible reasons might be the difference in the material. The wooden device was so hard that the patient often felt pain during training. A previous study reported that most patients felt pain during training and that the pain could affect adherence to training [17]. However, we used EVA sheets for a different purpose, which ensured a sustained load on the teeth at the insertion site during extended periods of training. Further studies involving more patients are necessary to investigate the benefits of this device and its effects on the teeth.

4. Conclusion

We effectively used a new device made of EVA in mouth-opening training in a patient with trismus due to bilateral mandibular fractures. The main advantage of this device is that it is not very hard, resulting in less stress on the teeth and less pain during training. Consequently, good adherence to training was achieved to improve the extent of mouth-opening. The oral function-related quality of life also improved with increase in the extent of mouth-opening.

Consent

Informed consent for publication was obtained from the patient using a patient consent form.

References

[1] D. Buchbinder, R. B. Currivan, A. J. Kaplan, and M. L. Urken, "Mobilization regimens for the prevention of jaw hypomobility in the radiated patient: a comparison of three techniques," *Journal of Oral and Maxillofacial Surgery*, vol. 51, no. 8, pp. 863–867, 1993.

[2] C. F. Baranano, E. L. Rosenthal, B. A. Morgan, N. L. McColloch, and J. S. Magnuson, "Dynasplint for the management of trismus after treatment of upper aerodigestive tract cancer: a retrospective study," *Ear, Nose, & Throat Journal*, vol. 90, no. 12, pp. 584–590, 2011.

[3] N. Pauli, B. Fagerberg-Mohlin, P. Andrell, and C. Finizia, "Exercise intervention for the treatment of trismus in head and neck cancer," *Acta Oncologica*, vol. 53, no. 4, pp. 502–509, 2014.

[4] K. Ichimura and T. Tanaka, "Trismus in patients with malignant tumours in the head and neck," *The Journal of Laryngology and Otology*, vol. 107, no. 11, pp. 1017–1020, 1993.

[5] K. Yamaguti, "Studies on the conservative treatment of condylar fracture of the mandible," *Journal of the Japanese Stomatological Society*, vol. 31, no. 9, pp. 2120–2134, 1985.

[6] T. Tashiro, N. Tanaka, T. Yanagisawa et al., "Evaluation of trismus after maxillomandibular fixation for mandibular fractures," *Journal of the Japanese Stomatological Society*, vol. 39, no. 11, pp. 1228–1233, 1993.

[7] M. R. DiMatteo, "Variations in patients' adherence to medical recommendations: a quantitative review of 50 years of research," *Medical Care*, vol. 42, no. 3, pp. 200–209, 2004.

[8] J. A. D. B. Campos, M. L. Zucoloto, F. S. S. Bonafé, and J. Maroco, "General Oral Health Assessment Index: a new evaluation proposal," *Gerodontology*, vol. 34, no. 3, pp. 334–342, 2017.

[9] K. Kunieda, T. Ohno, I. Fujishima, K. Hojo, and T. Morita, "Reliability and validity of a tool to measure the severity of dysphagia: the Food Intake Level Scale," *Journal of Pain and Symptom Management*, vol. 46, no. 2, pp. 201–206, 2013.

[10] D. H. Shulman, B. Shipman, and F. B. Willis, "Treating trismus with dynamic splinting: a cohort, case series," *Advances in therapy*, vol. 25, pp. 9–16, 2008.

[11] S. Hara, S. Shintani, T. Nagai, M. Mihara, K. I. Nakashiro, and H. Hamakawa, "A case of severe trismus due to cicatricial changes of the masseter muscle," *Journal of the Japanese Stomatological Society*, vol. 49, no. 7, pp. 466–469, 2003.

[12] W. H. Ren, H. W. Ao, Q. Lin, Z. G. Xu, and B. Zhang, "Efficacy of mouth opening exercises in treating trismus after maxillectomy," *Chinese Medical Journal*, vol. 126, no. 14, pp. 2666–2669, 2013.

[13] L. Yu-Hsuan, C. Wei-Chin, C. Tien-En, C. S. Lin, and Y. W. Chen, "Mouth-opening device as a treatment modality in trismus patients with head and neck cancer and oral submucous fibrosis: a prospective study," *Clinical Oral Investigations*, vol. 23, pp. 469–476, 2019.

[14] M. D. Stubblefield, L. Manfield, and E. R. Riedel, "A Preliminary Report on the Efficacy of a Dynamic Jaw Opening Device (Dynasplint Trismus System) as Part of the Multimodal Treatment of Trismus in Patients With Head and Neck Cancer," *Archives of physical medicine and rehabilitation*, vol. 91, no. 8, pp. 1278–1282, 2010.

[15] A. J. Gibbons and S. Abulhoul, "Use of a Therabite appliance in the management of bilateral mandibular coronoid hyperplasia," *British Journal of Oral and Maxillofacial Surgery*, vol. 45, no. 6, pp. 505-506, 2007.

[16] M. Jinnouchi, T. Ono, A. Oki et al., "Effect of prolonged stretching on prevention of range of motion limitation in rats," *Rigakuryoho Kagaku*, vol. 23, no. 1, pp. 169–173, 2008.

[17] L. J. Melchers, E. Van Weert, C. H. G. Beurskens et al., "Exercise adherence in patients with trismus due to head and neck oncology: a qualitative study into the use of the Therabite®," *International Journal of Oral and Maxillofacial Surgery*, vol. 38, no. 9, pp. 947–954, 2009.

20

Three-Layered Closure of Persistent Oroantral Fistula using Chin Graft, Buccal Fat Pad and Buccal Advancement Flap: A Case Report with Review of Literature

Shiv Prasad Sharma

Specialist Oral and Maxillofacial Surgeon, Zulfi General Hospital, Ministry of Health, King Abdulla Street, 11932, Saudi Arabia

Correspondence should be addressed to Shiv Prasad Sharma; shiv1412in@gmail.com

Academic Editor: Luis M. J. Gutierrez

Various techniques have been used for the repair of oroantral fistula (OAF) but majority of them have focused on the soft tissue closure alone, and most of the time, the osseous floor of the sinus was ignored. Existing literature supports that bone grafts supported by Buccal Fat Pad (BFP) heal well without undergoing significant resorption and necrosis. Through this case report, we wish to elaborate on the clinical success of using BFP and autogenous chin graft for simultaneous reconstruction of a large long-standing oroantral fistula with underlying osseous defect. The combination technique can prove beneficial for osseous regeneration of sinus floor and improve chances for future implant prosthetic rehabilitation.

1. Introduction

An oroantral fistula can develop as a sequel of dental extractions, infection, maxillary cyst/tumor excision, persistent infection/abscess, or radiotherapy [1, 2]. A small oroantral fistula < 3 mm can close spontaneously or by simple figure of eight suture, but large fistulae > 5 mm need more complicated surgical management [3–5]. It is shown that about 50% of patients with unattended OAF will develop maxillary sinus symptoms in 48 hours, and within 2 weeks, 90% will have maxillary sinusitis [6]. Early detection and management are advised to avoid further complications.

Management of established OAF can be classified into nonsurgical and surgical. Nonsurgical methods employ placing materials into the defect to act as a mechanical barrier without attempting flap closure. Synthetic graft materials, fibrin glue, xenograft, absorbable implants, and acrylic splints have all been used.

Surgical principle involves raising the adjacent or distant flap and advancing into the defect, for example, buccal flaps, palatal flaps, tongue flap, and nasolabial flaps [2]. All these methods have their own advantages and disadvantages.

The first clinical application of BFP was described by Egyedi in 1977 where he used it for reconstruction of palatal defect following tumor excision [7]. In recent years, Buccal Fat Pad (BFP) has been used successfully for closing oral defects due to its reliability and easy harvesting. With a proper technique of harvest, it can provide a 6 × 5 × 3 cm graft which can cover an area of 10 cm^2. The mean thickness is about 6 mm [8, 9]. Care should be taken while harvesting to avoid injury to the parotid duct and facial nerve branches.

Ignoring the underlying bony defect can have serious consequences with respect to prosthetic rehabilitation. Simultaneous use of autogenous bone graft for OAF closure is recommended to facilitate good prosthetic treatment. Bone grafts from different sites have been used. In 1969, Proctor reported the use of iliac crest graft for large OAF closure [10]. This of course had the disadvantage of a separate surgical procedure associated with unacceptable donor site morbidities sometimes. The chin area, retromolar area, tuberosity, and ramus of mandible and zygomatic bone are the preferred alternative donor sites [11]. All the previous studies have utilized the standard buccal flap (Rehrmann) to cover the graft. We would like to present the successful use of autogenous chin graft covered with BFP and closure with BAF in the reconstruction of OAF.

The use of chin grafts in OAF closure has been reported with successful outcomes. Haas et al. in their preliminary study showed successful results with chin grafts [12]. It is important to note that although chin grafts have been used with successful results in numerous applications, their use in OAF closure has been scarce or may be under reported. It provides high quality bone which is easy to harvest and can be used without any significant donor site morbidity. The grafts from different origins show varied rates of mineralization. In an interesting study by Schlegel et al., chin bone grafts were found to be superior in terms of mineralization over a 6-month period [13].

Several techniques have been utilized to reconstruct the bony defect. Most of the published articles are in the form of a case report or case series. There is a lack of large prospective randomized studies comparing the reliability and outcomes of these existing methods. Kapustecki et al. in their series of 20 cases used autogenous grafts from symphysis mandible (14 patients) and external oblique line (6 patients) covered with PRF (Platelet Rich Fibrin) membrane [14]. They observed successful fistula closure along with restoration of adequate alveolar width and height in preparation for future prosthetic solutions. In their series of 21 cases reconstructed with bone grafts from mandibular symphysis and retromolar areas, Watzak et al. realized a complication rate of 14.3% in the form of wound dehiscence, which healed by secondary intention [15].

Er et al. performed two-layered closure with simultaneous bone grafting using graft from different intraoral sites [16]. They noted wound dehiscence in 20% of their patients. It can be realized that wound breakdown can result from inadequate two-layered closure. Ahmed and Askar showed favorable results with the coverage of bone graft with buccal mucoperiosteal flap [17]. In a 10-month follow-up case, Weinstock et al. demonstrated the additional benefit of the three-layer closure with bone graft, buccal fat, and buccal advancement flap [18]. The two layers over the graft not only provide added support but also give a well vascularized bed for the success of the graft.

Table 1 summarizes various studies demonstrating the use of different modalities addressing the osseous defect associated with OAF.

2. Case Presentation

A 45-year-old male patient, chronic smoker, reported to us with the chief complain of leakage of liquids through his nose while drinking. Otherwise, he was asymptomatic. He underwent extraction of his tooth number 16 about 6 months back elsewhere. On clinical examination, there were no signs and symptoms suggestive of acute maxillary sinusitis. Intraorally, a fistulous opening round in shape with normal surrounding mucosa and an obvious bony defect was seen along the maxillary alveolus molar region (Figure 1). No active discharge was present.

Radiographic examination was done to define the underlying bony defect and also to rule out any foreign body (fractured root tip). The sinuses showed normal appearance. The bony defect of size 2 × 1.8 cm along the sinus floor was confirmed (Figure 2).

After correlating the clinical and radiographic findings, surgical closure using buccal advancement flap (BAF)+ BFP+autogenous bone graft from the chin was planned. Preoperatively, the patient was started on antral regime (Tab amoxicillin clavulanic 625 mg+metronidazole 500 mg+ Tab ibuprofen+Tab chlorpheniramine 4 mg + nasal decongestant) for 5 days.

The entire procedure was performed under local anesthesia (2% lignocaine with 1 : 80000 adrenaline) using Posterior Superior Alveolar block supplemented by infiltration+greater palatine nerve block. The fistulous tract was excised in a circumscribed manner along the defect. A modified buccal mucoperiosteal flap was elevated in trapezoidal outline starting from the mesial and distal end of the fistulous opening. The periosteum was incised along the posterior aspect of the flap to identify BFP. Gentle blunt dissection was done to harvest the BFP till we obtained the sufficient amount of fat to cover the graft and the defect. Next, the cortical bone graft was harvested from the chin of size matching the defect. The graft was press fit into the defect and did not require screw fixation. Then, the BFP was mobilized to cover the graft, and finally, the mucoperiosteal flap was repositioned and sutured in place (Figures 3 and 4). This way, 3-layered closures were performed to reconstruct the bony as well as soft tissue defect. The patient was put on nasogastric tube feed till the time of suture removal. Mucosalisation of the fat pad was noticed at follow-up visits after 1 week and 1 month later (Figures 5 and 6).

The patient was observed for signs of infection, dehiscence, and necrosis. Postoperative radiograph showed bone graft well in place (Figure 7). No significant complication was noted in the follow-up appointments. Both the primary site and the bone graft donor site healed without any dehiscence.

3. Discussion

The commonest cause for the development of OAF includes dental extractions of posterior teeth (molars, premolars) due to close proximity of the root apices to the sinus floor. Frequencies of such occurrences have been reported to be between 0.31% and 4.7% [19]. Based on its location, the fistula can be alveolosinusal, palatosinusal, or vestibulosinusal [20].

Ever since its first clinical use by Egyedi in 1977, BFP has gained popularity and rightly so because of its advantages: rapid epithelialization, excellent reliable blood supply, anatomically favorable position, ease of harvest, low rate of complications, and minimal to no donor site morbidity.

Problems that we can come across mainly at the time of harvesting BFP are perforation or shrinkage. Egyedi advocated covering the fat pad with split skin graft to overcome these issues, but Tideman et al. have shown that BFP was capable of self-epithelialization within 3-4 weeks of its inset [7, 21]. Nevertheless, covering the BFP might be essential in cases of large defects and where the amount of BFP may be inadequate. In such cases, buccal advancement flap is the best

TABLE 1: Summarizes various studies demonstrating the use of different modalities for OAF closure.

Author/year	Number of cases	Type of bone graft
(1) Waldrop TC et al. (1993)	1	Gelatin membrane+DFDBA+ePTFE
(2) Liversedge et al. (2002)	1	BFP+maxillary bone graft
(3) Haas et al. (2003) [12]	5	Chin graft+buccal flap
(4) Watzack G et al. (2005)	21	Retromolar/chin graft
(5) Delgado Galindez (2005)	22	Mandibular graft+mucoperiosteal flap
(6) Ogunsalu et al. (2005)	1	Bioss sandwiched between Biogide
(7) Scala M et al. (2007) bovine bone	3	Cryoplatelet gel+particulate bone maxilla+
(8) Penarrocha Diago M et al. (2007)	1	Zygomatic bone
(9) Lee BK (2008)	1	Ileac bone+palatal flap
(10) Doobrow JH et al. (2008)	1	Collagen matrix+FDB+$CaSO_4$
(11) Scattarella et al. (2010)	1	Autologous bone+particulate xenograft+PTFE
(12) Ahmed MS et al. (2011)	8	Chin/ramus graft+BAF
(13) Er et al. (2013) [16] wall (3)	10	Chin (3), buccal (1), tuberosity (2), ramus (1), maxillary
(14) Cottam JR et al. (2013)	1	Recombinant rhBMP-2+collagen matrix
(15) Pourdanesh F et al. (2013)	1	BFP+pedicled coronoid process+mucosa
(16) Weinstock RJ et al. (2014) [18]	1	Maxilla+BFP flap+buccal advancement flap
(17) De Biasi M et al. (2014)	20	BFP+hydroxyapatite crystals+collagen sheath
(18) Choi N et al. (2015)	1	Scapular tip free flap
(19) Kapustecki M et al. (2016) [14]	20	Mental protuberance (14)+oblique line (6)
(20) S Amroun et al. (2018)	1	Maxillary tuberosity+mucosal closure

Abbreviations: DFDBA: Decalcified Freeze-Dried Bone Allograft; ePTFE: extended polytetrafluoroethylene; BFP: Buccal Fat Pad; Biooss: bone graft material; Biogide: a resorbable membrane; FDB: Freeze-Dried Bone; $CaSO_4$: Calcium Sulphate; BAF: buccal advancement flap; rhBMP-2: recombinant human Bone Morphogenetic Protein-2.

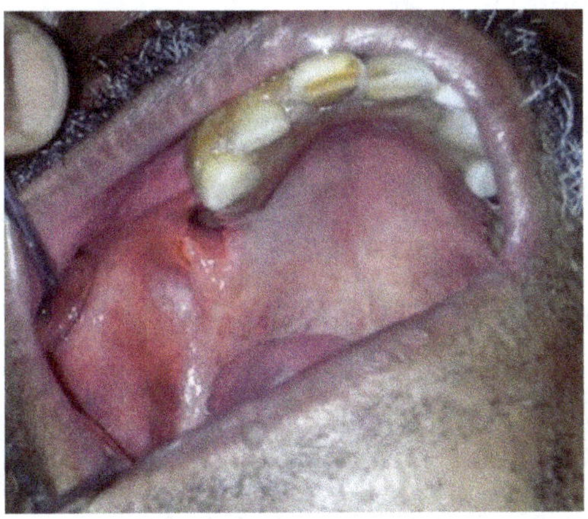

FIGURE 1: Clinical picture showing fistulous opening with identifiable bony defect.

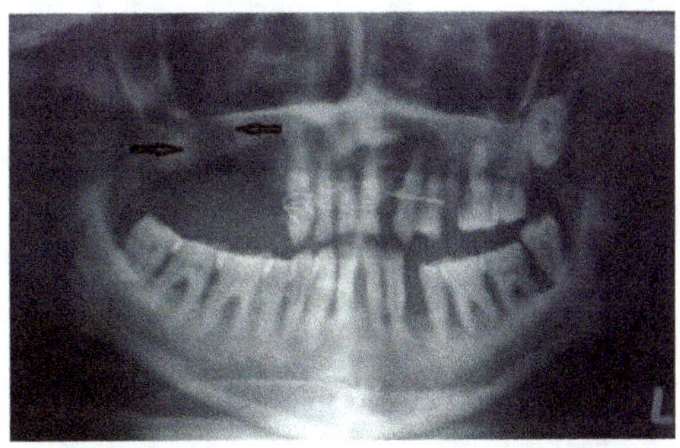

FIGURE 2: Panoramic X-ray demonstrating the underlying osseous defect.

option. This combination technique provides more stability and provides additional tissue for cover. In our case, this layered closure was needed to provide support to the bone graft and also to maintain a well vascularized environment for the graft take up.

Our idea of three-layer closure is supported by the studies of Er et al. and Weinstock et al. [16, 18]. Er et al. observed wound dehiscence in 20% of cases after two-layered closure. Weinstock et al. demonstrated additional benefit of the buccal flap covering the BFP over the graft in a study with a 10-month follow-up.

There is so much heterogeneity in the methods for OAF closure, and no particular technique is superior or inferior to other. Each case is at the discretion of the treating surgeon based on his experience and preference. The choice of the technique must be guided by 4 important assessment criteria: (a) size and type of defect, (b) presence or absence of sinus disease, (c) minimal donor site morbidity to the patient, and (d) prosthetic considerations. The described technique has the added advantage for graft support and minimizing the chance of graft resorption or wound dehiscence.

4. Conclusion

Repair of OAF is essential to prevent further complications related to the maxillary sinus. The routine flap based

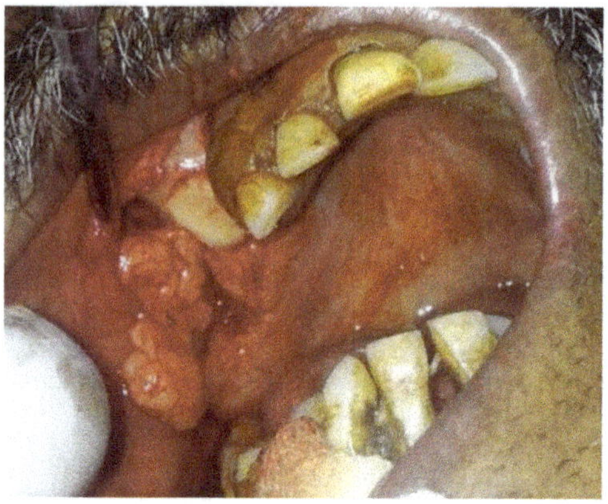

Figure 3: Harvested buccal fat+chin graft press fit into the bony defect.

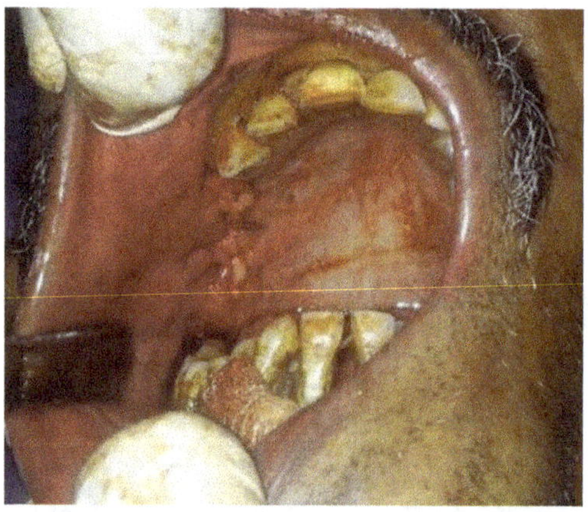

Figure 4: Three-layered closure achieved.

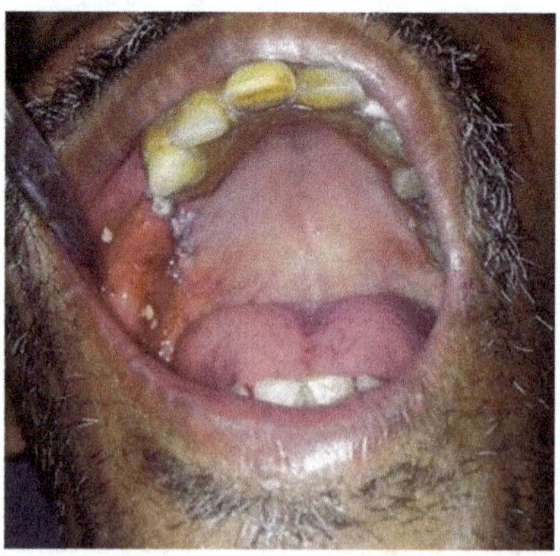

Figure 5: Mucosalisation of BFP noted at 1 week.

techniques will not be sufficient alone due to the continued demand and necessity for implant rehabilitation. Due consideration should be given to the underlying osseous defect as well.

Therefore, we used autogenous bone graft harvested from the chin for the closure of bone. BFP and chin graft may be

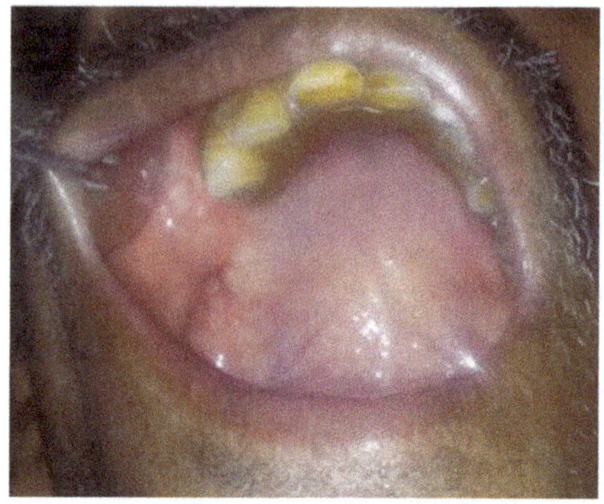

Figure 6: Complete healing after 1 month.

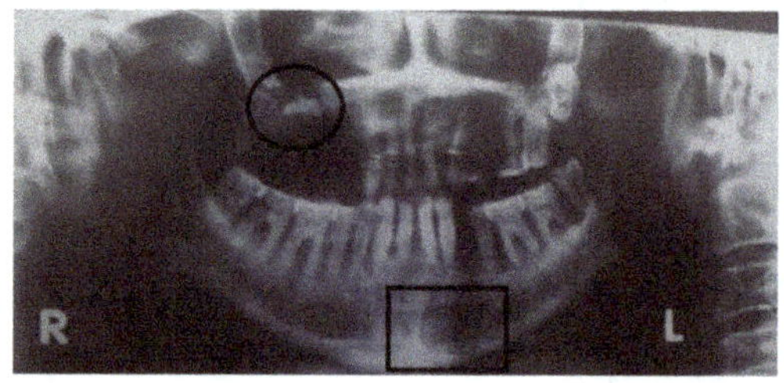

Figure 7: Radiograph showing chin graft well in place.

adequate to cover a large defect, but BAF may serve as an additional support and will help in minimizing any complication related to the grafts.

Acknowledgments

My sincere acknowledgement to Dr. Anuja Sharma, Private Dental Practitioner, for helping me in the drafting of this manuscript.

References

[1] T. Yilmaz, A. E. Suslu, and B. Gursel, "Treatment of oroantral fistula: experience with 27 cases," *American Journal of Otolaryngology*, vol. 24, no. 4, pp. 221–223, 2003.

[2] S. H. Visscher, B. van Minnen, and R. R. Bos, "Closure of oroantral communications: a review of the literature," *Journal of Oral and Maxillofacial Surgery*, vol. 68, no. 6, pp. 1384–1391, 2010.

[3] S. K. Lazow, "Surgical management of the oroantral fistula: flap procedures," *Operative Techniques in Otolaryngology-Head and Neck Surgery*, vol. 10, no. 2, pp. 148–152, 1999.

[4] R. Candamourty, M. K. Jain, K. Sankar, and M. R. Ramesh Babu, "Double-layered closure of oroantral fistula using buccal fat pad and buccal advancement flap," *Journal of Natural Science, Biology and Medicine*, vol. 3, no. 2, pp. 203–205, 2012.

[5] E. T. Daif, "Long-term effectiveness of the pedicled buccal fat pad in the closure of a large oroantral fistula," *Journal of Oral and Maxillofacial Surgery*, vol. 74, no. 9, pp. 1718–1722, 2016.

[6] H. Dym and J. C. Wolf, "Oroantral communication," *Oral and Maxillofacial Surgery Clinics of North America*, vol. 24, no. 2, pp. 239–247, 2012.

[7] P. Egyedi, "Utilization of the buccal fat pad for closure of oro-antral and/or oro-nasal communications," *Journal of Maxillofacial Surgery*, vol. 5, pp. 241–244, 1977.

[8] P. M. J. Tostevin and H. Ellis, "The buccal pad of fat: a review," *Clinical Anatomy*, vol. 8, no. 6, pp. 403–406, 1995.

[9] M.-K. Kim, W. Han, and S.-G. Kim, "The use of the buccal fat pad flap for oral reconstruction," *Maxillofacial Plastic and Reconstructive Surgery*, vol. 39, no. 1, article 5, 2017.

[10] B. Proctor, "Bone graft closure of large or persistent oro-maxillary fistula," *The Laryngoscope*, vol. 79, no. 5, pp. 822–826, 1969.

[11] M. Peñarrocha-Diago, B. Garcia, D. Gomez, and J. Balaguer, "Zygomatic bone graft for oral-antral communication closure and implant placement," *The Journal of Oral Implantology*, vol. 33, no. 5, pp. 305–309, 2007.

[12] R. Haas, G. Watzak, M. Baron, G. Tepper, G. Mailath, and G. Watzek, "A preliminary study of monocortical bone grafts for oroantral fistula closure," *Oral Surgery, Oral Medicine, Oral Pathology, Oral Radiology, and Endodontology*, vol. 96, no. 3, pp. 263–266, 2003.

[13] K. A. Schlegel, S. Schultze-Mosgau, J. Wiltfang, F. W. Neukam, S. Rupprecht, and M. Thorwarth, "Changes of mineralization of free autogenous bone grafts used for sinus floor elevation," *Clinical Oral Implants Research*, vol. 17, no. 6, pp. 673–678, 2006.

[14] M. Kapustecki, I. Niedzielska, H. Borgiel-Marek, and B. Różanowski, "Alternative method to treat oroantral communication and fistula with autogenous bone graft and platelet rich firbin," *Medicina Oral Patología Oral y Cirugia Bucal*, vol. 21, no. 5, pp. e608–e613, 2016.

[15] W. G, G. Tepper, W. Zechner, G. Monov, D. Busenlechner, and G. Watzek, "Bony press-fit closure of oro-antral fistulas: a technique for pre-sinus lift repair and secondary closure," *Journal of Oral and Maxillofacial Surgery*, vol. 63, no. 9, pp. 1288–1294, 2005.

[16] N. Er, H. Y. Tuncer, Ç. Karaca, and S. Çopuroğlu, "Treatment of oroantral fistulas using bony press-fit technique," *Journal of Oral and Maxillofacial Surgery*, vol. 71, no. 4, pp. 659–666, 2013.

[17] M. S. Ahmed and N. A. Askar, "Combined bony closure of oroantral fistula and sinus lift with mandibular bone grafts for subsequent dental implant placement," *Oral Surgery, Oral Medicine, Oral Pathology, Oral Radiology, and Endodontics*, vol. 111, no. 4, pp. e8–14, 2011.

[18] R. J. Weinstock, L. Nikoyan, and H. Dym, "Composite three-layer closure of oral antral communication with 10 months follow-up—a case study," *Journal of Oral and Maxillofacial Surgery*, vol. 72, no. 2, pp. 266.e1–266.e7, 2014.

[19] B. Gacic, L. Todorovic, V. Kokovic et al., "The closure of oroantral communications with resorbable PLGA-coated β-TCP root analogs, hemostatic gauze, or buccal flaps: A prospective study," *Oral Surgery, Oral Medicine, Oral Pathology, Oral Radiology, and Endodontology*, vol. 108, no. 6, pp. 844–850, 2009.

[20] A. E. Borgonovo, F. V. Berardinelli, M. Favale, and C. Maiorana, "Surgical options in oroantral fistula treatment," *The Open Dentistry Journal*, vol. 6, no. 1, pp. 94–98, 2012.

[21] H. Tideman, A. Bosanquet, and J. Scott, "Use of the buccal fat pad as a pedicled graft," *Journal of Oral and Maxillofacial Surgery*, vol. 44, no. 6, pp. 435–440, 1986.

21

Bone Augmentation Procedures in a Patient with Acromegaly

Laura Andreea Schiller,[1,2] **Albert Cristian Schiller**,[3,4] **Adalbert Schiller**,[5] **Aida Gabriela Dascalu**,[6] **and Silviu Brad**[1]

[1]*Department of Radiology "Victor Babes", University of Medicine and Pharmacy, Timisoara 300041, Romania*
[2]*Department of Oral Surgery, Stomdas Clinic (Private Practice), Bacau 600125, Romania*
[3]*Department of Prosthetic Dentistry "Victor Babes", University of Medicine and Pharmacy, Timisoara 300041, Romania*
[4]*Department of Endodontics, Stomdas Clinic (Private Practice), Bacau 600125, Romania*
[5]*Department of Nephrology "Victor Babes", University of Medicine and Pharmacy, Timisoara 300041, Romania*
[6]*Department of Orthodontics "Victor Babes", University of Medicine and Pharmacy, Timisoara 300041, Romania*

Correspondence should be addressed to Laura Andreea Schiller; dr.grosulaura@gmail.com

Academic Editor: Jose López-López

The objective of this clinical case is to evaluate if bone augmentation procedures can be successful in a patient with altered bone metabolism due to a systemic disease: acromegaly. Two guided bone regeneration procedures were made on the same patient: horizontal ridge augmentation with lateral wall approach sinus graft of the left maxilla and horizontal ridge augmentation of the front left maxilla. CBCT assessment of the new formed bone was made after a minimum of nine months and dental implants were placed. The results show that bone augmentation procedures can be successful in a patient with acromegaly, after pituitary adenoma removal, when autologous bone is not included in the grafting procedure.

1. Introduction

Acromegaly is a syndrome caused by growth hormone excess in adults and is due to a growth hormone-secreting pituitary adenoma in the vast majority of cases [1].

The facial features of patients with acromegaly are characteristic: the nose is broadened and thickened, the malar bone becomes prominent, the lips are thick, and the facial lines are marked. Jaw malocclusion is a common phenomenon in these patients as there is a tendency towards mandibular overgrowth with prognathism, macroglossia, and teeth separation. Cortical bone thickens, and its porosity is decreased [2].

Studies show that acromegaly has a negative influence on trabecular bone, but not on cortical bone. Unfortunately, these studies are based on investigations made on skeletal bones, other than the maxilla and mandible: radius [3] and tibia [4]. A direct comparison of the maxillary and mandibular trabecular bone pattern factor with those of skeletal sites is not useful and would lead to false conclusions because of the difference in orientation of the sectional planes to the cancellous trabeculae [5].

Based on these facts, we could assume that acromegaly might have a similar negative influence on autologous bone grafts and less influence on other types of graft materials like anorganic bovine-derived bone mineral (ABBM) and allografts.

ABBM is a deproteinized, sterilized, bovine cancellous bone that is osteoconductive and provides a favorable scaffold for bone formation. It incorporates into the newly formed bone and, since it is slowly resorbed, keeps the volume of the graft very stable [6, 7].

A bone allograft is an osseous, transplanted tissue from the same species as the recipient but of different genotype [8]. Mineralized cancellous bone allograft (MCBA) is an effective osteoconductive material because its highly porous structure maintains volume [6, 7].

The purpose of this case report is to present the treatment and outcome of a patient with acromegaly and deficient maxillary bone that was rehabilitated using ABBM and MCBA.

2. Case Report

A 39-year-old patient addressed our clinic for complex oral rehabilitation with dental implants. He was early diagnosed with acromegaly due to a pituitary adenoma. The patient was treated by a medical team from the Netherlands that surgically removed the tumor and stabilized his condition. We began the surgical procedures after we had their approval.

The pretreatment we applied consisted of dental impressions, study models, orthopantomography, cone beam computed tomography (CBCT) of the left maxilla and of the left and right mandible, and laboratory investigations. The blood workup revealed 25-hydroxyvitamin D3 (25-OH vitamin D3) deficiency (15.64 μg/L). We recommended vitamin D3 supplements (tablets 2000 U.I., 2/day, 60 days) until the values normalized. The initial image of orthopantomography is presented in Figure 1. The first stage of the treatment plan and workup was to reestablish oral health by removing old restorations, extracting unrestorable teeth (44, 45, 21, 22, 23, 24, 37, and 33) with addition of growth factors (Advanced Platelet-Rich Fibrin (A-PRF)), performing endodontic treatments, postcore restorations (15, 13, 12, and 11), and professional cleaning. The patient received provisional restorations: a fixed composite resin restoration with metal framework from tooth 15 to tooth 11 and a removable acrylic partial denture for the left maxilla.

The second stage of the treatment began 10 months later. The patient still suffered from 25-OH vitamin D3 deficiency (15.90 μg/L) so we recommended to continue vitamin D supplements (tablets 2000 U.I., 2/day, 60 days) until the values normalized, followed by a smaller daily dose for maintenance (500 U.I.). We performed horizontal ridge augmentation with lateral wall approach sinus graft. After the incision and the full thickness flap, we created the lateral-access window of the sinus wall with a Piezotome, and we uncovered a small cyst (visible on the pre-op CBCT) and aspirated its content. There was a small perforation of the sinus membrane right next to the antral septa that closed spontaneously after elevating it, but we applied a resorbable collagen membrane for safety reasons. The host site was prepared for the graft with small holes through the buccal cortical plate (Figure 2), and then, we released the buccal flap with a periosteal incision. We introduced particulate bovine bone graft mixed with 150 mg/mL clindamycin solution (0.8 mL) and sterile saline into the space created for the sinus graft [8]. The horizontal component of the defect was augmented using a mix of 50% particulate bovine bone graft, 50% particulate freeze-dried bone allograft, A-PRF membranes, and A-PRF exudate. A second layer of particulate bovine bone graft mixed with sterile saline was placed over the previous one. We covered everything with a resorbable collagen membrane which we secured with titanium pins on the buccal and with resorbable sutures on the palatal side. We could not stabilize the pins next to the alveolar ridge due to the thinness of the bone. First, we sutured the apical buccal periosteum to the palatal flap with resorbable sutures for further stabilization of the graft, and then, the surgical site was closed with nonresorbable monofilament sutures. Broad spectrum antibiotics and nonsteroidal anti-inflammatory drugs (NSAIDs) were prescribed. The post-op healing was uneventful, and the sutures were removed at 14 days.

The third stage of treatment followed 8 months later. The patient started treatment with Sandostatin LAR prescribed by the endocrinologist. After evaluating the new bone formation on a CBCT, we saw that the first operation was a success and we moved to the next step: horizontal ridge augmentation of the front left maxilla. After the incision and the full thickness flap, we were able to see the newly formed bone. The host site was prepared for the graft with small holes through the buccal cortical plate, and then, we released the buccal flap with a periosteal incision. The horizontal component of the defect was augmented using a mix of 50% particulate bovine bone graft, 50% particulate freeze-dried bone allograft, A-PRF membranes, and A-PRF exudate (Figure 2). A second layer of particulate bovine bone graft mixed with sterile saline was placed over the previous one. We covered everything with a resorbable collagen membrane which we secured with titanium pins on the buccal and on the palatal side. First, we sutured the apical buccal periosteum to the palatal flap with resorbable sutures for further stabilization of the graft, and then, the surgical site was closed with nonresorbable monofilament sutures. Broad spectrum antibiotics and NSAIDs were prescribed. The post-op healing was uneventful, and the sutures were removed at 14 days.

The next stage of treatment started one year later, when the patient was reevaluated with a post-op CBCT which showed sufficient bone formation for implant placement (Figure 3). The blood workup revealed normal values for 25-OH vitamin D3 (29.91 μg/L), and he was no longer on any medication. Unfortunately, there was a vertical bone loss due to the pressure from the removable provisional denture. Following the assessment of bone formation, we chose the dental implant sites and performed the implant placement: *22*: 3.5 × 11.5 mm, *24*: 4 × 13 mm, *26*: 4.5 × 13 mm, and *27*: 4.5 × 13 mm.

In Table 1, CBCT measurements show the amount of newly formed bone.

The patient returned after one year, and the implants were uncovered. He received an implant-supported composite resin restoration with metal framework for the left maxilla and a removable acrylic partial denture for the mandible (Figure 4). All the above treatment steps and clinical decisions are in accordance with the appropriate EQUATOR guidelines (CARE checklist) and with the ethical standards of the responsible committee on human experimentation (institutional and national) and with the Helsinki Declaration of 1975, as revised in 2000, approved by the local ethics committee no. 1/28.05.2015.

3. Discussion

The best treatment option to rehabilitate the maxilla and correct the crossbite would have been an overdenture, but the patient refused. He also refused orthognathic surgery to correct the malocclusion; therefore, the treatment plan for the maxilla was a fixed dental prosthesis for the right side and a fixed implant-supported prosthesis for the left side. We did

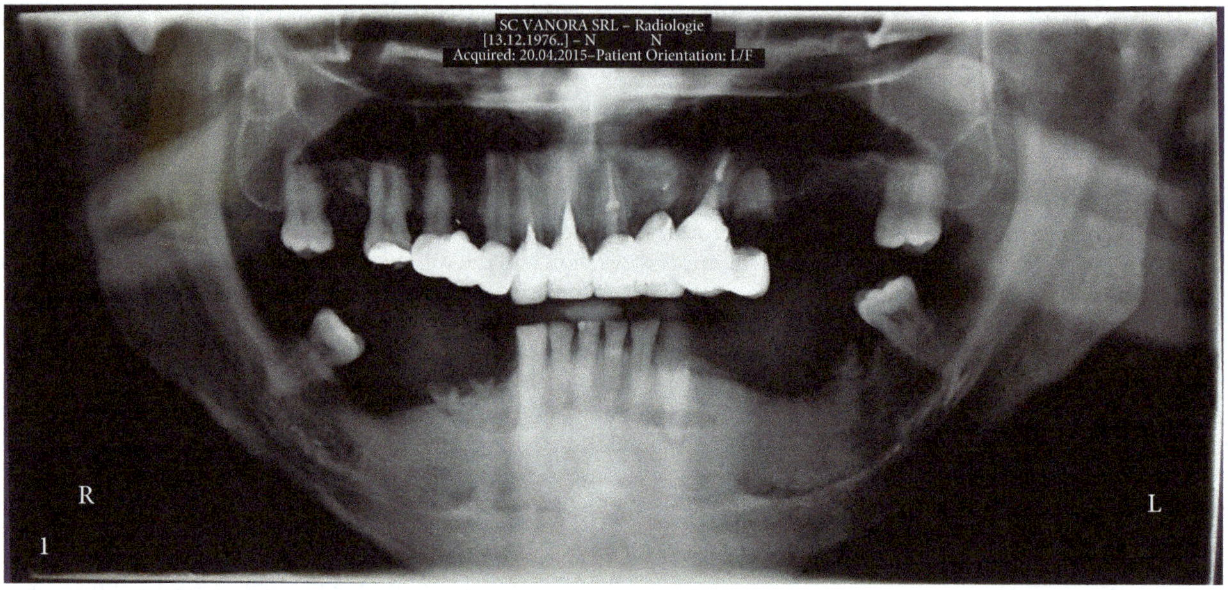

FIGURE 1: Initial orthopantomography.

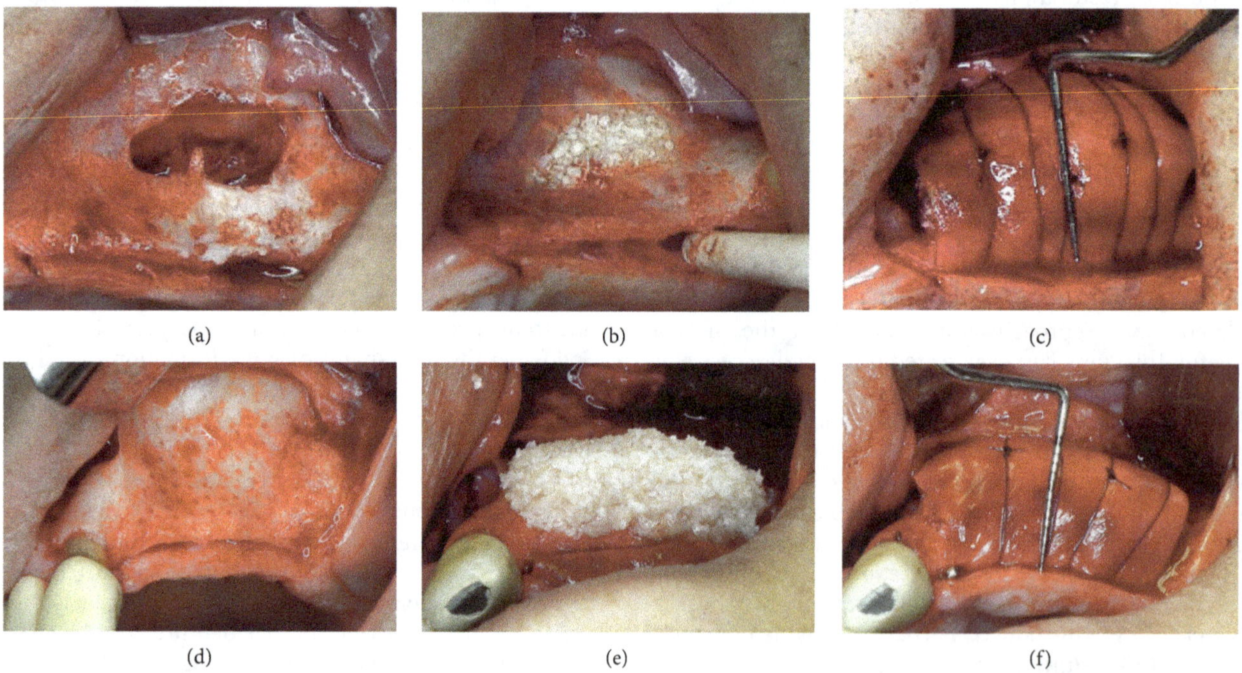

FIGURE 2: (a) Intraoral view of the elevated sinus membrane. (b) The sinus graft filling the space under the Schneiderian membrane. (c) Occlusal view of the horizontal ridge augmentation from the first surgery. (d) Labial view of the frontal defect, buccal perforations of the host bone, and, on the distal, the newly formed bone. (e) Occlusal view with the graft in place. (f) Occlusal view after stabilizing the graft with the resorbable membrane—second surgery.

not consider zygomatic implants as an option, because the patient still had many restorable teeth on the right side and we consider it is unethical to remove restorable teeth to replace them with implants.

In order to rehabilitate the left maxilla with a fixed implant-supported prosthesis, surgical modifications were needed to change the highly deficient maxillary bone. The main concern of our complex intervention was the unpredictability of the bone augmentation outcome since the published data about bone augmentation procedures in patients with acromegaly are scarce. We discussed this with the patient and began with the most predictable procedure: horizontal ridge augmentation with lateral wall approach sinus graft.

Even though autogenous bone [9, 10] is considered to be the gold standard for bone grafts, we decided not to include it in the augmentation procedure because it was highly probable that the patient's bone structure was affected by intense

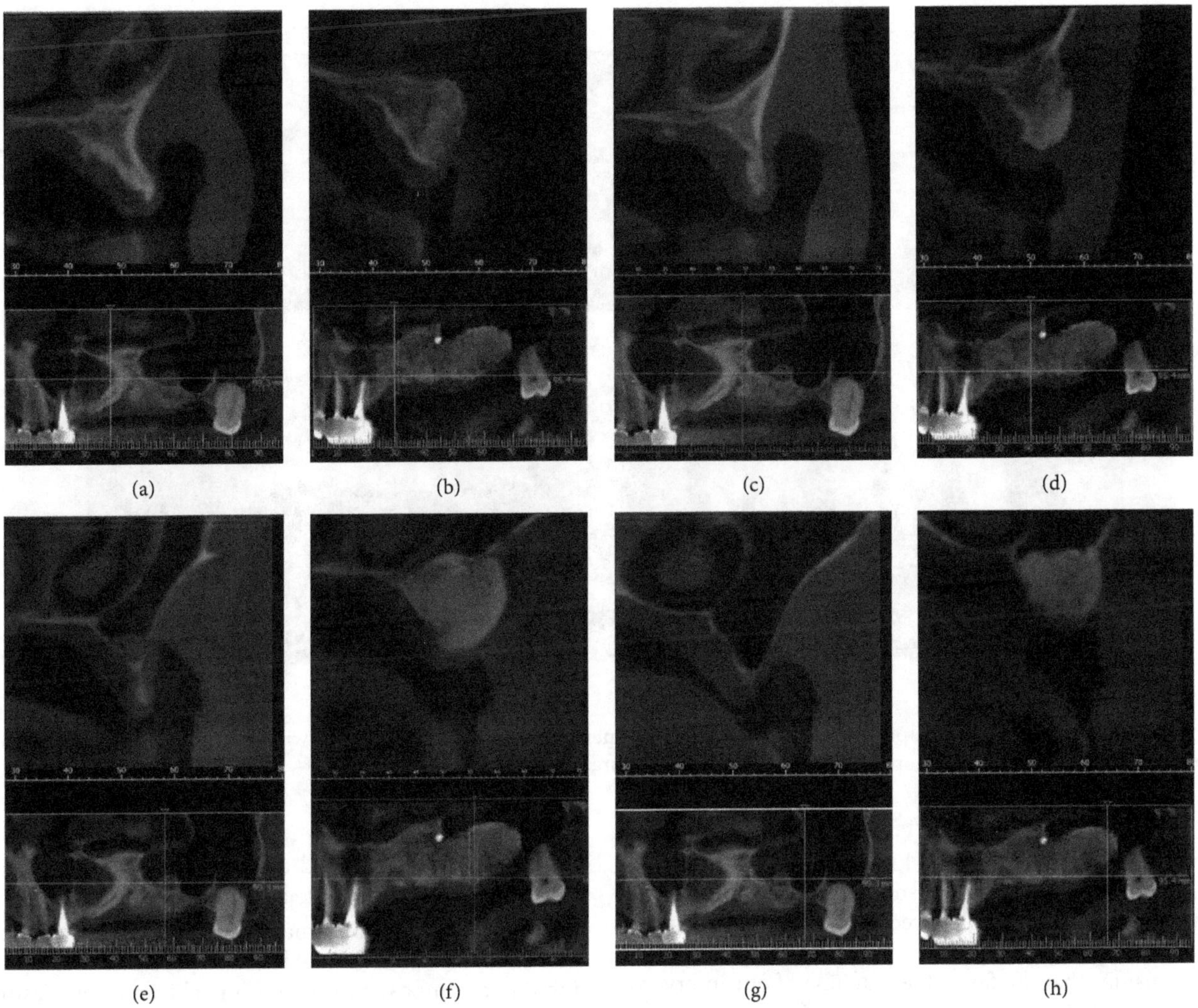

Figure 3: (a) Pre-op CBCT scan of the resorbed maxillary ridge on site 22. (b) Post-op CBCT scan of the newly formed bone on site 22. (c) Pre-op CBCT scan of the resorbed maxillary ridge on site 24. (d) Post-op CBCT scan of the newly formed bone on site 24. (e) Pre-op CBCT scan of the resorbed maxillary ridge on site 26. (f) Post-op CBCT scan of the newly formed bone on site 26. (g) Pre-op CBCT scan of the resorbed maxillary ridge on site 27. (h) Post-op CBCT scan of the newly formed bone on site 27.

Table 1: Evaluation of bone width on the CBCT.

Implant site	Before augmentation procedure (mm)	After augmentation procedure (mm)
22	1.6	6.0
24	2.2	7.0
26	1.4	7.9
27	2.3	8.6

remodeling due to his condition. We used anorganic bovine-derived bone mineral because is one of the most well-documented biomaterials and we mixed it with particulate freeze-dried bone allograft [11] to replace the autologous component. We took into consideration the fact that after a healing period of 9–10 months, the combination of deproteinized bovine bone mineral (DBBM) and a collagen membrane is an effective treatment option for horizontal bone augmentation before implant placement [12, 13].

The time between the stages of the treatment was longer than we would have wanted because the patient is not living in our country and came for therapy whenever possible. Furthermore, we made a removable provisional denture for the left maxilla at the patient's demand, only for aesthetic purposes. After each surgery, the denture was widely relieved and relined with soft material. The patient could not stay without denture for such a long time because of social reasons and that is why we decided not to reaugment the vertical discrepancy, considering that the result would have been the same. That is also the reason for which we did not use a different method. We were concerned that if we use a d-PTFE membrane [14, 15] with titanium reinforcement, bone block [16, 17] or bone shell [18, 19] techniques on a patient who is wearing a removable prosthesis over the grafted site, we would encounter graft exposure and infection. The fact that we could not see the patient on a regular basis because he lived in another country also influenced our decision-making. It might be possible that the bone formation would have been even better if the patient would not have worn a

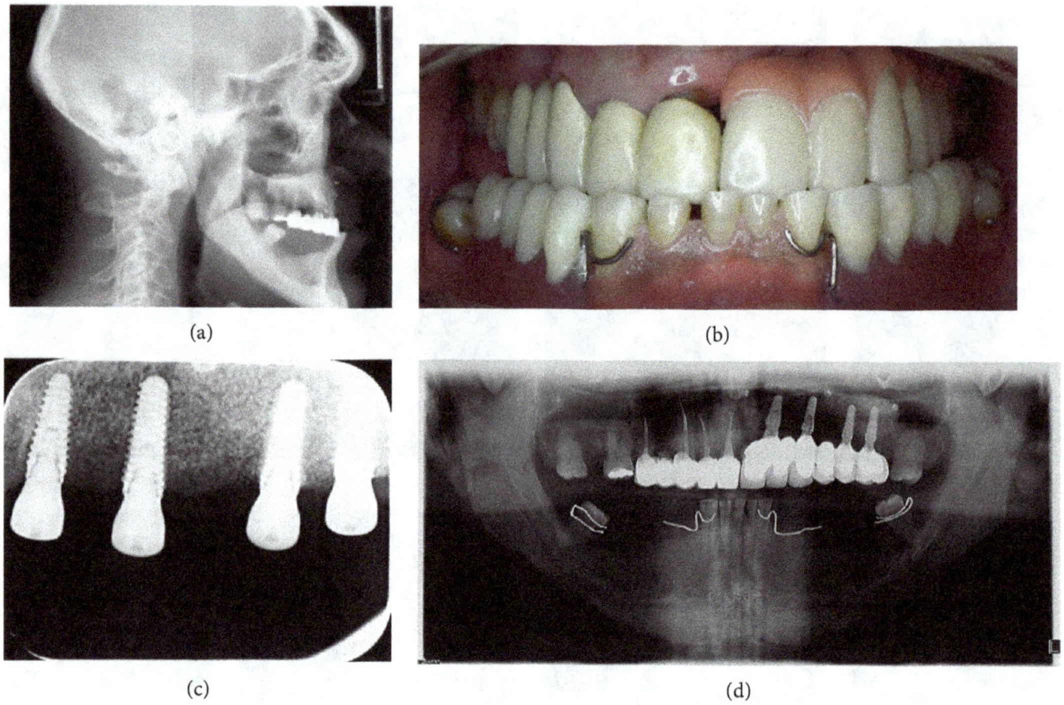

FIGURE 4: (a) Cephalometric radiograph made before implant placement. (b) Frontal intraoral view with the restorations. (c) Retroalveolar X-ray at implant uncovery. (d) Orthopantomography with the restorations.

removable partial denture. It is a known fact that one of the most important conditions for a successful bone graft is stability, which is negatively influenced by the inherent mobility of the removable appliance.

We consider that the favorable outcome of our interventions is also related to the stable condition of the patient after pituitary adenoma removal.

Due to the complex nature of the case and the sagittal intermaxillary relations, we anticipated a difficult prosthetic rehabilitation, by maintaining the crossbite (Figure 4), because the patient refused orthognathic surgery and the overdenture treatment option. Upper and lower restorations must be prepared in crossbite occlusion in order for the masticatory forces to be transmitted to the jaw in an appropriate angle. In centric occlusion, posterior teeth make an 80-degree angle with the frontal and horizontal planes. If the angle is smaller than 70 degrees, crossbite is inevitable [20].

Another challenge that we had was with the quality of the radiographs and CBCT images: due to the atypical anatomy of the patient, the alignment in the X-ray machine was less than ideal. That is why we had to do multiple exposures, so we could analyze the images to the best of our ability.

The initial treatment plan included vertical and horizontal bone augmentation procedures of the right and left mandible and fixed implant-supported restorations after bone formation, also replacing the provisional fixed dental prosthesis from the right maxilla with a definitive metal-ceramic one. The patient could not follow through with this option due to financial reasons; therefore, the removable acrylic partial denture and the fixed composite resin restoration with metal framework we made as provisional prostheses became definitive ones. We first made an implant-supported metal-ceramic restoration for the left maxilla, but ended up changing it to a composite resin with metal framework restoration due to the overall weight of the superstructure. Unfortunately, all of these changes lead to less than desirable aesthetics.

4. Conclusion

In this case report, we were able to show that guided bone regeneration procedures like horizontal ridge augmentation with lateral wall approach sinus graft and horizontal ridge augmentation of the front maxilla can be successful in a patient with acromegaly when autologous bone is not included in the grafting procedure and the patient has a stable condition after pituitary adenoma removal. Unfortunately, the follow-up period of the augmented bone is not very long (two and a half years for the first surgery) and we do not have any follow-up after the delivery of the restoration.

For now, we have a reason to say that in the presented report, bone regeneration procedures were successful, but we cannot make any statement about implant survival in the augmented bone. More research is needed in order to improve the predictability of this type of interventions.

References

[1] H. Godara, A. Hirbe, M. Nassif, H. Otepka, and A. Rosenstock, *The Washington Manual of Medical Therapeutics*, PA: Wolters Kluwer/Lippincott Williams & Wilkins, Philadelphia, 34th edition, 2014.

[2] B. S. Mahesh, S. Padmashree, H. John, and J. Rema, "Acromegaly: oral diagnostician's role in diagnosis: a case report," *IJSS Case Reports & Reviews*, vol. 2, no. 8, pp. 8–11, 2016.

[3] F. Jockenhövel, S. Rohrbach, S. Deggerich, D. Reinwein, and C. Reiners, "Differential presentation of cortical and trabecular peripheral bone mineral density in acromegaly," *European Journal of Medical Research*, vol. 1, no. 8, pp. 377–382, 1996.

[4] M. Madeira, L. V. Neto, F. de Paula Paranhos Neto et al., "Acromegaly has a negative influence on trabecular bone, but not on cortical bone, as assessed by high-resolution peripheral quantitative computed tomography," *The Journal of Clinical Endocrinology and Metabolism*, vol. 98, no. 4, pp. 1734–1741, 2013.

[5] G. Watzek, *Implants in Qualitatively Compromised Bone*, Quintessence Publishing Co, Ltd, New Malden, UK, 2004.

[6] I. Urban, *Vertical and Horizontal Ridge Augmentation*, Quintessence Publishing Co, Ltd, New Malden, UK, 2017.

[7] C. Maiorana, M. Beretta, S. Salina, and F. Santoro, "Reduction of autogenous bone graft resorption by means of Bio-Oss coverage: a prospective study," *The International Journal of Periodontics & Restorative Dentistry*, vol. 25, no. 1, pp. 19–25, 2005.

[8] C. E. Misch, *Contemporary Implant Dentistry*, Mosby Elsevier, St. Louis, Missouri, 2008.

[9] A. Sakkas, F. Wilde, M. Heufelder, K. Winter, and A. Schramm, "Autogenous bone grafts in oral implantology-is it still a "gold standard"? A consecutive review of 279 patients with 456 clinical procedures," *International Journal of Implant Dentistry*, vol. 3, no. 1, p. 23, 2017.

[10] H. H. Horch and C. Pautke, "Regeneration statt reparation," *Mund-, Kiefer- und Gesichtschirurgie*, vol. 10, no. 4, pp. 213–220, 2006.

[11] J. T. Mellonig and R. G. Triplett, "Guided tissue regeneration and endosseous dental implants," *The International Journal of Periodontics & Restorative Dentistry*, vol. 13, no. 2, pp. 108–119, 1993.

[12] C. H. Hämmerle, R. E. Jung, D. Yaman, and N. P. Lang, "Ridge augmentation by applying bioresorbable membranes and deproteinized bovine bone mineral: a report of twelve consecutive cases," *Clinical Oral Implants Research*, vol. 19, no. 1, pp. 19–25, 2008.

[13] G. Mendoza-Azpur, A. Fuente, E. Chavez, E. Valdivia, and I. Khouly, "Horizontal ridge augmentation with guided bone regeneration using particulate xenogenic bone substitutes with or without autogenous block grafts: a randomized controlled trial," *Clinical Implant Dentistry and Related Research*, vol. 21, no. 4, pp. 521–530, 2019.

[14] I. A. Urban, J. L. Lozada, S. A. Jovanovic, H. Nagursky, and K. Nagy, "Vertical ridge augmentation with titanium-reinforced, dense-PTFE membranes and a combination of particulated autogenous bone and anorganic bovine bone-derived mineral: a prospective case series in 19 patients," *The International Journal of Oral & Maxillofacial Implants*, vol. 29, no. 1, pp. 185–193, 2014.

[15] D. Buser, U. Brägger, N. P. Lang, and S. Nyman, "Regeneration and enlargement of jaw bone using guided tissue regeneration," *Clinical Oral Implants Research*, vol. 1, no. 1, pp. 22–32, 1990.

[16] T. von Arx and D. Buser, "Horizontal ridge augmentation using autogenous block grafts and the guided bone regeneration technique with collagen membranes: a clinical study with 42 patients," *Clinical Oral Implants Research*, vol. 17, no. 4, pp. 359–366, 2006.

[17] V. Chappuis, Y. Cavusoglu, D. Buser, and T. von Arx, "Lateral ridge augmentation using autogenous block grafts and guided bone regeneration: a 10-year prospective case series study," *Clinical Implant Dentistry and Related Research*, vol. 19, no. 1, pp. 85–96, 2017.

[18] F. Khoury and T. Hanser, "Three-dimensional vertical alveolar ridge augmentation in the posterior maxilla: a 10-year clinical study," *The International Journal of Oral & Maxillofacial Implants*, vol. 34, no. 2, pp. 471–480, 2019.

[19] F. Khoury, "The bony lid approach in pre-implant and implant surgery: a prospective study," *European Journal of Oral Implantology*, vol. 6, no. 4, pp. 375–384, 2013.

[20] O. F. Karaalioğlu and Z. Yeşil Duymuş, "Prosthetic restoration of a patient with acromegaly - a case report," *Atatürk Üniv Diş Hek Fak Derg*, vol. 19, no. 1, pp. 41–46, 2009.

22

Glandular Odontogenic Cyst in Dentigerous Relationship: An Uncommon Case Report

Jean Carlos Barbosa Ferreira,[1] Eneida Franco Vêncio,[2] Rodrigo Tavares de Sá,[1] and Giovanni Gasperini[1]

[1]*Department of Oral and Maxillofacial Surgery, Clinical Hospital, Federal University of Goiás, Goiânia, Brazil*
[2]*Department of Oral Medicine (Oral Pathology), Dental School, Federal University of Goiás, Goiânia, Brazil*

Correspondence should be addressed to Giovanni Gasperini; gasperinibuco@gmail.com

Academic Editor: Roberto Sacco

Glandular odontogenic cyst (GOC) is an uncommon cyst of the jaw. Less than 200 cases are reported in the literature, and only 22 cases are associated with an unerupted tooth (dentigerous relationship). Although it is an asymptomatic lesion, it can be destructive and has high recurrence rates. The diagnosis can be especially challenging due to the lack of distinct diagnostic clinic-radiological criteria and nonspecific microscopic features, mimicking benign and malignant lesions. Conservative surgical treatment has been the choice for most surgeons, but marginal or partial jaw resection has been reported. This report describes a rare case of GOC in a dentigerous relationship, which was treated with enucleation and peripheral osteotomy.

1. Introduction

Glandular odontogenic cysts (GOCs) are uncommon jawbone cysts of odontogenic origin which were firstly described in 1987 by Padayachee and Van Wyk [1] as a "botryoid" odontogenic cyst with glandular component and denominated "sialo-odontogenic cyst." Gardner et al. [2] in 1988 established this cyst as a distinct entity-denominated glandular odontogenic cyst, which was classified as an odontogenic cyst by the WHO in 1992 [3].

To the best of our knowledge, there are 196 GOCs in the English literature [4–14]. Clinically, GOCs are small and usually appear as an asymptomatic swelling, though a few cases have presented with pain and paresthesia. The most common site is the mandible, particularly the anterior region. The cyst shows no sex predilection and mostly affects middle-aged individuals, between 45 and 50 years old; however, there are also reports in pediatric patients [4, 15]. According to Kaplan et al. [16], its recurrence rate is around 35.9%, particularly when conservative surgical treatment is chosen.

Radiographically, it presents as a uni- or multilocular cystic lesion, with well-defined margins, though some lesions exhibit scalloped borders. Other findings include loss of cortical integrity, root resorption, and association with unerupted teeth [15]. Some cases show a dentigerous, lateral periodontal, and "globulomaxillary" relationship [17].

Microscopically, the diagnosis of GOC can be challenging, given the rarity of the lesion and the fact that the differential diagnosis includes benign and malignant lesions, such as botryoid cysts, surgical ciliated cysts, radicular or dentigerous cysts with metaplastic changes, and low-grade mucoepidermoid carcinoma (MEC) [14, 16, 17]. Histopathological features for the GOC have been described, but the exact microscopic criteria necessary for diagnosis have not been universally accepted. These features include a nonkeratinized stratified squamous lining epithelium with focal thickening (plaques) in the cystic lining, eosinophilic

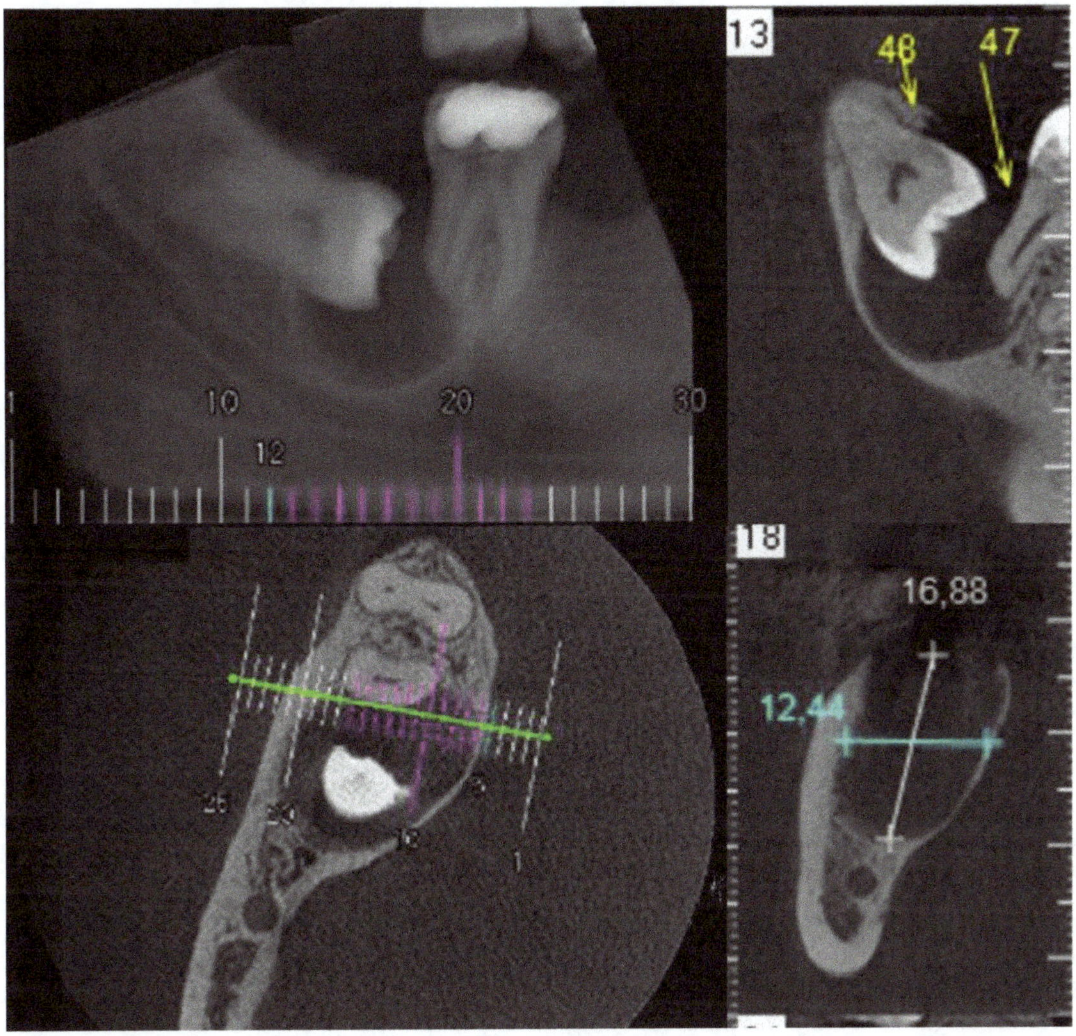

FIGURE 1: Preoperative CBCT showing well-defined unilocular radiolucency associated with an impacted right third molar extending to the distal root of the second molar.

cuboidal or ciliated columnar cells, mucous cells, and interepithelial gland-like structures [1–3, 16].

Several treatment modalities have been indicated for the GOCs, including conservative approaches, such as enucleation with or without curettage, marsupialization, peripheral ostectomy and chemical cauterization with Carnoy's solution, and marginal resection/partial jaw resection [4]. This report documents an uncommon case of GOC in a dentigerous relationship (GOC-DR), which was treated with enucleation and peripheral osteotomy.

2. Case Report

A 36-year-old male, with no medical history, was referred to the Clinical Hospital of the Federal University of Goiás, Goiânia, Goiás, Brazil, for evaluation of an asymptomatic radiolucent lesion in the posterior mandible region. Cone-beam computed tomography (CBCT) scan showed a well-defined unilocular radiolucency associated with an impacted right third molar, extending to the distal root of the second molar, measuring 17 × 12.5 mm (Figure 1). Intraoral examination revealed signs of healthy gingiva; absence of teeth 16, 36, 37, and 46; and absence of bone expansion. However, clinical attachment loss in the distal root of tooth 47 with pulp vitality was verified. Previous aspiration was negative and previous diagnosis of dentigerous cyst was made. Due to the small size of the lesion, the treatment choice included tooth removal, enucleation, and peripheral osteotomy. A thick cystic wall was evident during the surgical procedures.

The histopathological examination revealed cyst wall lining by nonkeratinized stratified squamous epithelium with varied thickness (Figure 2(a)). Duct-like structures surrounded by cuboidal cells and numerous mucous cells were also identified (Figures 2(b) and 2(c)). The superficial layer of the epithelium showed columnar ciliated and eosinophilic cuboidal cells, also called "hobnail cells" (Figure 2(d)).

Glycogen-rich and mucin-secreting cells were highlighted by periodic acid-Schiff (PAS), periodic acid-Schiff diastase

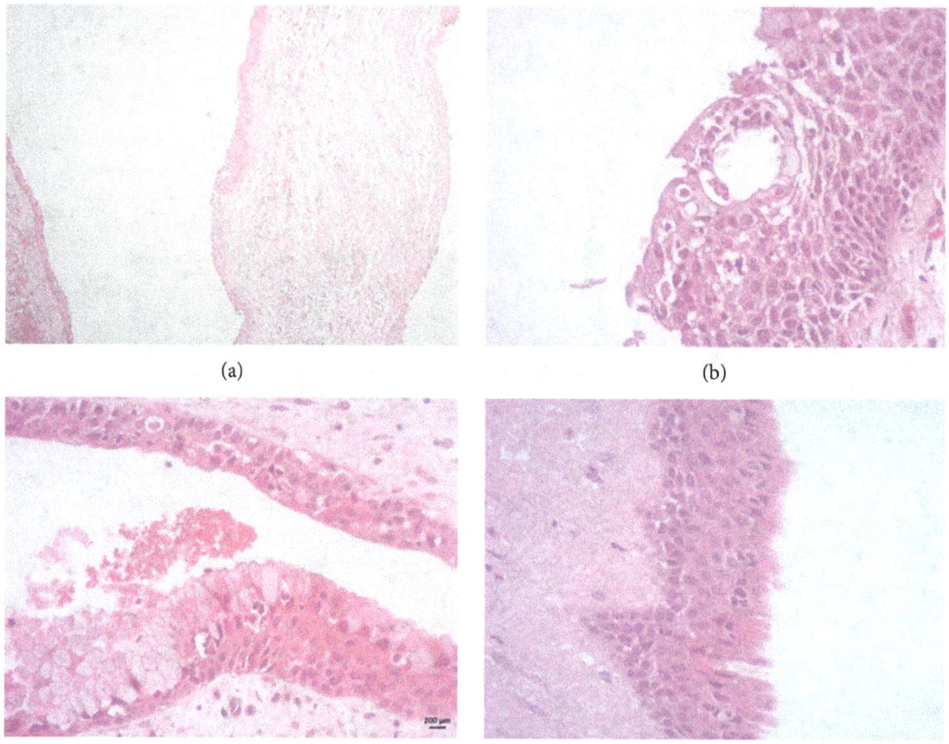

FIGURE 2: Microscopic features of the GOC. (a) Cystic cavity lined by nonkeratinized stratified squamous epithelium of varying thickness. (b) Duct-like structures observed in the cystic lining. (c) Presence of numerous goblet cells. (d) Note the presence of eosinophilic cuboidal cells. Slides stained with haematoxylin and eosin. Original magnifications: 50x and 400x.

(PAS-D) (Figures 3(a)–3(c)), and mucicarmine staining (Figure 3(d)). A final diagnosis of GOC was made following the criteria established by Fowler et al. [17]. The postoperative orthopantomogram (OPG) revealed no recurrence one year postsurgery (Figure 4).

3. Discussion

Our study reports an uncommon case of GOC associated with an unerupted third molar mimicking a dentigerous cyst. This characteristic was defined by Fowler et al. [17] as a "dentigerous relationship." In the English literature, only 22 similar cases have been documented [18–22].

Table 1 [17–27] summarizes previous published cases of GOC-DR. Complete clinical data was not be available in all cases. Males were more often affected (male : female ratio, 3 : 1) and age ranged from 21 to 62 years old (mean 38 years old). The mandible was affected in 53.8% of cases, in which 57.1% involved the unerupted third molar and 42.8% the canine. Swelling was the most common clinical presentation with 85.7%, followed by pain (28.5%), and numbness (14.2%). Unilocular radiolucency was described in 10 cases (76.9%). Half of the cases were treated with enucleation, followed by curettage (41.6%) and block resection (8.3%). In the present case, a 36-year-old male presented an asymptomatic mandibular lesion detected incidentally by routine radiological examination treated with enucleation and peripheral osteotomy [4, 16, 18, 21, 22]. It should be noted that unlike classic GOC, GOC-DR has a strong predilection for the male sex and posterior mandible.

Clinical diagnosis of GOC is challenging. The differential diagnosis includes radicular and dentigerous cysts, odontogenic keratocysts, and ameloblastoma. Although Krishnamurthy et al. [19] suggest that a preoperative aspiration biopsy may be helpful in diagnosing GOC, in our case, it was negative, as reported by Momeni Roochi et al. [23]. Distinct fluids have been reported in the literature, including clear with low viscosity, creamy high-viscosity, and brownish-red liquids [19, 23, 28, 29]. Another interesting clinical finding in our case was the presence of a thick cystic wall, contrary to findings shown by Thor et al. [30].

The histopathological diagnosis of GOC also remains a challenge. Microscopic features include focal epithelial thickening, epithelial plaques, and glycogen-rich epithelial cells, which are also observed in botryoid and lateral periodontal cysts. The presence of ciliated epithelium and duct-like spaces with mucous cells and eosinophilic cuboidal cells located in the epithelial surface support the diagnosis of GOC [17, 31]. According to Fowler et al. [17], the presence of microcysts, clear cells, and epithelial spheres may be helpful in distinguishing GOC-DR from dentigerous cyst with metaplastic changes. The most important and difficult distinction according to Kaplan et al. [16] is the differentiation of low-grade MEC from GOC, especially its multicystic

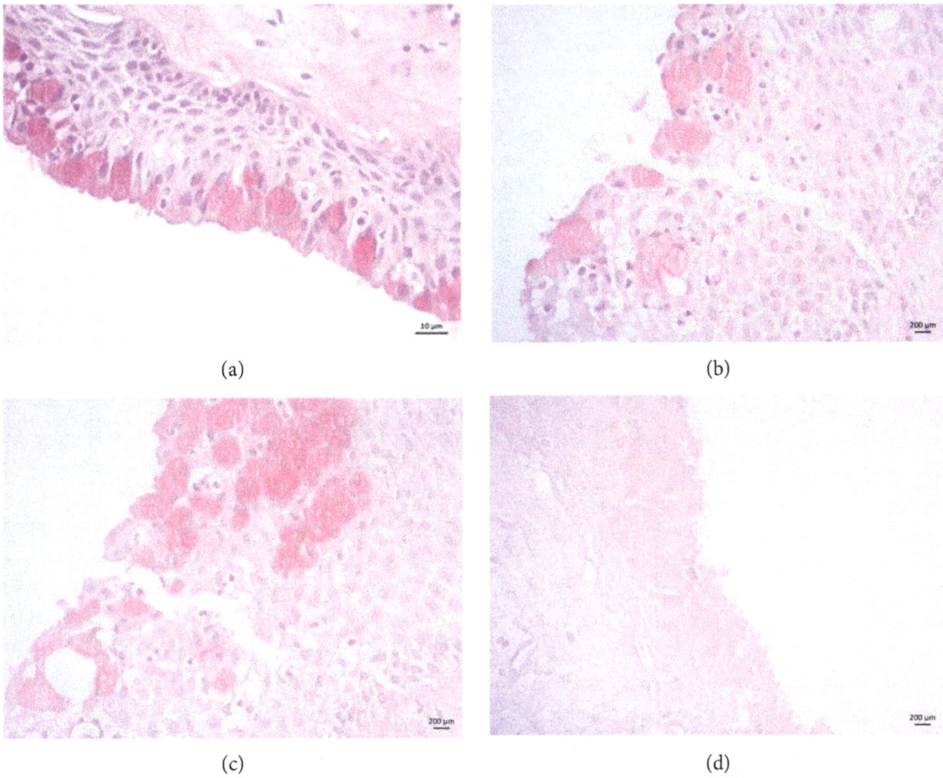

FIGURE 3: Special stains for GOC. (a, b) Periodic acid-Schiff- (PAS-) and periodic acid-Schiff diastase- (PAS-D-) positive goblet cells showing glycogen-rich cells. (c) Note the glandular-like structure stained by PAS-D. Mucin-secreting cells were also identified.

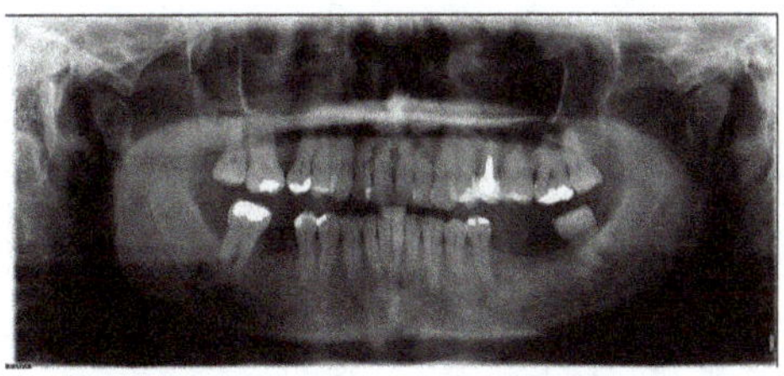

FIGURE 4: Patient's orthopantomogram (OPG) showing bone healing after a 2-year follow-up.

variant. Ciliated cells, superficial cuboidal cells, epithelial whorls, and intraepithelial microcyst or duct-like structures are not typical for low-grade MEC, which can help in the differentiation. Immunostain for MASPIN, Ki-67, and CKs 18 and 19 may be helpful to distinguish GOC from low-grade MEC [14].

Due to the overlapping of histological features with others lesions, Fowler et al. [17] suggested 10 microscopic parameters for diagnosing GOC: surface eosinophilic cuboidal cells or "hobnail cells", intraepithelial microcysts or duct-like spaces lined by a single layer of cuboidal to columnar cells, apocrine snouting of hobnail cells, clear or vacuolated cells, variable thickness in the cyst lining, papillary projections or "tufting" into the cyst lumen, mucous goblet cells, epithelial spheres, or plaque-like thickening cilia, and multiple compartments. According to the authors, the presence of seven or more microscopic parameters is highly predictive of a diagnosis of GOC. In our case, only multiple compartments and papillary projections were not evidenced.

Minor surgical procedures, such as enucleation with or without curettage and peripheral ostectomy, are the most common treatment modalities reported in the literature [4, 32]. In this study, enucleation associated with peripheral osteotomy was performed due to three factors: patient choice, clinical and radiological diagnosis of a dentigerous cyst, and lesion size (17 × 12.5 mm). On the other hand, radical treatments, such as marginal resection, can sometimes be considered due to the biological behavior of GCO, particularly due to local aggressiveness and recurrence rates around 21-55% [15, 19, 33]. Some reports suggest that recurrence is more common in larger lesions, with cortical bone perforation and multilocular radiographic appearance [30, 32]. In the present case, neither of these characteristics was evident and no recurrence was detected after two years follow-up.

4. Conclusion

This report describes an uncommon case of GOC-DR mimicking other lesions in the oral cavity. These lesions tend to most commonly affect the posterior mandible and younger male patients.

TABLE 1: Clinical and radiological data of GOC in dentigerous relationship.

Year	Author	Number of cases	Age/gender	Site	Clinical presentation	Radiologic features	Treatment	Follow-up (year)
2019	Ferreira et al. (our case)	1	36/M	Mandibular right third molar	Asymptomatic	Unilocular radiolucency	Enucleation/peripheral osteotomy	1
2015	Momeni Roochi et al. [23]	1	62/M	Mandibular right canine impacted	Swelling	Unilocular radiolucency	Enucleation	3
2012	Cano et al. [18]	1	54/M	Mandibular right third molar (ramus/body)	Swelling	Multilocular radiolucent, large and well-defined	Enucleation and curettage, reconstruction	3
2011	Fowler et al. [17]	8	NS	NS	NS	NS	NS	NS
2009	Krishnamurthy et al. [19]	1	21/M	Mandibular left third molar	Swelling	Multilocular radiolucency	En bloc resection	2
2006	Kasaboglu et al. [24]	1	45/M	Mandibular left canine	Swelling and numbness	Unilocular radiolucency with a well-defined border	Enucleation	0.5
2006	Shen et al. [25]	2	Case 1: 40/M; case 2: NS	Case 1: maxillary tooth-like structures; case 2: NS	Case 1: NS; case 2: NS	Case 1: unilocular radiolucency; case 2: NS	Case 1: NS; case 2: NS	NS
2006	Yoon et al. [20]	1	66/F	Mandibular right third molar	Swelling and painful	Unilocular radiolucency, thin sclerotic margin, root resorption	Enucleation	1
2005	Qin et al. [26]	5*	Case 1: 28/M; case 2: 40/M; case 3: 25/M; case 4: 22/M; case 5: 52/F	Case 1: maxilla L (21-27); case 2: maxilla R (11-16); case 3: maxilla R (13-16); case 4: maxilla L (21-23); case 5: maxilla (16-25)	Case 1: NS; case 2: NS; case 3: NS; case 4: NS; case 5: NS	Case 1: Unilocular radiolucency; case 2: unilocular radiolucency, irregular borders; case 3: unilocular radiolucency, irregular borders; case 4: unilocular radiolucency; case 5: multilocular radiolucency	Case 1: curettage; case 2: curettage; case 3: curettage; case 4: curettage; case 5: curettage	NS
2005	Kaplan et al. [21, 22]	1	49/M	Mandibular left third molar	Swelling and painless	Unilocular radiolucency	Enucleation, peripheral ostectomy, reconstruction with iliac crest & alloplast bone graft	4
1996	Ide et al. [27]	1	54/F	Mandibular right canine	Asymptomatic	Unilocular radiolucent definite contained the crown of the horizontally impacted right canine	Enucleation	1

Legend: NS: not specified; M: male; F: female; L: left; R: right. *Case 2 shown in the work of Shen et al. [25].

Consent

The patient has given his consent for the use of his pictures in this article.

Acknowledgments

This report was funded by Coordenação de Aperfeiçoamento de Pessoal de Nível Superior (CAPES/BRASIL; process number: 88887.295564/2018-00) and Fundação de Amparo à Pesquisa do Estado de Goiás (FAPEG).

References

[1] A. Padayachee and C. W. Van Wyk, "Two cystic lesions with features of both the botryoid odontogenic cyst and the central mucoepidermoid tumour: sialo-odontogenic cyst?," *Journal of Oral Pathology and Medicine*, vol. 16, no. 10, pp. 499–504, 1987.

[2] D. G. Gardner, H. P. Kessler, R. Morency, and D. L. Schaffner, "The glandular odontogenic cyst: an apparent entity," *Journal of Oral Pathology and Medicine*, vol. 17, no. 8, pp. 359–366, 1988.

[3] I. R. H. Kramer, J. J. Pindborg, and M. Shear, "The WHO histological typing of odontogenic tumors. A commentary on the second edition," *Cancer*, vol. 70, no. 12, pp. 2988–2994, 1992.

[4] M. Faisal, S. A. Ahmad, and U. Ansari, "Glandular odontogenic cyst – literature review and report of a paediatric case," *Journal of Oral Biology and Craniofacial Research*, vol. 5, no. 3, pp. 219–225, 2015.

[5] B. Chandolia, M. Bajpai, and M. Arora, "Glandular odontogenic cyst," *Journal of the College of Physicians Surgeons Pakistan*, vol. 27, no. 3, pp. 23–25, 2017.

[6] M. Alaeddini, N. Eshghyar, and S. Etemad-Moghadam, "Expression of podoplanin and TGF-beta in glandular odontogenic cyst and its comparison with developmental and inflammatory odontogenic cystic lesions," *Journal of Oral Pathology & Medicine*, vol. 46, no. 1, pp. 76–80, 2017.

[7] İ. Akkaş, O. Toptaş, F. Özan, and F. Yılmaz, "Bilateral glandular odontogenic cyst of mandible: a rare occurrence," *Journal of Maxillofacial and Oral Surgery*, vol. 14, no. S1, pp. 443–447, 2015.

[8] N. R. Figueiredo, A. D. Dinkar, and M. M. Khorate, "Glandular odontogenic cyst of the maxilla: a case report and literature review," *The Pan African Medical Journal*, vol. 25, p. 116, 2016.

[9] A. A. Shah, A. Sangle, S. Bussari, and A. V. Koshy, "Glandular odontogenic cyst: a diagnostic dilemma," *Indian Journal of Dentistry*, vol. 7, no. 1, pp. 38–43, 2016.

[10] K. L. S. Kumar, S. Manuel, B. J. Nair, and S. Vinod Nair, "An ambiguous asymptomatic swelling in the maxillary anterior region - a case report," *International Journal of Surgery Case Report*, vol. 23, pp. 65–69, 2016.

[11] E. Bulut, B. Baş, D. Dinçer, and Ö. Günhan, "Treatment of maxillary glandular odontogenic cyst involving the same place of previously treated traumatic bone cyst," *Journal of Craniofacial Surgery*, vol. 27, no. 2, pp. e150–e153, 2016.

[12] S. Chandra, E. S. Reddy, K. Sah, and A. Srivastava, "Maxillary glandular odontogenic cyst: an uncommon entity at an unusual site," *Archives of Iranian Medicine*, vol. 19, no. 3, pp. 221–224, 2016.

[13] A. Mittal, V. Narang, G. Kaur, and N. Sood, "Glandular odontogenic cyst of mandible: a rare entity," *Journal of Clinical and Diagnostic Research*, vol. 9, no. 12, pp. 9-10, 2015.

[14] M. Mascitti, A. Santarelli, A. Sabatucci et al., "Glandular odontogenic cyst: review of literature and report of a new case with cytokeratin-19 expression," *The Open Dentistry Journal*, vol. 8, no. 1, pp. 1–12, 2014.

[15] J. A. Regezi, "Odontogenic cysts, odontogenic tumors, fibroosseous and giant cell lesions of the jaws," *Modern Pathology*, vol. 15, no. 3, pp. 331–341, 2002.

[16] I. Kaplan, Y. Anavi, and A. Hirshberg, "Glandular odontogenic cyst: a challenge in diagnosis and treatment," *Oral Diseases*, vol. 14, no. 7, pp. 575–581, 2008.

[17] C. B. Fowler, R. B. Brannon, H. P. Kessler, J. T. Castle, and M. A. Kahn, "Glandular odontogenic cyst: analysis of 46 cases with special emphasis on microscopic criteria for diagnosis," *Head and Neck Pathology*, vol. 5, no. 4, pp. 364–375, 2011.

[18] J. Cano, D. M. Benito, J. Montáns, J. F. Rodríguez-Vázquez, J. Campo, and C. Colmenero, "Glandular odontogenic cyst: two high-risk cases treated with conservative approaches," *Journal of Cranio-Maxillofacial Surgery*, vol. 40, no. 5, pp. e131–e136, 2012.

[19] A. Krishnamurthy, H. J. Sherlin, K. Ramalingam et al., "Glandular odontogenic cyst: report of two cases and review of literature," *Head and Neck Pathology*, vol. 3, no. 2, pp. 153–158, 2009.

[20] J. H. Yoon, S. G. Ahn, S. G. Kim, and J. Kim, "An unusual odontogenic cyst with diverse histologic features," *Yonsei Medical Journal*, vol. 47, no. 1, pp. 122–125, 2006.

[21] I. Kaplan, Y. Anavi, R. Manor, J. Sulkes, and S. Calderon, "The use of molecular markers as an aid in the diagnosis of glandular odontogenic cyst," *Oral Oncology*, vol. 41, no. 9, pp. 895–902, 2006.

[22] I. Kaplan, G. Gal, Y. Anavi, R. Manor, and S. Calderon, "Glandular odontogenic cyst: treatment and recurrence," *Journal of Oral and Maxillofacial Surgery*, vol. 63, no. 4, pp. 435–441, 2005.

[23] M. Momeni Roochi, I. Tavakoli, F. M. Ghazi, and A. Tavakoli, "Case series and review of glandular odontogenic cyst with emphasis on treatment modalities," *Journal of Cranio-Maxillofacial Surgery*, vol. 43, no. 6, pp. 746–750, 2015.

[24] O. Kasaboglu, Z. Basal, and A. Usubütün, "Glandular odontogenic cyst presenting as a dentigerous cyst: a case report," *Journal of Oral and Maxillofacial Surgery*, vol. 64, no. 4, pp. 731–733, 2006.

[25] J. Shen, M. Fan, X. Chen, S. Wang, L. Wang, and Y. Li, "Glandular odontogenic cyst in China: report of 12 cases and immunohistochemical study," *Journal of Oral Pathology & Medicine*, vol. 35, no. 3, pp. 175–182, 2006.

[26] X.-N. Qin, J.-R. Li, X.-M. Chen, and X. Long, "The glandular odontogenic cyst: clinicopathologic features and treatment of 14 cases," *Journal of Oral and Maxillofacial Surgery*, vol. 63, no. 5, pp. 694–699, 2005.

[27] F. Ide, T. Shimoyama, and N. Horie, "Glandular odontogenic cyst with hyaline bodies: an unusual dentigerous presentation," *Journal of Oral Pathology & Medicine*, vol. 25, no. 7, pp. 401–404, 1996.

[28] H. H. Araújo de Morais, R. José de Holanda Vasconcellos, T. de Santana Santos, L. M. Guedes Queiroz, and É. J. Dantas da Silveira, "Glandular odontogenic cyst: case report and

review of diagnostic criteria," *Journal of Cranio-Maxillofacial Surgery*, vol. 40, no. 2, pp. e46–e50, 2012.

[29] H. S. Koppang, S. Johannessen, L. K. Haugen, H. R. Haanaes, T. Solheim, and K. Donath, "Glandular odontogenic cyst (sialo-odontogenic cyst): report of two cases and literature review of 45 previously reported cases," *Journal of Oral Pathology & Medicine*, vol. 27, no. 9, pp. 455–462, 1998.

[30] A. Thor, G. Warfvinge, and R. Fernandes, "The course of a long-standing glandular odontogenic cyst: marginal resection and reconstruction with particulated bone graft, platelet-rich plasma, and additional vertical alveolar distraction," *Journal of Oral and Maxillofacial Surgery*, vol. 64, no. 7, pp. 1121–1128, 2006.

[31] P. Speinght, C. B. Fowler, and H. Kessler, "Odontogenic and non-odontogenic developmental cysts," in *WHO Classification of Head and Neck Tumours*, A. K. El-Naggar, C. JKC, J. R. Grandis, T. Takata, and P. J. Slootweg, Eds., Reed IARC, Lyon, 4th edition, 2017.

[32] P. Boffano, E. Cassarino, E. Zavattero, P. Campisi, and P. Garzino-Demo, "Surgical treatment of glandular odontogenic cysts," *Journal of Craniofacial Surgery*, vol. 21, no. 3, pp. 776–780, 2010.

[33] M. C. N. Lyrio, A. F. de Assis, A. R. Germano, and M. de Moraes, "Treatment of mandibular glandular odontogenic cyst with immediate reconstruction: case report and 5-year follow-up," *British Journal of Oral & Maxillofacial Surgery*, vol. 48, no. 8, pp. 651–653, 2010.

23

Traumatic Dental Injuries: Clinical Case Presentation and a 10-Year Epidemiological Investigation in an Italian Dental Emergency Service

Alberto Murri Dello Diago, Luigi Generali, Roberto Apponi, Vittorio Colombini, and Vittorio Checchi

Department of Surgery, Medicine, Dentistry and Morphological Sciences-Unit of Dentistry and Oral-Maxillo-Facial Surgery, University of Modena and Reggio Emilia, Modena, Italy

Correspondence should be addressed to Alberto Murri Dello Diago; alberto.murridellodiago@gmail.com

Academic Editor: Leandro Napier de Souza

Traumatic dental injuries (TDIs) are very common in the world population, and international literature reports several studies which helped in the definition of international guidelines. The aim of this study is to present two clinical cases of TDI and to investigate epidemiological and etiological aspects of TDIs in patients treated in Modena, Italy, between January 2010 and December 2020. The presented case reports are two explicative clinical cases of successful TDI management with a long-term follow-up. The epidemiological analysis was performed on patients who visited the Dental Emergency Service of the Dentistry and Oral-Maxillo-Facial Surgery Unit of Modena (Italy) over a period of 10 years. Data relating to age, gender, type of trauma, and place of accident were collected. Five-hundred-sixty-five TDIs that occurred to patients from 1 to 68 years old were reported, with a total of 860 injured teeth. The peak age at which TDIs are most represented varies between 2 and 3 years old, and they occurred frequently from 1 up to 7 years old. 57.5% were male, while 42.5% were female. The most common trauma resulted to be the uncomplicated crown fracture (20%), immediately followed by lateral luxation (19%), intrusive luxation (18%), avulsion (17%), and complicated crown fracture (15%). TDIs occurred at home in 44% of cases. The need for more prevention training must be highlighted, due to the fact that many TDIs occur at home and in a preschool age.

1. Introduction

Traumatic dental injuries (TDIs) are common in the worldwide population. Although the oral cavity represents a small component of the human body, TDIs represent 5% of all health injuries and up to 17% in pediatric patients [1]. A recent study shows that more than one billion living people have had TDIs [1]. Scientific literature shows a great variability regarding the incidence and prevalence of TDIs in the world population [2–4]. Although the International Association of Dental Traumatology (IADT) had codified precise guidelines [5–7], this variability is related to several reasons, such as the diversity in TDI classification methods and parameter recording, and the different cultural and social contexts in which the various studies had been performed.

TDIs mainly affect the pediatric population, with a high percentage of preschool children and adolescents, and hardly concern elderly patients, if not in a small percentage [1]. The most frequent TDIs in patients with deciduous teeth are periodontal injuries and luxation, while hard tissue injuries and consequent crown fractures are more specific and related to patients with permanent dentition [7]. Trauma such as avulsion and complicated fractures determine functional and esthetic issues that could affect social relationships; numerous studies have shown how TDIs could lead to relationship difficulties and therefore be the reason for personal, domestic, and social issues [3, 8, 9].

The aim of this article is to present two explicative clinical cases of TDI management and to investigate TDI frequency, patterns, and causes in patients treated in Modena, Italy, between January 2010 and December 2020.

2. Case Presentation

Making use of a digital clinical chart archiving system, TDI cases that occurred at the Dental Emergency Service of the Dental Clinic of Modena University, between 1 January 2010 and 31 December 2020, were selected. All patients have been treated according to the protocols established by the IADT guidelines [5–7], enhanced with photographic documentation, radiographic examination, pulp status evaluation, and instrumental investigations. According to the principle of minimum invasiveness and with the aim of optimizing the oral health-related quality of life, individualized treatment plans for each patient were implemented in line with scientific evidence [10–14].

All the anamnestic questionnaires and the TDI-related information were collected, and the following data were obtained: demographic data (gender and age); causes of trauma (sports injuries, accidents at work, collisions, violence and abuse, unintentional falls, and road accidents); location of the trauma (home, school, leisure activities, sports environment, and work); type of trauma, classified according to IADT classification [5–7]; and teeth involved (permanent or deciduous, maxillary or mandibular, and anterior or posterior). All data were registered into Microsoft Excel version 14.1.0 for Macintosh.

Among all selected TDIs, the management of two explicative and challenging clinical cases is described, following CARE reporting guidelines for case reports.

2.1. Clinical Case #1. A 15-year-old female patient was referred due to traumatic avulsion of her right upper central incisor that occurred during a volleyball game (Figure 1).

This tooth had been kept in an extraoral dry environment for two hours and had a mature apex, and for this reason, nonviable soft tissues were removed from the root with a gauze and endodontic therapy was carried out prior to replantation. After local anesthesia administration, the socket was irrigated with saline solution and carefully checked to exclude the presence of bony fractures. The tooth was then replanted applying slight but firm pressure. The correct position of the tooth was verified clinically and radiographically, and it was stabilized through a passive flexible splint made by a 0.4 mm diameter metal wire bonded to the tooth and to adjacent teeth (Figure 2).

Postoperative instructions included antibiotic therapy with amoxicillin, soft diet for 2 weeks, and soft-bristle toothbrush and chlorhexidine 0.12% mouth rinses, twice a day for 2 weeks. The splint was kept in place for 2 weeks, and the patient was visited after 2, 3, and 6 months and yearly. At the 3-year follow-up visit, the tooth appeared asymptomatic, with physiological mobility, no sensitivity to percussion, and normal percussion sound. No radiotransparency and no radiographic evidence of root resorption were detected (Figure 3).

At the 8-year follow-up visit instead, the tooth presented no mobility, metallic percussion sound, and clinical infraposition. Radiographically, there was evidence of ankylosis-related resorption (Figure 4).

2.2. Clinical Case #2. A 20-year-old male patient was referred due to traumatic root fracture of his left upper central incisor after a bike accident (Figure 5).

A passive and flexible buccal splint with metal stainless steel wire and composite patches was immediately performed and kept for 4 weeks, aimed at stabilizing the mobile coronal segment and maintaining the vitality of the tooth. Soft diet was suggested for 1 week and oral hygiene instructions were delivered, brushing with a soft-bristle toothbrush and rinsing with chlorhexidine 0.12% mouthwash to prevent accumulation of plaque and biofilm.

However, after one month, the tooth still did not respond to electrometric and thermal pulp testing, due to plausible pulp necrosis development. For this reason, an endodontic treatment of the coronal tooth segment to the fracture line had to be performed (Figure 6).

After a further 4 weeks, the patient still referred pain and discomfort of the area, and the decision for a surgical approach had to be taken. An apicectomy with a retrograde canal obturation was performed in order to remove the symptomatology and obtain a complete healing of the area (Figure 7).

Postsurgical instructions included prevention of further injury by avoidance of contact sports, meticulous oral hygiene, and rinsing with an antibacterial agent such as chlorhexidine gluconate 0.12%.

Healing was uneventful, and the patient did not refer pain nor swelling. At the 4-year follow-up visit, clinical and radiographic analysis showed a healed area with a good ossification of the periradicular bone (Figure 8).

2.3. Epidemiological Results. Out of a total of 26355 patients who accessed the Dental Emergency Service unit in the period from January 2010 to December 2020, 565 TDIs were registered. Patients' age varied from 0 to 68 years, and the peak age at which TDIs were most represented varied between 2 and 3 years old; however, it was highly represented from 1 up to 7 years old.

In 40% of the cases, only one tooth was involved, in 38% two teeth, in 15% three teeth, and in 7% four teeth, for a total of 860 injured teeth.

The most frequent injury resulted in an uncomplicated crown fracture (20% of cases), immediately followed by lateral luxation. Successively, this was followed by 18% of intrusive luxation, 17% of avulsion, and 15% of complicated crown fracture (Figure 9). Crown-root fractures were represented in the 2% of the cases. The 57.5% of affected patients were male, while 42.5% were female. The most frequent TDI among males resulted in uncomplicated crown fracture, while the most frequent TDI among females resulted in lateral luxation.

TDIs involved permanent dentition in 63% of patients: maxillary anterior teeth involvement was observed in 55.5% of cases, mandibular anterior in 6.5%, while posterior teeth

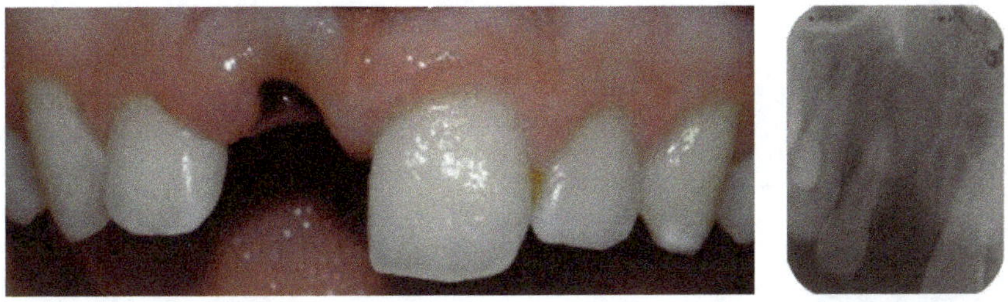

(a) (b)

FIGURE 1: Posttraumatic (a) clinical and (b) radiographic view showing the absence of the upper right central incisor.

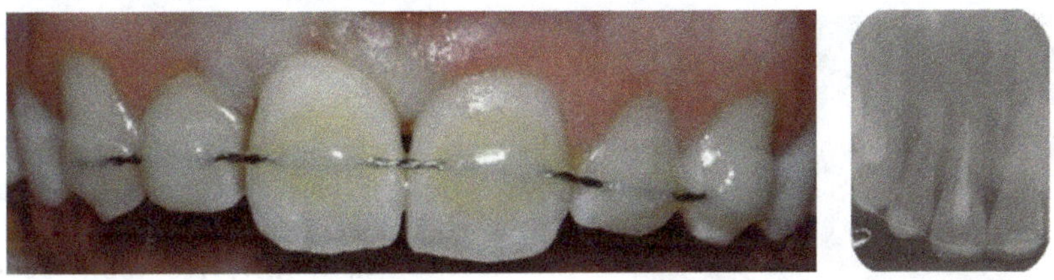

(a) (b)

FIGURE 2: (a) Clinical and (b) radiographic view of the upper incisor after reimplantation and splint.

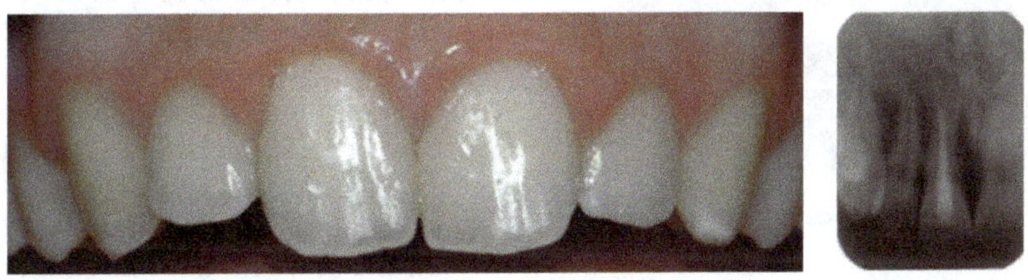

(a) (b)

FIGURE 3: (a) Clinical and (b) radiographic view of the upper incisor at the 3-year follow-up visit.

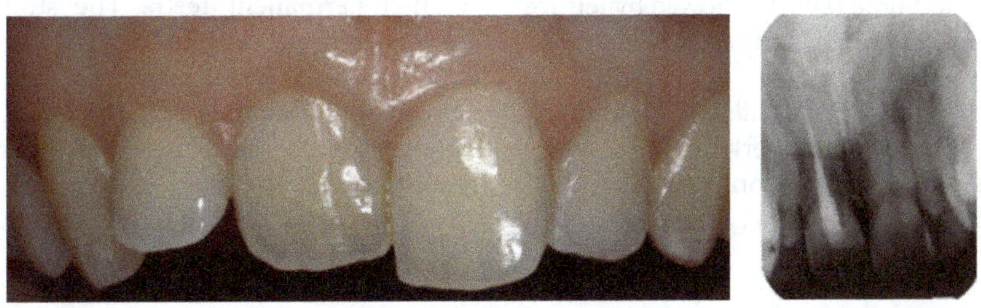

(a) (b)

FIGURE 4: (a) Clinical and (b) radiographic view of the upper incisor at the 8-year follow-up visit: tooth infraposition and root resorption are evident.

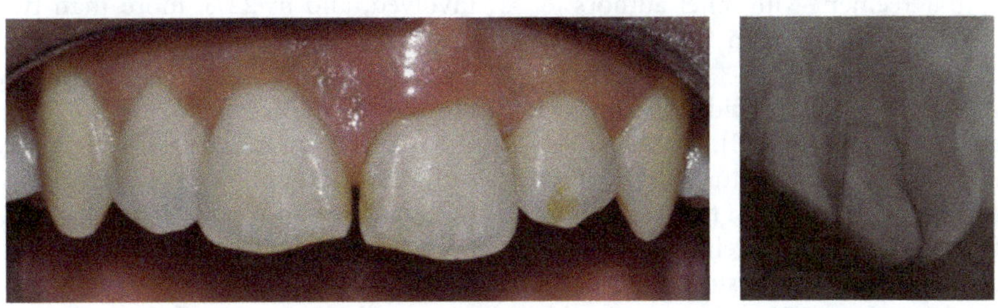

(a) (b)

FIGURE 5: Posttraumatic (a) clinical and (b) radiographic view. Gingival tissues around the upper left central incisor are swollen and red, while a horizontal root fraction is detectable from the periapical X-ray.

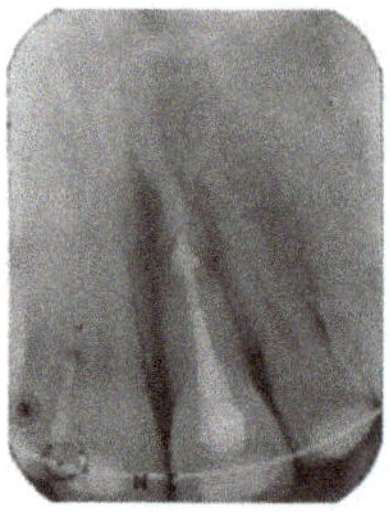

FIGURE 6: Radiographic view of the upper left central incisor after endodontic treatment.

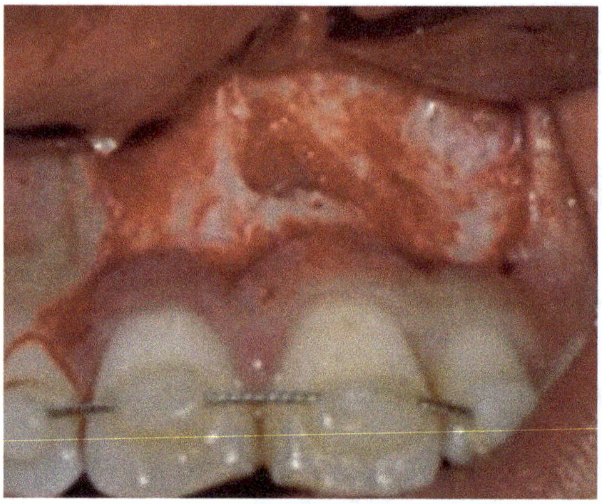

FIGURE 7: Surgical view of the upper left central incisor during apicectomy.

were involved in only 1% of the cases. The remaining 37% involved deciduous teeth.

TDIs occurred mainly at home (44%), followed by leisure activities (23.5%), school (19.5%), and workplace (9%) (Figure 10).

Trauma was caused by unintentional falls in 72% of cases, by road accidents in 8%, by accidents at work in 7%, by sports injuries in 7%, by consequences of collision in 5.5%, and by violence and abuse in the remaining 0.5% (Figure 11).

3. Discussion

In the present epidemiological analysis, avulsions were found in 17% of the total population. When related to deciduous teeth, these represented 11.6%, while in permanent teeth these represented 5.4%, in agreement with other authors [6, 15], but proportionally slightly higher than the percentage reported by Andreasen et al. (4%) [16].

In a recent comprehensive review, guidelines for the treatment of avulsed teeth were published [6]. In these cases, the choice of treatment is related to the maturity of the root (open or closed apex) and to the condition of the periodontal ligament (PDL) cells. The survival of these cells is dependent on the time out of the mouth and on the storage liquid in which the avulsed tooth is kept, since PDL cells are nonviable after an extraalveolar dry time of 30 minutes [6]. In Clinical Case #1, the total extraoral dry time had been more than 60 minutes, and therefore, the PDL cells were likely to be nonviable. Literature demonstrated that delayed replantation has a poor long-term prognosis and that the periodontal ligament becomes necrotic, is not expected to regenerate, and the expected outcome is ankylosis-related root resorption [6]. The goal of replantation in Clinical Case #1 was to restore, although temporarily, esthetics and function while maintaining alveolar bone height, width, and contour.

The possibility of replacing avulsed tooth in a growing patient with implant-prosthetic rehabilitations through mini-implants has proved to be an effective therapeutic option [17–22].

In this epidemiological analysis, luxation occurred in 41% of the total cases: 27.2% in deciduous teeth and 13.9% in permanent teeth. Lateral luxation represented 20% and intrusive luxation 18%, while extrusive luxation occurred only in 3% of the sample. These data represent a high frequency if compared with Andreasen et al.'s results who reported 9% frequency for nonspecific luxations [16]. Treatment usually involves tooth reposition and semiflexible splinting, as documented by the IADT guidelines [5–7].

Similarly to Andreasen et al.'s results [16], the present epidemiological analysis reported that complicated crown fractures occurred in 15% of the cases, showing a higher frequency than other studies [3, 23]. The most represented TDI was the uncomplicated crown fracture, observed in 20% of the cases, while other authors reported different frequencies, such as 13% [23], 86% [24], 94% [6], and 50% [16]. In these cases, a therapeutic approach with a direct composite reconstruction should be preferably performed.

In the present data collection, crown-root fractures were represented in 2% of the cases: 0.3% concerned deciduous teeth and 1.7% concerned permanent teeth. Root fractures were 3%: 0.2% concerned deciduous teeth and 2.8% concerned permanent teeth. The study by Andreasen et al. instead reports different results, such as 9% of crown-root fractures and 7% of root fractures [16]. The treatment of crown-root fractures depends on the level of the fracture along the root, and therefore different kinds of therapies could be addressed.

In accordance with Glendor et al., it was observed that in 55% of the cases, the involved teeth were permanent maxillary incisors, while in 6.5%, those involved were the permanent mandibular ones [3, 8]. Deciduous teeth were involved in 37% of the cases, according to Piovesan et al.'s results that reported rates between 9.4% and 41% [24, 25]. In 40% of the cases, only one tooth was involved; in 36%, two teeth were involved; and in 22%, more than two teeth were involved. This was different from Andreasen et al.'s study that reported a greater difference in cases involving one (80%) and two (18%) teeth [16].

A recent comprehensive review gave useful indications for the treatment of root fractures [5]. In detail, no endodontic treatment should be started at the emergency visit since pulp necrosis and infection could develop later and usually in the coronal fragment only [5]. If endodontic therapy is requested, treatment of the only coronal segment is indicated, and apexification may be needed if the determination of the root canal length may be challenging due to oblique fracture lines [5]. In Clinical Case #2, root canal therapy

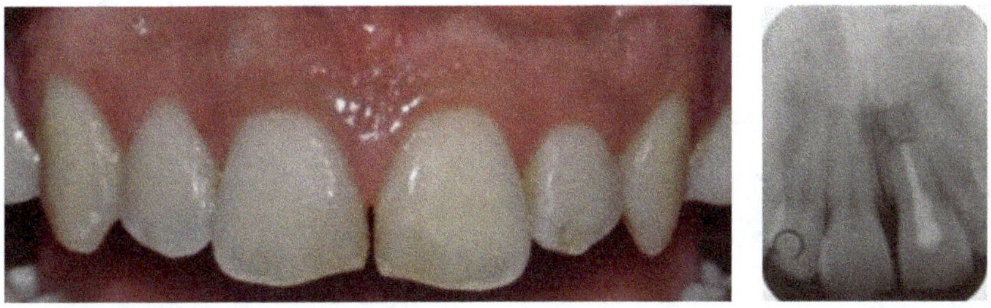

(a) (b)

FIGURE 8: (a) Clinical and (b) radiographic view 4 years after the surgical therapy.

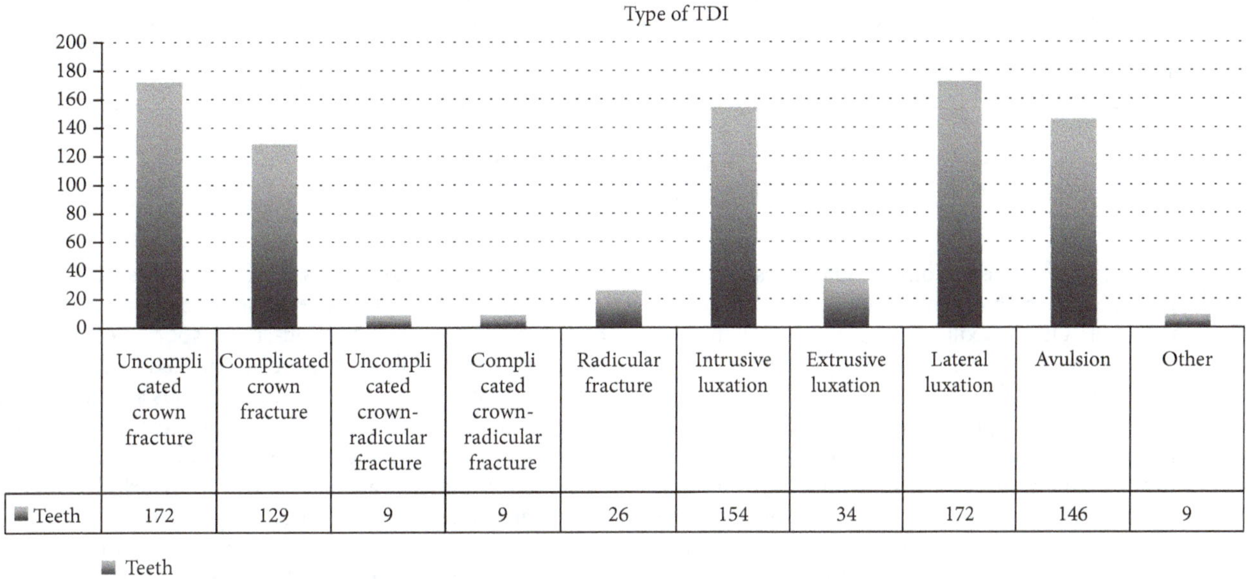

FIGURE 9: TDI frequency based on the type of injury.

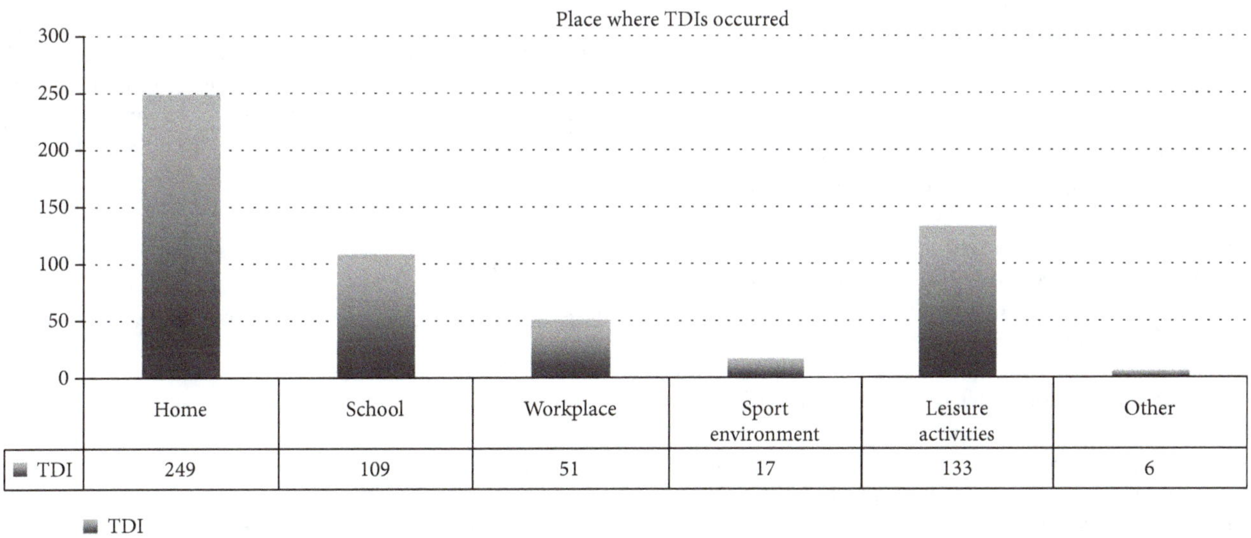

FIGURE 10: TDI frequency based on the place where injuries occurred.

had to be performed after one month since the tooth did not respond to thermal pulp testing nor electrometric test. Following IADT guidelines, only the coronal part of the fractured tooth was treated. However, after another month, a surgical approach had to be chosen in order to solve the patient's symptomatology that was still present.

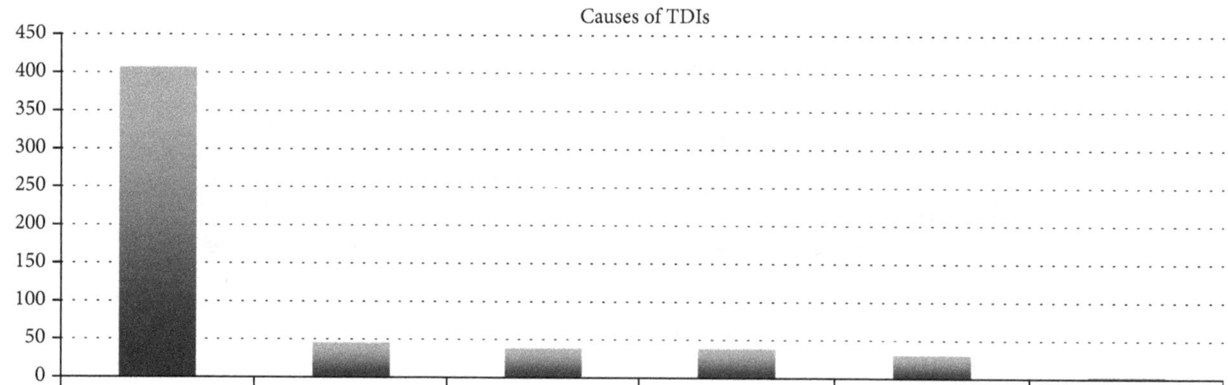

	Unintentional falls	Road accident	Accident at work	Sport injuries	Collision	Violence and abuse
TDI	407	46	39	39	31	3

■ TDI

FIGURE 11: TDI frequency based on the cause of injury.

The results of this epidemiological analysis show that TDI frequency treated in the Dental Emergency Service of the Dentistry and Oral-Maxillo-Facial Surgery Unit of Modena, Italy, are in line with what is recorded in other national and international data.

Concerning a patient's age, the results of this epidemiological investigation are only partially in agreement with previous researches that, although with a larger population sample, revealed a TDI average age incidence of about 15 years [3, 8]. In our case, the peak diagnosis of TDIs has been observed between 2 and 3 years old. The mobility skills of a child between 2 and 3 years of age are still to be developed since they must still acquire an adult confidence. However, the desire to overcome personal limits often pushes the child to test himself, thus risking his own safety, and these aspects could explain the TDI peak incidence in this age group. Other possible causes, such as lack of supervision or child abuse, have to be considered.

In accordance with previous studies [3, 8, 9], about 46% of TDIs were however found in the age group between 1 and 7 years (preschool). At this stage of life, children are very dynamic and sports activities are increasingly practiced, leading to TDIs being consequently much more frequent.

As demonstrated by several studies [3, 8, 9], a prevalence of TDI has been observed among male subjects (57.5%), rather than female (42.5%). This prevalence appears equal to the findings of Glendor et al.'s results that show a 2 : 1 ratio of TDIs between males and females [7].

Concerning TDI reasons, it emerged that the main cause was an unintentional fall, especially in preschool age, which most frequently caused luxation and avulsion. Domestic falls and accidental impacts against objects, in particular interior furnishings such as tables, chairs, and sinks, were recorded in 72% of total cases.

Road accidents, which range from falling from a bicycle or moped to, more rarely, car accidents, were reported in 8% of the cases. According to these data, accidents at work are also frequent along with sports injuries, causing a significant incidence of avulsions. Different types of TDIs can be observed based on the type of sport activity and therefore of the impact dynamic. High-speed sports seem to lead to bone fractures, while low-speed sports lead to dental injuries. These data are in agreement with previous studies on the etiology of trauma [22, 26–33]. In fact, sports injuries have been observed in patients aged 12 to 32, road accidents have been observed in patients aged 17 to 62, and workplace accidents have been observed only in adult patients, as well as collisions. In a similar way, in a recent study, the majority of TDI patients were adolescents (27.9%), or younger than 10 years (23.2%). The main cause of TDI was cycling (43.5%), followed by sports such as football and baseball [34].

Although there are well-coded international prevention guidelines, TDIs are still very relevant in pediatric patients. Therefore, there is a need for the development of training and prevention programs for TDI, organizing adequate emergency services, and planning awareness campaigns.

Disclosure

The funding source has no role in conceiving and performing the study.

References

[1] S. Petti, U. Glendor, and L. Andersson, "World traumatic dental injury prevalence and incidence, a meta-analysis—one billion living people have had traumatic dental injuries," *Dental Traumatology*, vol. 34, no. 2, pp. 71–86, 2018.

[2] S. Petti, J. O. Andreasen, U. Glendor, and L. Andersson, "The fifth most prevalent disease is being neglected by public health organizations," *The Lancet Global Health*, vol. 6, no. 10, pp. e1070–e1071, 2018.

[3] U. Glendor, "Epidemiology of traumatic dental injuries—a 12 year review of the literature," *Dental Traumatology*, vol. 24, no. 6, pp. 603–611, 2008.

[4] GBD 2015 Disease and Injury Incidence and Prevalence Collaborators, "Global, regional, and national incidence, prevalence, and years lived with disability for 310 diseases and injuries, 1990-2015: a systematic analysis for the Global Burden of Disease Study 2015," *Lancet*, vol. 388, no. 10053, pp. 1545–1602, 2016.

[5] C. Bourguignon, N. Cohenca, E. Lauridsen et al., "International Association of Dental Traumatology guidelines for the management of traumatic dental injuries: 1. Fractures and luxations," *Dental Traumatology*, vol. 36, no. 4, pp. 314–330, 2020.

[6] A. F. Fouad, P. V. Abbott, G. Tsilingaridis et al., "International Association of Dental Traumatology guidelines for the management of traumatic dental injuries: 2. Avulsion of permanent teeth," *Dental Traumatology*, vol. 36, no. 4, pp. 331–342, 2020.

[7] P. F. Day, M. T. Flores, A. C. O'Connell et al., "International Association of Dental Traumatology guidelines for the management of traumatic dental injuries: 3. Injuries in the primary dentition," *Dental Traumatology*, vol. 36, no. 4, pp. 343–359, 2020.

[8] R. Lam, "Epidemiology and outcomes of traumatic dental injuries: a review of the literature," *Australian Dental Journal*, vol. 61, Suppl 1, pp. 4–20, 2016.

[9] U. Glendor, "Aetiology and risk factors related to traumatic dental injuries—a review of the literature," *Dental Traumatology*, vol. 25, no. 1, pp. 19–31, 2009.

[10] L. Giannetti, A. Murri Dello Diago, G. Silingardi, and E. Spinas, "Superficial infiltration to treat white hypomineralized defects of enamel: clinical trial with 12-month follow-up," *Journal of Biological Regulators and Homeostatic Agents*, vol. 32, no. 5, pp. 1335–1338, 2018.

[11] M. Mazur, S. Westland, F. Guerra et al., "Objective and subjective aesthetic performance of icon treatment for enamel hypomineralization lesions in young adolescents: a retrospective single center study," *Journal of Dentistry*, vol. 68, pp. 104–108, 2018.

[12] L. Giannetti, A. Murri Dello Diago, E. Corciolani, and E. Spinas, "Deep infiltration for the treatment of hypomineralized enamel lesions in a patient with molar incisor hypomineralization: a clinical case," *Journal of Biological Regulators and Homeostatic Agents*, vol. 32, no. 3, pp. 751–754, 2018.

[13] K. Bakes, S. Amend, J. Priller, C. Zamek, T. Stamm, and N. Krämer, "Changes in oral health-related quality of life after treatment of hypersensitive molar incisor hypomineralization-affected molars with a sealing," *Clinical Oral Investigations*, 2021.

[14] A. Murri Dello Diago, M. Cadenaro, R. Ricchiuto et al., "Hypersensitivity in molar incisor hypomineralization: superficial infiltration treatment," *Applied Sciences*, vol. 11, no. 4, p. 1823, 2021.

[15] L. Giannetti and A. Murri, "Clinical evidence and literature to compare two different therapeutic protocols in tooth avulsion," *European Journal of Paediatric Dentistry*, vol. 7, no. 3, pp. 122–130, 2006.

[16] J. O. Andreasen, F. M. Andreasen, and L. Andersson, *Textbook and Color Atlas of Traumatic Injuries to the Teeth*, Wiley-Blackwell, 4th edition, 2013, ISBN: 978-1-118-69990.

[17] L. Giannetti, A. Murri Dello Diago, F. Vecci, and U. Consolo, "Mini-implants in growing patients: a case report," *Pediatric Dentistry*, vol. 32, no. 3, pp. 239–244, 2010.

[18] J. B. Cope and D. McFadden, "Temporary replacement of missing maxillary lateral incisors with orthodontic miniscrew implants in growing patients: rationale, clinical technique, and long-term results," *Journal of Orthodontics*, vol. 41, Suppl. 1, pp. 62–74, 2014.

[19] L. Giannetti, R. Apponi, A. Murri Dello Diago, and F. Mintrone, "Rehabilitation of a patient with mini-implants after avulsion of the upper incisors: a 13-year follow up," *Dental Traumatology*, vol. 37, no. 2, pp. 354–359, 2021.

[20] D. Re, D. Augusti, G. Paglia, G. Augusti, and E. Cotti, "Treatment of traumatic dental injuries: evaluation of knowledge among Italian dentists," *European Journal of Paediatric Dentistry*, vol. 15, no. 1, pp. 23–28, 2014.

[21] E. Spinas, M. Aresu, F. Canargiu, and L. Giannetti, "Preventive treatment of post-traumatic dental infraocclusion: study on the knowledge of dental decoronation in a sample of Italian dental students and dentists," *European Journal of Paediatric Dentistry*, vol. 16, no. 4, pp. 279–283, 2015.

[22] E. Spinas, L. Generali, A. Mameli, C. Demontis, D. Martinelli, and L. Giannetti, "Delayed tooth replantation and inflammatory root resorption in childhood and adolescence," *Journal of Biological Regulators and Homeostatic Agents*, vol. 33, no. 2, pp. 623–627, 2019.

[23] D. Locker, "Prevalence of traumatic dental injury in grade 8 children in six Ontario communities," *Canadian Journal of Public Health*, vol. 96, no. 1, pp. 73–76, 2005.

[24] C. Piovesan, R. S. Guedes, L. Casagrande, and T. M. Ardenghi, "Socioeconomic and clinical factors associated with traumatic dental injuries in Brazilian preschool children," *Brazilian Oral Research*, vol. 26, no. 5, pp. 464–470, 2012.

[25] C. Piovesan, C. Abella, and T. M. Ardenghi, "Child oral health-related quality of life and socioeconomic factors associated with traumatic dental injuries in schoolchildren," *Oral Health & Preventive Dentistry*, vol. 9, no. 4, pp. 405–411, 2011.

[26] J. Traebert, M. A. Peres, V. Blank, S. Böell Rda, and J. A. Pietruza, "Prevalence of traumatic dental injury and associated factors among 12-year-old school children in Florianópolis, Brazil," *Dental Traumatology*, vol. 19, no. 1, pp. 15–18, 2003.

[27] E. Spinas, M. Aresu, and L. Giannetti, "Use of mouth guard in basketball: observational study of a group of teenagers with and without motivational reinforcement," *European Journal of Paediatric Dentistry*, vol. 15, no. 4, pp. 392–396, 2014.

[28] D. Stanbouly, R. Stanbouly, K. C. Lee, and S. K. Chuang, "Prevalence of dentofacial injuries and concussions among college athletes and their perceptions of mouthguards," *Journal of Craniofacial Surgery*, vol. 32, no. 4, pp. 1600–1603, 2021.

[29] E. Spinas, A. Mameli, and L. Giannetti, "Traumatic dental injuries resulting from sports activities; immediate treatment and five years follow-up: an observational study," *The Open Dentistry Journal*, vol. 12, no. 1, pp. 1–10, 2018.

[30] G. Shirani, M. H. Kalantar Motamedi, A. Ashuri, and P. S. Eshkevari, "Prevalence and patterns of combat sport related maxillofacial injuries," *Journal of Emergencies, Trauma, and Shock*, vol. 3, no. 4, pp. 314–317, 2010.

[31] E. Spinas, L. Giannetti, A. Mameli, and D. Re, "Dental injuries

in young athletes, a five-year follow-up study," *European journal of paediatric dentistry*, vol. 19, no. 3, pp. 187–193, 2018.

[32] Y. Z. Tan, L. Levin, W. Guo, and Y. Chen, "Dental injuries at the Xi'an, China Stomatological Hospital: a retrospective study," *Dental Traumatology*, vol. 36, no. 5, pp. 505–509, 2020.

[33] M. Oliveira Werlich, L. R. Honnef, J. V. Silva Bett et al., "Prevalence of dentofacial injuries in contact sports players: a systematic review and meta-analysis," *Dental Traumatology*, vol. 36, no. 5, pp. 477–488, 2020.

[34] H. K. Park, J. Y. Park, N. R. Choi, U. K. Kim, and D. S. Hwang, "Sports-related oral and maxillofacial injuries: a 5-year retrospective study, Pusan National University Dental Hospital," *Journal of Oral and Maxillofacial Surgery*, vol. 79, 2021.

Cavernous Sinus Involvement and Near Miss Mediastinitis following Mandibular Tooth Infection Treated during the COVID-19 Pandemic: Clinical Diagnosis and Treatment

Alessio Danilo Inchingolo,[1] Sabino Ceci,[1] Luisa Limongelli,[1] Alberto Corriero,[2] Luigi Curatoli,[3] Daniela Azzollini,[1] Pietro Paolo Mezzapesa,[1] Grazia Marinelli,[1] Giuseppina Malcangi,[1] Giovanni Coloccia,[1] Mario Ribezzi,[2] Maria Massaro,[4] Ioana Roxana Bordea,[5] Antonio Scarano,[6] Felice Lorusso,[6] Nicola Brienza,[2] Gianfranco Favia,[1] Nicola Quaranta,[3] and Francesco Inchingolo[1]

[1]*Department of Interdisciplinary Medicine, Section of Dental Medicine, University of Bari "Aldo Moro", 70124 Bari, Italy*
[2]*Unit of Anesthesia and Resuscitation, Department of Emergencies and Organ Transplantations, Aldo Moro University, Bari, Italy*
[3]*Department Neurosciences & Sensory Organs & Musculoskeletal System, University of Bari "Aldo Moro", 70124 Bari, Italy*
[4]*Azienda Ospedaliero-Universitaria Consorziale Policlinico di Bari, Bari, Italy*
[5]*Department of Oral Rehabilitation, Faculty of Dentistry, Iuliu Haţieganu University of Medicine and Pharmacy, 400012 Cluj-Napoca, Romania*
[6]*Department of Innovative Technologies in Medicine and Dentistry, University of Chieti-Pescara, 66100 Chieti, Italy*

Correspondence should be addressed to Ioana Roxana Bordea; roxana.bordea@ymail.com, Antonio Scarano; ascarano@unich.it, Felice Lorusso; drlorussofelice@gmail.com, and Francesco Inchingolo; francesco.inchingolo@uniba.it

Academic Editor: Rui Amaral Mendes

Odontogenic infections represent a frequent condition that in some cases, if not treated promptly, can spread quickly to the rest of the body and turn into life-threatening infections. In this work, the case is reported of a 59-year-old woman, diabetic and overweight, who presented to the Odontostomatology and Otolaryngology Section of the Policlinic of Bari with mandibular tooth infection that had developed into a deep neck space infection leading to the involvement of cavernous sinuses and near mediastinum. The diagnosis, the surgical drainage of the phlegmon and removal of infection foci, appropriate control of the airways, and a correct antibiotic therapy made it possible to avoid a potentially fatal condition. Prompt management and early diagnosis of deep space neck infections, such as phlegmon and/or necrotizing fasciitis, with the auxilium of CT scans and tools such as LRINEC (Laboratory Risk Indicator for Necrotizing Fasciitis), NLR (Neutrophil-to-Lymphocyte Ratio), and LRINECxNLR scores (Laboratory Risk Indicator for Necrotizing Fasciitis and Neutrophil to Lymphocyte Ratio), are advised to evade delays and complications that could potentially worsen the patient's outcome.

1. Introduction

Severe deep neck abscess secondary to an odontogenic cause is often reported in the literature and is a cause for concern for the patient's life [1, 2]. Deep neck space infections (DNSIs) are bacterial infections that involve different spaces in the neck, starting from the upper aerodigestive tract [3]. Dental infections are the most common cause of DNSIs [4], followed by pharyngeal and tonsillar origin [5] and upper airway infections [6]. Generally, the source of infection is in the odontogenic periapical of the mandibular second or third molar teeth [7], which is able to invade the cortical bone. The progression of infection is often unpredictable, largely depending on the causal tooth and the head and neck anatomy of the individual. In fact, the infection may spread downward, establishing DNSI and causing mediastinitis or pericarditis, pleural empyema, jugular vein thrombosis, and septic shock. Alternatively, the infection may spread upward to the brain and cause brain abscess, cavernous sinus thrombosis, or meningitis [8, 9]. Different authors suggest the denomination descending necrotizing mediastinitis (DNM) to indicate a serious complication of the spread of cervical necrotizing fasciitis (CNF) down to the mediastinum and thorax. CNF is an aggressive and potentially lethal deep neck infection where necrosis of soft tissues such as fascia, muscle, and cervical fat is observed [10]. Nowadays, DNIs are usually more significantly decreased than in the preantibiotic era. At that time, the major part of DNIs (70%) arose from pharyngitis or tonsillitis, while today, although tonsillitis remains the most common cause in children [11], poor dental hygiene has become the most common nonsurgical cause of DNIs in adults, followed by infections of unknown origin and foreign body ingestion [12]. In this article, we report the rare case of a 59-year-old diabetic, overweight female with a bilateral phlegmonous neck collection starting from a lower right molar abscess leading to bilateral parotid gland and bilateral cavernous sinus involvement and a near miss mediastinitis. A peculiarity is the presence of gas bubbles in both cavernous sinuses and in the right half of the face.

2. Case Report

The present study reports the case of a retired 59-year-old female, overweight (BMI 29.3 kg/m^2), with decompensated type two diabetes mellitus (DM) and hypercholesterolaemia, under drug therapy (ezetimibe with simvastatin 1 tbt/day and metformin hydrochloride 1000 mg 1 tbt twice a day), no coronary artery disease or herpetic virus liver disease, previous appendectomy surgery under general anaesthesia, and common childhood rashes. The patient was treated during the COVID-19 period, and all indicated measures according to the scientific literature were taken to protect all medical workers and the patient. Seven days prior to emergency room (ER) admission, she reported swelling in the right mandibular region which showed progressive volumetric increase with spontaneous and on-palpation pain. She started a nonbetter-specified antibiotic therapy with no benefits at all so that a subsequent dysphonia and liquid and solid dysphagia developed. On ER physical examination, the patient presented a voluminous right half-face abscess, inability to speak correctly due to trismus, and oedema of the tongue and mouth floor (Figure 1). Optical fiber video exploration of the upper respiratory tract showed mucosal oedema and hyperaemia of both the hypopharynx and the larynx. Complete blood count and laboratory tests (the most relevant values are reported in Table 1), Sars-CoV2 swab (negative), orthopantomography (OPG) X-ray (Figure 2), computed tomographies (CT) of the head-neck (Figures 3 and 4), and chest (Figure 5) were performed. Skull CT underlined the presence of gas bubbles in both the cavernous sinuses, possible odontogenic focus on tooth 4.7, part of a prosthetic bridge (4.7–4.5); neck CT was positive for huge phlegmon and gas bubbles affecting the right half of the face and platysma, the right parotid gland posteriorly, extending up to the contralateral parotid capsule and sternocleidomastoid muscle medially and the thyroid space inferiorly; chest CT showed no pathological findings. Emergency surgical laterocervical abscess drainage appeared to be mandatory and was performed together with the homolateral submandibular gland sialoadenectomy. The patient also underwent a surgical tracheostomy, according to the previous optic fibre video evaluation, in order to secure the airways and ensure proper ventilation (Figure 6). Antibiotic therapy with Teicoplanin 400 mg and Levofloxacin 500 mg was prescribed (Targosid 400 (Teicoplanina) mg Endovein at 12 : 00 and 22 : 00 with Rocefin (Ceftriaxone) 2 g Endovein at 8 : 00 and 20 : 00, and Desometasone 8 MG at 8 : 00 and 22 : 00 + gastroprotectives.)

The day after the emergency surgery, neurosurgical signs (negative) and infectious disease (new antibiotic therapy: piperacillin/tazobactam 4.5 g and linezolid 600 mg) consultations were requested. Urgent head and neck-chest computed tomography (CT) scans were performed. Presence of bilateral gas bubbles in correspondence to the cavernous sinuses was revealed. At the level of the neck, a large phlegmonous collection was present with a considerable contextual air share located mainly in the right half of the face, the platysma, and the ipsilateral parotid gland capsule. Medially, it extended to the buccal floor to the left submandibular lodge and the sternocleidomastoid fascia. C-reactive protein value was reduced but still high. On the third day of hospitalization, the patient was admitted to the intensive care unit because septic shock had developed due to the patient requiring vasopressors to maintain a mean arterial pressure higher than 65 mmHg and presenting a serum lactate level greater than 2 mmol/L. SOFA score was 9, and fever was present (38.2 degrees C). Neck-chest CT showed increased phlegmonous collection, especially on the left side (extended to the left parotid gland), on the anterior region of the neck, and down to the superior mediastinal region in the retrosternal site. Head CT revealed almost complete reabsorption of the gaseous collections at the level of the cavernous sinuses on both sides; only a small gas bubble remained in the right cavernous sinus. Emphysema in the neck was also moderately reabsorbed. There were no signs of venous thrombosis of the cerebral vessels or neck. Thoracic surgery consultation revealed no need for emergency surgery and neck-thorax CT with contrast medium after 48 hours and revaluation. The patient proceeded to surgery (Figure 7). After local anaesthesia (mepivacaine 3%) without vasoconstrictor, tooth 1.7 was removed because of a periapical lesion with necrosis; afterwards, the prosthetic bridge 4.5-4.7 was sectioned with rotating instruments in order to save the 4.5. Tooth 4.7 was extracted together with the pontic 4.6. Since a radiopacity spot in area 4.8 was seen on the skull-CT, a surgical revision in this site was also carried out. Alveolar curettage was performed using Volkmann spoons, and two specimens of exudate, collected in the postextraction site (4.7) and in 4.8 area, were sent for histological and microbiological examination; after washing with physiological solution and rifamicine topic antibiotic, haemostis with oxidized regenerated cellulose gauzes (Tabotamp®) was performed.

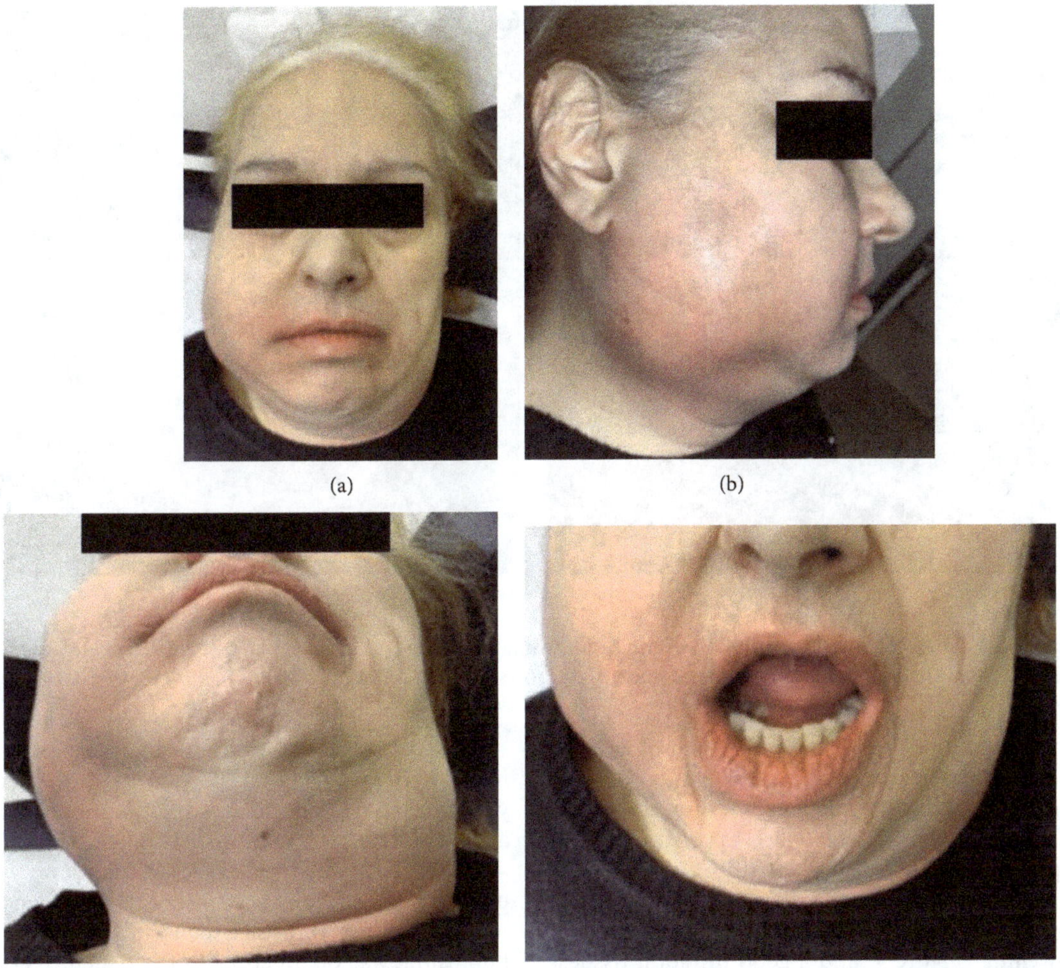

(a) (b) (c) (d)

Figure 1: (a–d) Patient photos at ER presentation 13/02/2021: front (a); right side (b); inferior (c); open mouth (d). Evident swelling of the medial and inferior third of the right side of the face (a, b). Trismus, oedema of the tongue and mouth floor (d).

Table 1: Most relevant values of the complete blood count.

	Laboratory tests
Uraemia	105 mg/dL
Glycaemia	414 mg/dL
eGFR	68 mL/min
Albumin	2.3 g/dL
CRP	389 mg/L
Fibrinogen	1279 mg/dL
D-dimers	1068 μg/L
pO2	70 mmHg

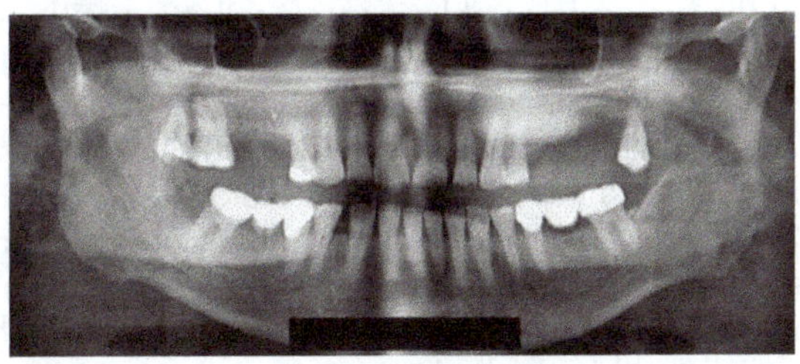

Figure 2: Initial orthopantomography (OPG) X-ray 13/02/2021: partial edentulism; outcomes of conservative and orthodontic therapy, prosthetic rehabilitation.

The day after surgery, the patient was kept sedated and under controlled mechanical ventilation; SOFA score dropped from 9 to 8, and haemodynamic stability was achieved through vasopressors (noradrenaline). Fever was still present. In the following days, as the SOFA score dropped to 0 and discontinuation from amine support transpired, fever resolved, and the patient initiated successful weaning that resulted in disconnection from the ventilator on the 9th day of hospitalization. ENT (ear, nose, and throat) consultation revealed a thorough surgical treatment and suggested surgical wound dressing, washing with H_2O_2 and physiological solution through the drains. In addition, dentistry and thoracic surgery consultations were required. A new neck-thorax CT with contrast medium showed unchanged bilateral neck abscess and involvement of the anterior part of the neck down to the superior mediastinal region in the retrosternal site that did not require surgical treatment. After 10 days of hospitalization, chest X-ray did not show any variation compared to the previous evaluation,

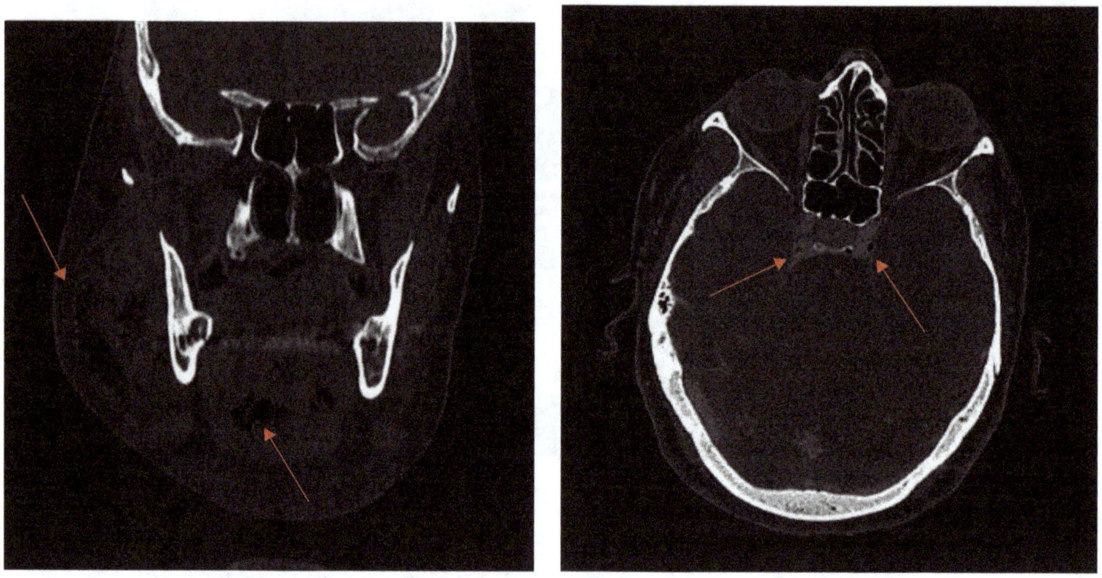

(a) (b)

Figure 3: (a, b) Initial computed tomography (CT) of the head: frontal plane (a); transverse plane (b). Presence of gas bubbles in both cavernous sinuses, the right half of the face and buccal floor (red arrows) (13/02/2021).

and the patient's condition was stable, being neurologically well oriented, hemodynamically stable, and with good gas exchange. On the 12th day, the patient was moved to the ENT ward. Patient discharge took place approximately 1 month after performing neck and chest CTs (Table 2 and Figure 8).

Check-up 3 months after discharge revealed no externally visible swelling (Figure 9) and a good intraoral tissues healing (Figure 10). Control OPG (Figure 11); CTs of head-neck and chest were requested and checked.

Neck-chest CT (13/02/2021): presence of bilateral gas bubbles in correspondence to the cavernous sinuses. At the level of the neck, a large phlegmonous collection with a considerable contextual air share located mainly in the right half face, the platysma, and the ipsilateral parotid gland capsule. Medially, it extended to the buccal floor to the left submandibular lodge and the sternocleidomastoid fascia.

Chest X-ray (bedridden) (14/02/2021): presence of tracheostomy tube with distal end in place; raised right hemidiaphragm with ipsilateral basal dysventilation; heart substantially within the limits.

CT neck-chest (15/02/2021): increase of the known phlegmon, especially on the left side (where it also extends to the left parotid gland) and also to the anterior region of the neck and down to the superior mediastinal region in the retrosternal site.

Cranial CT (15/02/2021): almost complete reabsorption of the gaseous collections at the level of the cavernous sinuses on both sides; currently, only a small gas box remains in the right cavernous sinus. Emphysema in the neck is also moderately reabsorbed; no signs of venous thrombosis of the cerebral vessels and neck.

Ct neck and thorax with contrast medium (17/02/2021): the known abscess collection in the neck bilaterally unchanged, especially on the left. It also extends to the anterior region of the neck and down to the superior mediastinal region in the retrosternal site; filiform the lumen of the pharynx and larynx. The pharyngolaryngeal spaces are obliterated. The remaining finds unchanged.

Chest X-ray bedridden (22/02/2021): no variation compared to the previous.

The written informed consent for the study and case publishing was obtained from the patient recruited.

3. Results and Discussion

Infections of dental origin are common and are well-controlled by antibiotic prescription. Nevertheless, when not controlled, these infections could spread into the cervical and maxillofacial region, thus risking a myriad of possible complications including Ludwig's angina, respiratory obstruction, facial deep neck abscesses, cellulitis, NCF, aspiration pneumonia, septicaemia, thoracic empyema, descending mediastinitis, pleuropulmonary suppuration, brain abscess, endocarditis, pericarditis, pneumothorax, jugular thrombophlebitis and abscess of the carotid sheath, hematogenous dissemination to distant organs, fulminant state of disseminated intravascular coagulation (DIC), and coagulation abnormalities which could all eventually result in mortality [9, 13, 14]. DNSIs are infections involving the pharyngeal and neck spaces [15–19]. The most frequent sources of infection are oral cavity, in particular teeth, and pharynx [6, 20], although in 25% of cases, there is no clear source [5]. The location frequency is as follows: 36% submandibular, 13% sublingual, 12% parapharyngeal, and 3% retropharyngeal [5]. Bacteria from different locations such as oral cavity, pharynx, blood, and tonsils can cause abscesses and phlegmon (a suppurative inflammation of the subcutaneous connective tissue) [21], spreading along the connective tissues and fascial spaces. DNSIs are a quite common and

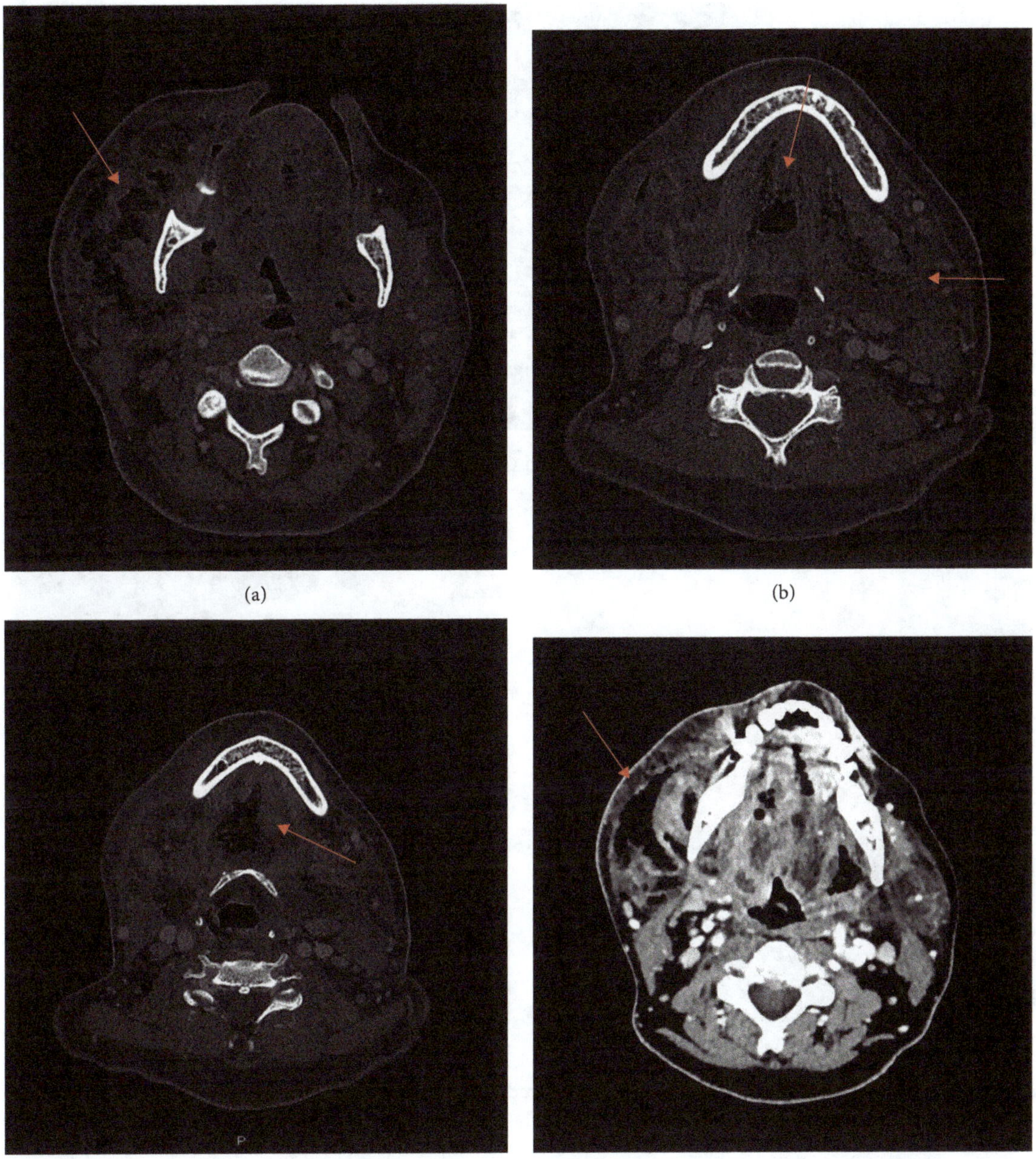

(a) (b) (c) (d)

FIGURE 4: (a–d) Initial CT of the neck (transverse plane) highlighting the presence of gas bubbles (red arrows): at the right parotid gland posteriorly (a); oral floor extending up to the contralateral parotid capsule (b); sternocleidomastoid muscle medially and the thyroid space inferiorly (c); at the right parotid gland in a different cutting plane height (d) (13/02/2021).

potentially life-threating entity, related to high rates of hospitalisation, complications, and eventually death. Prompt medical, and often surgical, treatment is mandatory in order to avoid fatal outcomes [22]. If a correct diagnosis and surgical treatment are carried out within the first twelve hours, the mortality rate drops [23, 24]. A first strength in the treatment of the patient in this case report was certainly the rapid laterocervical surgical drainage, tracheostomy, and administration of a correct and adequate antibiotic therapy. In fact, treatment of these infections is complex and includes broad-spectrum antibiotics, airway management (including tracheostomy), and surgical intervention. Furthermore, a surgical drainage of the abscess may be necessary in the first place [4, 6]. Life-threatening complications are airway compromise, mediastinitis, pericarditis, intracranial involvement, and arterial erosion [25–29]. Another grave complication is descending necrotizing mediastinitis (DNM) [1], a serious and progressive infection involving the neck and the chest, in which an odontogenic, pharyngeal, or cervical infection spreads rapidly through the subcutaneous tissue and cervical fascia to the thoracic cavity causing tissue necrosis, with a high death rate (10-40%) by sepsis and organic failure if not treated quickly and appropriately [30, 31]. Almost 60-70% of DNM cases are due to descending odontogenic infections, first of all, when they are caused by second and third lower molar necrosis [32]. Therefore, a second

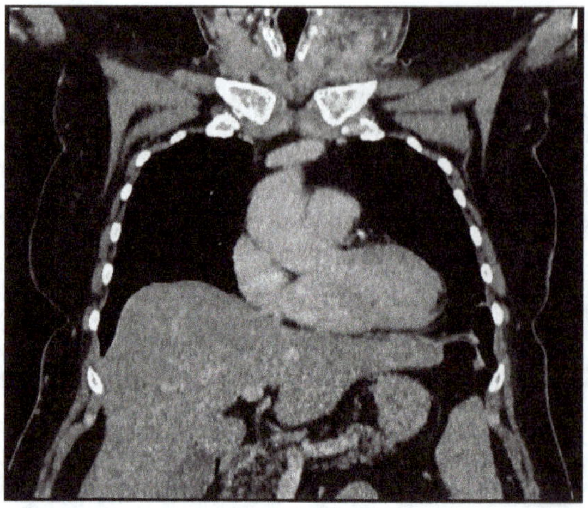

FIGURE 5: Initial CT of the chest.

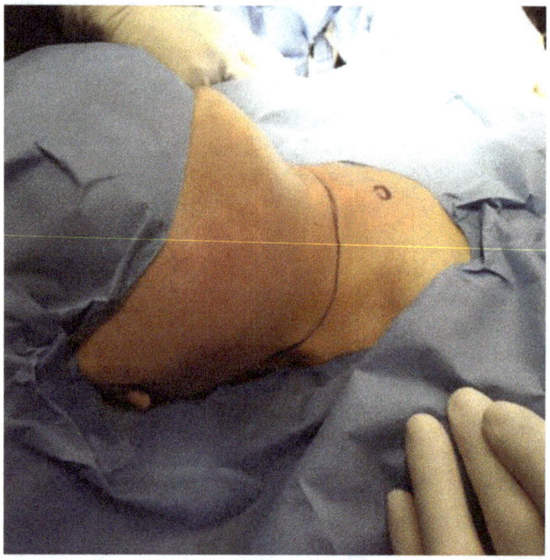

(a)

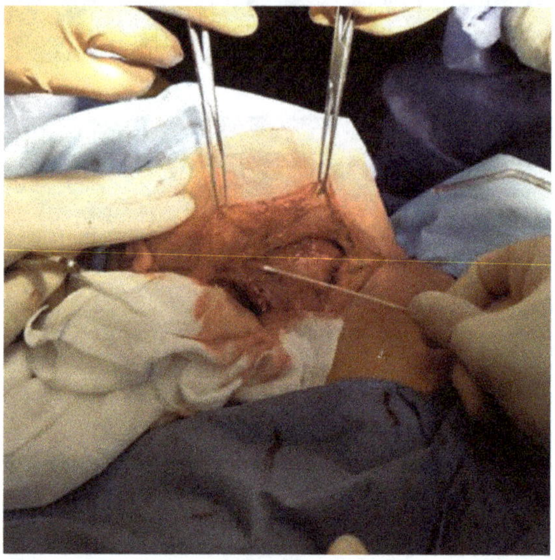

(b)

FIGURE 6: (a, b) Emergency surgery at ER: surgical procedure preparation (a); laterocervical abscess drainage (b).

strength in the present case is certainly the avoidance of fatal mediastinitis, a "near miss" mediastinitis, because the patient was treated quickly and properly. Another important aspect to consider is the presence of comorbidities or other clinical conditions. The patient reported in this article suffers from diabetes and is overweight. DM, liver cirrhosis, alcoholism, hypertension, chronic renal insufficiency, and malignancy are necrotizing fasciitis (NF) predisposing factors [33]. DM is the most frequently encountered comorbidity, and it greatly increases the risk of complications of DNSI and mortality [34]. In a study of 263 cases, a high number of subjects with DNSI had associated systemic diseases, such as primary arterial hypertension, coronary heart disease, DM, and HIV infection [4, 35]. The impact of body mass index (BMI) in the development of DNSI is remarkable: in fact, if it increases, it is clear that acute phlegmonous laryngitis as etiological agent, phlegmon of the neck as localization, and complications augment [35].

A notable aspect in this case was the presence of gas bubbles at the level of the cavernous sinus, as highlighted by CT. This scan is a very accurate tool, with 79% sensitivity and 94% specificity, which is why it is requested on patient admission and during hospitalization [36, 37]. Presence of gas bubbles resulting from bacterial fermentation is not uncommon in a wide range of important infections. The microbiota is also an important aspect that can influence the evolution of a patient. A particular pathological event, necrotizing fasciitis (NF), a term introduced by Wilson in 1952 [38] to indicate an inflammatory process of soft tissues, determining a fascial necrosis, can allow an easy and wide spread of the infection along the laterocervical bands and thus through locus minoris resistentiae, reaching the mediastinum and causing descending necrotizing mediastinitis (DNM). The greatest incidence of NF is in the 30-50 age group, although no age group is excluded [39–46], and it is characterized by a high mortality rate [3]. The oral cavity

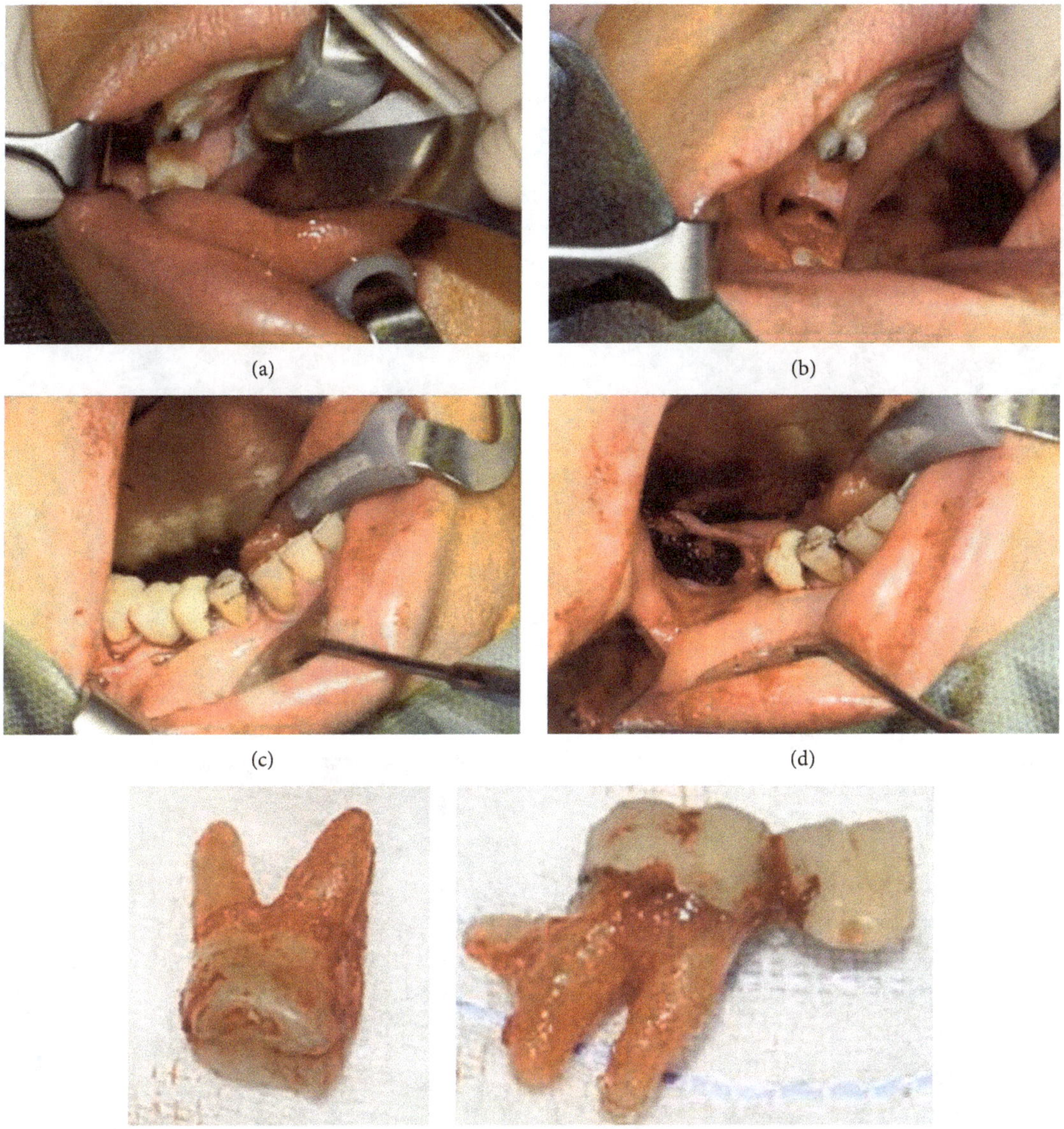

(a) (b)

(c) (d)

(e) (f)

FIGURE 7: (a–f) Extraction of 1.7 (a, b); extraction of 4.7 plus pontic (c, d); extracted 1.7 (e) and 4.7 (f).

TABLE 2: Data regarding the patient evaluation.

Study timeline	
13-02-2021	E.R. admission, emergency surgery, airway management
15-02-2021	I.C.U. admission: oral surgery procedure
24-02-2021	E.N.T. admission
15-03-2021	Discharge
17-06 2021	Check-up

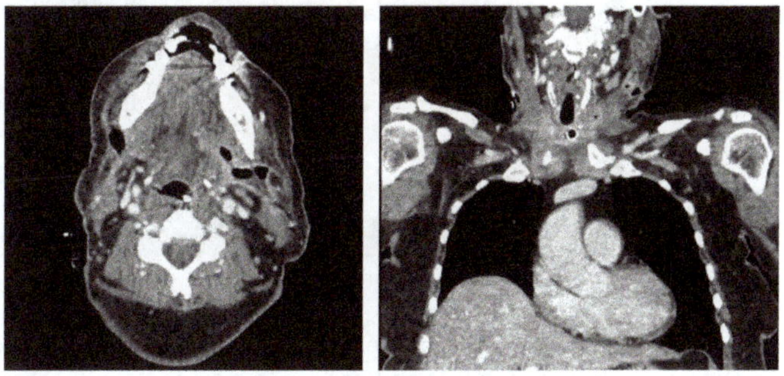

FIGURE 8: Final CT neck and chest 01/03/2021.

is the most frequent starting location of the infection [39, 41, 47–55]. Cervical necrotizing fasciitis (CNF) indicates necrosis involvement of the neck tissues, especially less vascularized tissues, i.e., fascia, but also fat and muscles [46, 56, 57]. Only 3.5% of DNSIs are CNF, but the mortality rate is 7-22%, 41% if there is thoracic involvement, and 64% with DNM and complications caused by sepsis [58]. There are 2 different forms of CNF: suppurative and gaseous. The first one is characterized by purulent fluid collection; the second by gas formation [10]. Sakai et al. [59] analysed six patients

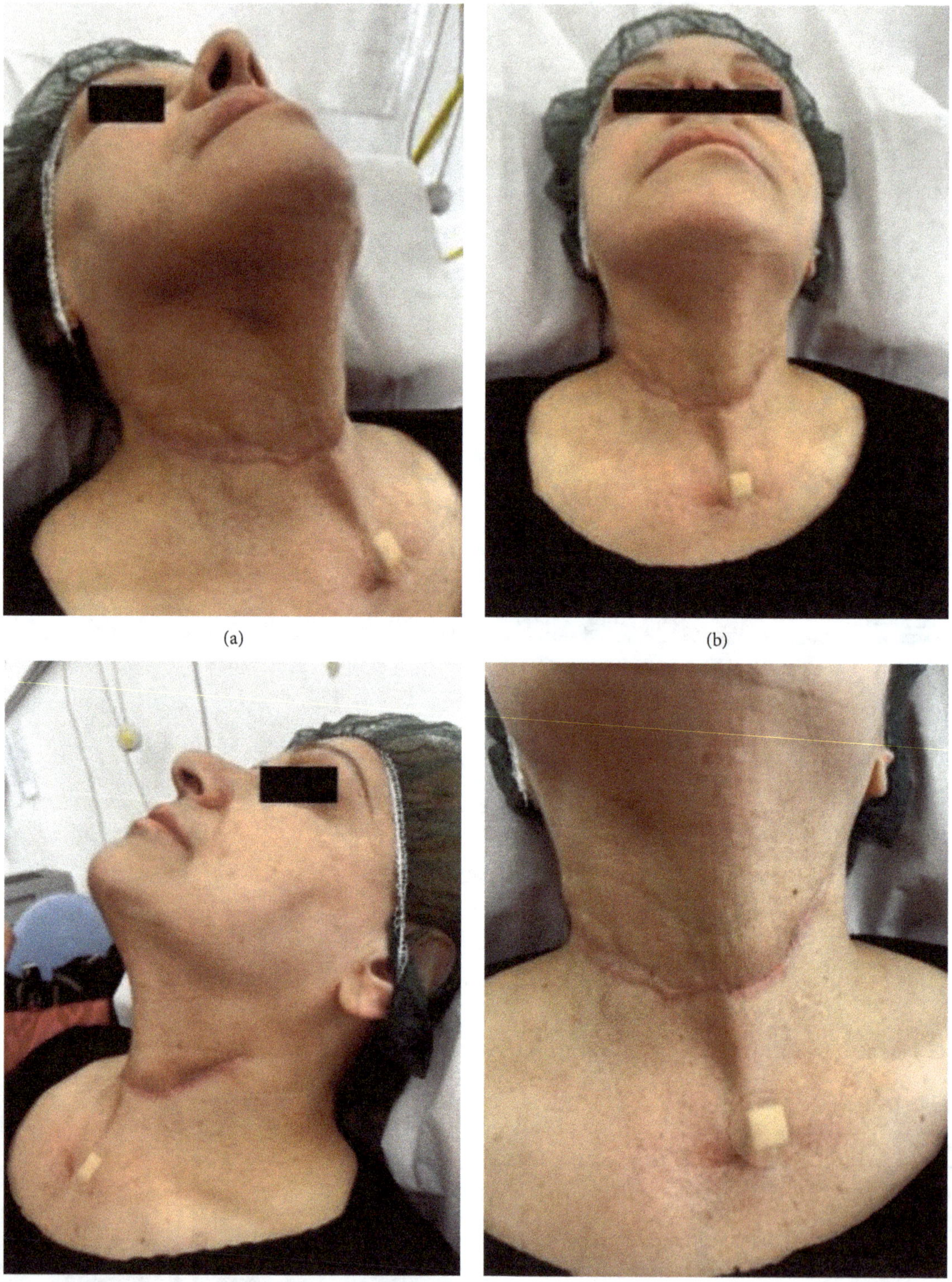

(a) (b) (c) (d)

Figure 9: (a–d) Final patient photos: right side (a); front (b); left side (c); neck scar detail (d). Presence of scarring outcomes on the neck; absence of swelling of the face and neck.

with DNM caused by pharyngolaryngeal and odontogenic infection which required broad-spectrum antibiotic therapy, aggressive drainage, and thoracic surgery. Four of these patients had polymicrobial infections (aerobic and anaerobic bacteria including *Streptococcus anginosus* group SAG) and all of them showed gas bubbles on chest TC. Ng et al. [60] reported the case of a 66-year-old man with Emphysematous aortitis from Clostridial infection of the thoracic aorta with presence of gas bubbles along the aortic wall. These findings were visible in the CT scan of the chest. After proliferation in necrotic or anoxic areas, Clostridia can release toxins and enzymes (hyaluronidase and hemolysin), producing gas

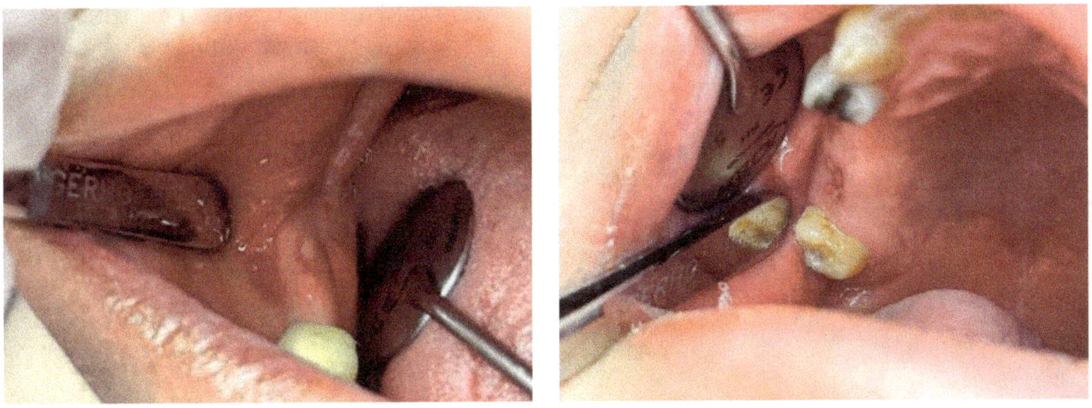

(a) (b)

FIGURE 10: (a, b) Final intraoral photos: after extraction site of 4.7 (a); after extraction site of 1.7 (b). Good tissue healing on the extraction sites of 4.7 (blue arrow) and 1.7 (green arrow).

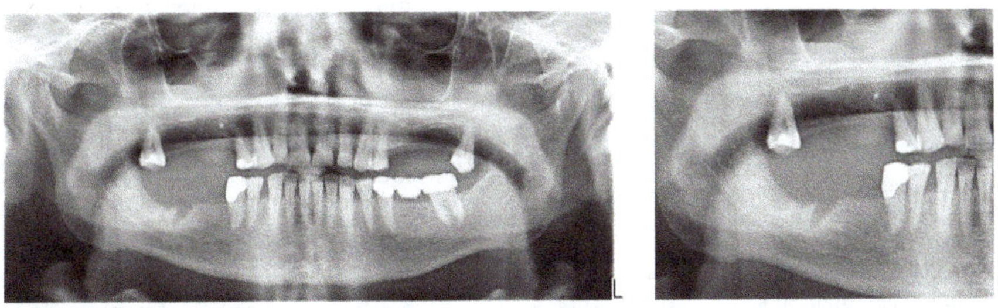

(a) (b)

FIGURE 11: (a, b) Final OPG X-ray (17/06/2021): no relevant findings on the extraction sites (magnification (b)).

gangrene infection. In another article, Xing et al. [61] described a case of emphysematous pyelonephritis (EPN), a lethal necrotic infection of the kidney with collection of gas in the renal parenchyma, and/or perinephric tissues [62]. Point-of-care ultrasound (POCUS) detected gas bubbles in the hepatorenal space. *E. coli* and other *Enterobacteriaceae* are the most frequent causes of EPN, and they produce gas by fermentation of glucose and lactate in necrotic tissues [63]. Richards et al. [64] reported a 64-year-old woman who presented to the emergency department with a 6-day history of dental pain and significant right-sided facial swelling. A panoramic radiograph showed periapical radiolucencies associated with her carious lower right first premolar (LR5) and second molar (LR7) which led to a diagnosis of rapidly progressing odontogenic abscess. CT revealed an extensive abscess with gas pockets adjacent to the right mandible which was indicative of the severity of the infection. In the case of the patient mentioned in the present article, the microbiological examination of the exudate taken from the postextraction site was performed, which gave a negative result. In literature, the evaluation of exudate from the abscess site or from the gangrenous necrosis region frequently provides negative feedback [65, 66] and is not considered of fundamental importance. On other occasions, it provides uncertain results, multiple etiology [42, 47, 50, 51, 65–72], or the finding of saprophytic or symbiont microorganisms. It can be useful to administer a specific antibiotic treatment if it is possible to highlight certain bacterial strains and/or fungi. An additional strength in the management of this clinical case was the empirical antibiotic therapy, developed by combining an antibiotic active against gram negative and one active against gram positive as this is frequently found in the literature [49, 66, 67, 73–77]. It is important to define and use some reliable tools to quickly detect and identify DNSI complications such as CNF, DNM, and systemic sepsis. There are some clinical signs and symptoms useful for identifying CNF but they have only 67% of sensitivity [78]. On the other hand, there are no specific laboratory studies proven to be predictive of the NF diagnosis [79], although Fiorella et al. propose the use of Laboratory Risk Indicator for Necrotizing Fasciitis (LRINEC) score (Table 3), the neutrophil-to-lymphocyte ratio (NLR), and LRINEC × NLR scores as predictive tools to early evaluate septic complications and the risk of CNF during DNSI. Indicator LRINEC×NLR was proposed by Fiorella et al. to enhance the predictive value of the analysis [80]. LRINEC score was introduced by Wong et al. to help clinicians access for NF checking on serum: white blood cell count, haemoglobin, sodium, glucose, creatinine, and C-reactive protein. NLR has an important meaning especially during the initial and last phases of sepsis [81]. It was initially proposed by Baglam et al. as a predictive factor for DNSI [82]. Patient LRINEC score, calculated on the parameters shown in Table 2, was 6. This indicated a medium risk of developing NF according to Wong et al. and Chen et al. [58, 81] with 94% of sensitivity and specificity according to Sandner et al. [36]. NLR score was 8.9 predicting systemic septic involvement (sensitivity and specificity rate of 74.2%

Table 3: LRINEC scores.

Variable, unit	Score
C-reactive protein (CRP), mg/L	
<150	0
≥ 150	4
Haemoglobin, g/dL	
>13.5	0
11-13.5	1
<11	2
Total white cell count, per mm^3	
<15	0
15-25	1
>25	2
Sodium, mmol/L	
≥ 135	0
<135	2
Creatinine, μmol/L	
≤ 141	0
>141	2
Glucose, mg/dL	
≤ 180	0
>180	1

LRINEC scores: low risk (probability less than 50%) for LRINEC-score 5; medium risk (probability of 50-75%) for LRINEC-score between 6 and 7; high risk (probability more than 75%) for LRINEC – score ≥ 8.

and 61.5% above value of 8.2) and LRINEC×NLR score 53.4 indicating an important risk of CNF having a sensitivity of 90.9% above values of 43.5 according to Fiorella et al. [80]. In this case report, it is possible to see how failure to apply the LRINEC score to early detect a rapidly developing necrotizing failure could potentially lead to either a mediastinitis or a life-threatening infection in the cranial fossae: the patient should have been screened in the emergency room and correctly directed into an intensive care ward rather than ENT ward to establish proper care, which happened only after 48 hours from hospitalization.

4. Conclusions

Early treatment of any odontogenic infection should be taken care of since a missed or late diagnosis of deep space neck infection could potentially cause serious complications. Surgical drainage within the first hours, early extraction of the odontogenic focuses, proper airway management, and broad-spectrum antibiotic treatment decreased the number of hospitalization days and the recovery period, without increasing complications.

Take home messages:

(1) Correct early treatment of odontogenic infections

(2) LRINEC, NLR, and LRINEC×NLR scores should be assessed quickly to direct the patient to the best diagnostic/therapeutic path

(3) Collaboration between different specialities regarding the treatment of this type of case is mandatory

Authors' Contributions

Alessio Danilo Inchingolo, Sabino Ceci, Luisa Limongelli, Alberto Corriero, and Luigi Curatoli contributed equally to this work as co-first authors. Nicola Brienza, Gianfranco Favia, Nicola Quaranta, and Francesco Inchingolo contributed equally to this work as co-last authors.

References

[1] A. K. Tormes, M. M. De Bortoli, R. M. Júnior, and E. S. Andrade, "Management of a severe cervicofacial odontogenic infection," *The Journal of Contemporary Dental Practice*, vol. 19, no. 3, pp. 352–355, 2018.

[2] S. Kinzer, J. Pfeiffer, S. Becker, and G. J. Ridder, "Severe deep neck space infections and mediastinitis of odontogenic origin: clinical relevance and implications for diagnosis and treatment," *Acta Oto-Laryngologica*, vol. 129, no. 1, pp. 62–70, 2009.

[3] S. Priyamvada and G. Motwani, "A study on deep neck space infections," *Indian Journal of Otolaryngology and Head & Neck Surgery*, vol. 71, Supplement 1, pp. 912–917, 2019.

[4] S. Prabhu and E. Nirmalkumar, "Acute fascial space infections of the neck: 1034 cases in 17 years follow up," *Annals of Maxillofacial Surgery*, vol. 9, no. 1, pp. 118–123, 2019.

[5] J. Velhonoja, M. Lääveri, T. Soukka, H. Irjala, and I. Kinnunen, "Deep neck space infections: an upward trend and changing characteristics," *European Archives of Oto-Rhino-Laryngology*, vol. 277, no. 3, pp. 863–872, 2020.

[6] T.-T. Huang, T.-C. Liu, P.-R. Chen, F.-Y. Tseng, T.-H. Yeh, and Y.-S. Chen, "Deep neck infection: analysis of 185 cases," *Head & Neck*, vol. 26, no. 10, pp. 854–860, 2004.

[7] P. Boscolo-Rizzo, M. Stellin, E. Muzzi et al., "Deep neck infections: a study of 365 cases highlighting recommendations for management and treatment," *European Archives of Oto-Rhino-Laryngology*, vol. 269, no. 4, pp. 1241–1249, 2012.

[8] M. Pesis, E. Bar-Droma, A. Ilgiyaev, and N. Givol, "Deep neck infections are life threatening infections of dental origin: a presentation and management of selected cases," *The Israel Medical Association Journal*, vol. 21, no. 12, pp. 806–811, 2019.

[9] N. Montemurro, P. Perrini, W. Marani et al., "Multiple brain abscesses of odontogenic origin. May oral microbiota affect their development? A review of the current literature," *Applied Sciences*, vol. 11, no. 8, 2021.

[10] A. Karkas, K. Chahine, S. Schmerber, P.-Y. Brichon, and C. A. Righini, "Optimal treatment of cervical necrotizing fasciitis associated with descending necrotizing mediastinitis," *British Journal of Surgery*, vol. 97, no. 4, pp. 609–615, 2010.

[11] P.-K. Blankson, G. Parkins, M. O. Boamah et al., "Severe odontogenic infections: a 5-year review of a major referral hospital in Ghana," *The Pan African Medical Journal*, vol. 32, p. 71, 2019.

[12] G. Marioni, R. Rinaldi, C. Staffieri et al., "Deep neck infection with dental origin: analysis of 85 consecutive cases (2000-2006)," *Acta Oto-Laryngologica*, vol. 128, no. 2, pp. 201–206, 2008.

[13] D. Opitz, C. Camerer, D.-M. Camerer et al., "Incidence and management of severe odontogenic infections–a retrospective analysis from 2004 to 2011," *Journal of Cranio-Maxillo-Facial Surgery*, vol. 43, no. 2, pp. 285–289, 2015.

[14] E. Zawiślak and R. Nowak, "Odontogenic head and neck region infections requiring hospitalization: an 18-month retrospective analysis," *BioMed Research International*, vol. 2021, Article ID 7086763, 8 pages, 2021.

[15] J. M. Coticchia, G. S. Getnick, R. D. Yun, and J. E. Arnold, "Age-, site-, and time-specific differences in pediatric deep neck abscesses," *Archives of Otolaryngology – Head & Neck Surgery*, vol. 130, no. 2, p. 201, 2004.

[16] D. J. Kirse and D. W. Roberson, "Surgical management of retropharyngeal space infections in children," *The Laryngoscope*, vol. 111, no. 8, pp. 1413–1422, 2001.

[17] J. E. McClay, A. D. Murray, and T. Booth, "Intravenous antibiotic therapy for deep neck abscesses defined by computed tomography," *Archives of Otolaryngology – Head & Neck Surgery*, vol. 129, no. 11, pp. 1207–1212, 2003.

[18] W. D. Miller, I. M. Furst, G. K. B. Sàndor, and M. A. Keller, "A prospective, blinded comparison of clinical examination and computed tomography in deep neck infections," *The Laryngoscope*, vol. 109, no. 11, pp. 1873–1879, 1999.

[19] M. Nagy, M. Pizzuto, J. Backstrom, and L. Brodsky, "Deep neck infections in children: a new approach to diagnosis and treatment," *The Laryngoscope*, vol. 107, no. 12, pp. 1627–1634, 1997.

[20] A. K. Koç, W. M. Alakhras, H. Acıpayam, H. E. Koçak, and F. T. Kayhan, "Seven years of experience in 160 patients with deep neck infection," *Imaging (MRI)*, vol. 5, p. 4, 2016.

[21] L. Simion and S. Dumitru, "Phlegmon of the oral floor. Contradictions in diagnosis and treatment," *The Moldovan Medical Journal*, vol. 61, no. 1, pp. 42–48, 2018.

[22] F. Vieira, S. M. Allen, R. M. S. Stocks, and J. W. Thompson, "Deep neck infection," *Otolaryngologic Clinics of North America*, vol. 41, no. 3, pp. 459–483, 2008.

[23] J. K. Muhammad, H. Almadani, B. A. Al Hashemi, and M. Liaqat, "The value of early intervention and a multidisciplinary approach in the management of necrotizing fasciitis of the neck and anterior mediastinum of odontogenic origin," *Journal of Oral and Maxillofacial Surgery*, vol. 73, no. 5, pp. 918–927, 2015.

[24] P. Cruz Toro, À. Callejo Castillo, J. Tornero Saltó, X. González Compta, A. Farré, and M. Maños, "Cervical necrotizing fasciitis: report of 6 cases and review of literature," *European Annals of Otorhinolaryngology, Head and Neck Diseases*, vol. 131, no. 6, pp. 357–359, 2014.

[25] W.-L. Chan, V. B. Fernandes, and M. G. Carolan, "Retropharyngeal abscess on a Ga-67 scan: a case report," *Clinical Nuclear Medicine*, vol. 24, no. 12, pp. 942–944, 1999.

[26] Y. Abba, H. Hassim, H. Hamzah, and M. M. Noordin, "Antiviral activity of resveratrol against human and animal viruses," *Advances in Virology*, vol. 2015, Article ID 184241, 7 pages, 2015.

[27] H.-J. Kim, E. D. Park, J. H. Kim, E. G. Hwang, and S. H. Chung, "Odontogenic versus nonodontogenic deep neck space infections: CT manifestations," *Journal of Computer Assisted Tomography*, vol. 21, no. 2, pp. 202–208, 1997.

[28] C. M. Ursic, S. V. Shah, and A. Kaviani, "Neck abscess after blunt cervical trauma," *The Journal of Trauma: Injury, Infection and Critical Care*, vol. 51, no. 1, pp. 146–148, 2001.

[29] Z. Waggie, M. Hatherill, A. Millar, H. France, A. Van Der Merwe, and A. Argent, "Retropharyngeal abscess complicated by carotid artery rupture," *Pediatric Critical Care Medicine*, vol. 3, no. 3, pp. 303-304, 2002.

[30] H. M. Prado-Calleros, E. Jiménez-Fuentes, and I. Jiménez-Escobar, "Descending necrotizing mediastinitis: systematic review on its treatment in the last 6 years, 75 years after its description," *Head & Neck*, vol. 38, no. S1, pp. E2275–E2283, 2016.

[31] C. Benedetto, V. N. Tanzariello, A. Militi et al., "Catastrophic descending necrotizing mediastinitis of the anterior and posterior compartments: a case report," *Radiology Case Reports*, vol. 15, no. 10, pp. 1832–1836, 2020.

[32] H. Sakamoto, T. Aoki, Y. Kise, D. Watanabe, and J. Sasaki, "Descending necrotizing mediastinitis due to odontogenic infections," *Oral Surgery, Oral Medicine, Oral Pathology, Oral Radiology, and Endodontology*, vol. 89, no. 4, pp. 412–419, 2000.

[33] J.-M. Wang and H.-K. Lim, "Necrotizing fasciitis: eight-year experience and literature review," *Brazilian Journal of Infectious Diseases*, vol. 18, no. 2, pp. 137–143, 2014.

[34] D. Bross-Soriano, J. R. Arrieta-Gómez, H. Prado-Calleros, J. Schimelmitz-Idi, and S. Jorba-Basave, "Management of Ludwig's angina with small neck incisions: 18 years experience," *Otolaryngology and Head and Neck Surgery*, vol. 130, no. 6, pp. 712–717, 2004.

[35] A. Adoviča, L. Veidere, M. Ronis, and G. Sumeraga, "Deep neck infections: review of 263 cases," *Otolaryngologia Polska*, vol. 71, no. 5, pp. 37–42, 2017.

[36] A. Sandner, S. Moritz, S. Unverzagt, S. K. Plontke, and D. Metz, "Cervical necrotizing fasciitis–the value of the laboratory risk indicator for necrotizing fasciitis score as an Indicative parameter," *Journal of Oral and Maxillofacial Surgery*, vol. 73, no. 12, pp. 2319–2333, 2015.

[37] A. J. Thomas and T. K. Meyer, "Retrospective evaluation of laboratory-based diagnostic tools for cervical necrotizing fasciitis," *The Laryngoscope*, vol. 122, no. 12, pp. 2683–2687, 2012.

[38] B. Wilson, "Necrotizing fascitis," *The American Surgeon*, vol. 18, pp. 416–431, 1952.

[39] P. C. Valko, S. M. Barret, and J. P. Campbell, "Odontogenic cervical necrotizing fasciitis," *Annals of Emergency Medicine*, vol. 19, no. 5, pp. 568–571, 1990.

[40] A. R. Gillis and T. M. Gillis, "Necrotizing cervical fasciitis of unknown origin," *The Journal of Otolaryngology*, vol. 21, no. 3, pp. 171–173, 1992.

[41] S. Kantu and G. Har-El, "Cervical necrotizing fasciitis," *The Annals of Otology, Rhinology, and Laryngology*, vol. 106, no. 11, pp. 965–970, 1997.

[42] L. M. Isaacs, B. Kotton, M. M. Peralta et al., "Fatal mediastinal abscess from upper respiratory infection," *Ear, Nose, & Throat Journal*, vol. 72, no. 9, pp. 620–631, 1993.

[43] H. K. Chua, C. B. Segar, R. Krishnan, and C. K. Ho, "Cervical necrotising fasciitis consequent to mastoid infection," *The Medical Journal of Malaysia*, vol. 57, no. 1, pp. 104–107, 2002.

[44] M. A. Safak, I. Haberal, D. Kiliç, and H. Göçmen, "Necrotizing fasciitis secondary to peritonsillar abscess: a new case and review of eight earlier cases," *Ear, Nose, & Throat Journal*, vol. 80, no. 11, pp. 824–833, 2001.

[45] K. C. Ndukwe, O. A. Fatusi, and V. I. Ugboko, "Craniocervical necrotizing fasciitis in Ile-Ife, Nigeria," *British Journal of Oral and Maxillofacial Surgery*, vol. 40, no. 1, pp. 64–67, 2002.

[46] N. Skitarelić, R. Mladina, and M. Morović, "Cervical necrotizing fasciitis: sources and outcomes," *Infection*, vol. 31, no. 1, pp. 39–44, 2003.

[47] L. J. H. Greinwald, J. F. Wilson, and P. G. Haggerty, "Peritonsillar abscess: an unlikely cause of necrotizing fasciitis," *The Annals of Otology, Rhinology, and Laryngology*, vol. 104, no. 2, pp. 133–137, 1995.

[48] R. J. Balcerak, J. M. Sisto, and R. C. Bosack, "Cervicofacial necrotizing fasciitis: report of three cases and literature review," *Journal of Oral and Maxillofacial Surgery*, vol. 46, no. 6, pp. 450–459, 1988.

[49] A. S. Helmy, M. A. Salah, H. A. Nawara, H. Khatab, H. A. Khalaf, and N. Abd el-Maguid, "Life-threatening cervical necrotizing fasciitis," *Journal of the Royal College of Surgeons of Edinburgh*, vol. 42, no. 6, pp. 410–413, 1997.

[50] R. H. Maisel and R. Karlen, "Cervical necrotizing fasciitis," *The Laryngoscope*, vol. 104, no. 7, p. 795???798, 1994.

[51] T. De Backer, M. Bossuyt, and J. Schoenaers, "Management of necrotizing fasciitis in the neck," *Journal of Cranio-Maxillofacial Surgery*, vol. 24, no. 6, pp. 366–371, 1996.

[52] D. M. Dohan Ehrenfest, M. Del Corso, F. Inchingolo, and J.-B. Charrier, "Selecting a relevant in vitro cell model for testing and comparing the effects of a Choukroun's platelet-rich fibrin (PRF) membrane and a platelet-rich plasma (PRP) gel: tricks and traps," *Oral Surgery, Oral Medicine, Oral Pathology, Oral Radiology, and Endodontics*, vol. 110, no. 4, pp. 409–411, 2010, author reply 411-413.

[53] F. Inchingolo, F. S. Martelli, C. Gargiulo Isacco et al., "Chronic periodontitis and immunity, towards the implementation of a personalized medicine: a translational research on gene single nucleotide polymorphisms (SNPs) linked to chronic oral dysbiosis in 96 Caucasian patients," *Biomedicines*, vol. 8, no. 5, 2020.

[54] I. A. Charitos, A. Ballini, L. Bottalico et al., "Special features of SARS-CoV-2 in daily practice," *World Journal of Clinical Cases*, vol. 8, no. 18, pp. 3920–3933, 2020.

[55] V. H. Pham, C. Gargiulo Isacco, K. C. D. Nguyen et al., "Rapid and sensitive diagnostic procedure for multiple detection of pandemic Coronaviridae family members SARS-CoV-2, SARS-CoV, MERS-CoV and HCoV: a translational research and cooperation between the Phan Chau Trinh University in Vietnam and University of Bari 'Aldo Moro' in Italy," *European Review for Medical and Pharmacological Sciences*, vol. 24, no. 12, pp. 7173–7191, 2020.

[56] C. Lin, F.-L. Yeh, J.-T. Lin et al., "Necrotizing fasciitis of the head and neck: an analysis of 47 cases," *Plastic and Reconstructive Surgery*, vol. 107, no. 7, pp. 1684–1693, 2001.

[57] I. Mohammedi, P. Ceruse, S. Duperret, J.-M. Vedrinne, and P. Boulétreau, "Cervical necrotizing fasciitis: 10 years' experience at a single institution," *Intensive Care Medicine*, vol. 25, no. 8, pp. 829–834, 1999.

[58] L. L. Chen, B. Fasolka, and C. Treacy, "Necrotizing fasciitis: a comprehensive review," *Nursing*, vol. 50, no. 9, pp. 34–40, 2020.

[59] T. Sakai, A. Sano, Y. Azuma, S. Koezuka, H. Otsuka, and A. Iyoda, "Streptococcus anginosus group infection as a predictor for the progression of descending necrotizing mediastinitis," *Annals of Palliative Medicine*, vol. 10, no. 4, pp. 4008–4016, 2021.

[60] T. G. Ng, U. Trivedi, K. Shah, and P. Maldjian, "Clostridial mycotic aneurysm leading to emphysematous aortitis," *Cureus*, vol. 13, no. 3, p. e14136, 2021.

[61] Z.-X. Xing, H. Yang, W. Zhang et al., "Point-of-care ultrasound for the early diagnosis of emphysematous pyelonephritis: a case report and literature review," *WJCC*, vol. 9, no. 11, pp. 2584–2594, 2021.

[62] Y. Song and X. Shen, "Diabetic ketoacidosis complicated by emphysematous pyelonephritis: a case report and literature review," *BMC Urology*, vol. 20, no. 1, 2020.

[63] S. S. Ubee, L. McGlynn, and M. Fordham, "Emphysematous pyelonephritis," *BJU International*, vol. 107, no. 9, pp. 1474–1478, 2011.

[64] C. Richards, T. W. Walker, S. Girgis, and S. Colbert, "'Bubble sign': gas-forming bacteria from an odontogenic infection," *BML Case Reports*, vol. 13, no. 6, article e233946, 2020.

[65] D. Mathieu, R. Neviere, C. Teillon, J. L. Chagnon, N. Lebleu, and F. Wattel, "Cervical necrotizing fasciitis: clinical manifestations and management," *Clinical Infectious Diseases*, vol. 21, no. 1, pp. 51–56, 1995.

[66] P. Gidley, B. Ghorayeb, and C. Stiernberg, "Contemporary management of deep neck space infections☆☆☆," *Otolaryngology-Head and Neck Surgery*, vol. 116, no. 1, pp. 16–22, 1997.

[67] Y. Rapoport, M. Z. Himelfarb, D. Zikk, and J. Bloom, "Cervical necrotizing fasciitis of odontogenic origin," *Oral Surgery, Oral Medicine, Oral Pathology*, vol. 72, no. 1, pp. 15–18, 1991.

[68] J. A. Freischlag, G. Ajalat, and R. W. Busuttill, "Treatment of necrotizing soft tissue infections: the need for a new approach," *The American Journal of Surgery*, vol. 149, no. 6, pp. 751–755, 1985.

[69] Y. P. Krespi, W. Lawson, S. M. Blaugrund, and H. F. Biller, "Massive necrotizing infections of the neck," *Head & Neck*, vol. 3, no. 6, pp. 475–481, 1981.

[70] R. M. Moss, S. Kunpittaya, and A. Sorasuchart, "Cervical necrotizing fasciitis: an uncommon sequela to dental infection," *Annals of Otology, Rhinology & Laryngology*, vol. 99, no. 8, pp. 643–646, 1990.

[71] L. Santacroce, I. A. Charitos, A. Ballini et al., "The human respiratory system and its microbiome at a glimpse," *Biology*, vol. 9, no. 10, p. 318, 2020.

[72] A. Ballini, A. Gnoni, D. De Vito et al., "Effect of probiotics on the occurrence of nutrition absorption capacities in healthy children: a randomized double-blinded placebo-controlled pilot study," *European Review for Medical and Pharmacological Sciences*, vol. 23, no. 19, pp. 8645–8657, 2019.

[73] M. Bahna and R. F. Canalis, "Necrotizing fasciitis (streptococcal gangrene) of the face: report of a case and review of the literature," *Archives of Otolaryngology-Head and Neck Surgery*, vol. 106, no. 10, pp. 648–651, 1980.

[74] A. J. F. Beerens, L. J. Bauwens, and C. R. Leemans, "A fatal case of craniofacial necrotizing fasciitis," *European Archives of Oto-Rhino-Laryngology*, vol. 256, no. 10, pp. 506–509, 1999.

[75] M. E. Lang, W. Vaudry, and J. L. Robinson, "Case report and literature review of late-onset group B streptococcal disease manifesting as necrotizing fasciitis in preterm infants: is this a new syndrome?," *Clinical Infectious Diseases*, vol. 37, no. 9, pp. e132–e135, 2003.

[76] I. L. Feinerman, H. K. K. Tan, D. W. Roberson, R. Malley, and M. A. Kenna, "Necrotizing fasciitis of the pharynx following

adenotonsillectomy," *International Journal of Pediatric Otorhinolaryngology*, vol. 48, no. 1, pp. 1–7, 1999.

[77] J. Skorina and D. Kaufman, "Necrotizing fasciitis originating from pinna perichondritis," *Otolaryngology-Head and Neck Surgery*, vol. 113, no. 4, pp. 467–473, 1995.

[78] E. J. C. Goldstein, D. A. Anaya, and E. P. Dellinger, "Necrotizing soft-tissue infection: diagnosis and management," *Clinical Infectious Diseases*, vol. 44, no. 5, pp. 705–710, 2007.

[79] E. Moskowitz and T. Schroeppel, "Necrotizing fasciitis following abdominal gunshot wound," *Trauma Surgery & Acute Care Open*, vol. 3, no. 1, article e000163, 2018.

[80] M. L. Fiorella, P. Greco, L. M. Madami, O. V. Giannico, V. Pontillo, and N. Quaranta, "New laboratory predictive tools in deep neck space infections," *Acta Otorhinolaryngologica Italica*, vol. 40, no. 5, pp. 332–337, 2020.

[81] C.-H. Wong, L.-W. Khin, K.-S. Heng, K.-C. Tan, and C.-O. Low, "The LRINEC (laboratory risk indicator for necrotizing fasciitis) score: a tool for distinguishing necrotizing fasciitis from other soft tissue infections," *Critical Care Medicine*, vol. 32, no. 7, pp. 1535–1541, 2004.

[82] T. Baglam, A. Binnetoglu, A. C. Yumusakhuylu, F. Gerin, B. Demir, and M. Sari, "Predictive value of the neutrophil-to-lymphocyte ratio in patients with deep neck space infection secondary to acute bacterial tonsillitis," *International Journal of Pediatric Otorhinolaryngology*, vol. 79, no. 9, pp. 1421–1424, 2015.

25

Molar Incisor Hypomineralization (MIH) in a Child with Congenital Chronic Intestinal Pseudoobstruction (CIPO)

Mohammed Zameer[1] **Syed Ali Peeran**[1] **Syed Nahid Basheer,**[2] **Syed Wali Peeran**[3] **Sameen Badiujjama Birajdar,**[4] **Faisal Mohammad Alzahrani,**[1] **and Ali Mohammed A. Alkhayrat**[5]

[1]*Armed Forces Hospital, Jazan, Saudi Arabia*
[2]*Department of Restorative Dentistry, College of Dentistry, Jazan, Saudi Arabia*
[3]*Department of Periodontology & Oral Implantology, Faculty of Dentistry, University of Sebha, Sebha, Libya*
[4]*Sanjeevani Dental Clinic, Raichur, India*
[5]*College of Dentistry, Jazan, Saudi Arabia*

Correspondence should be addressed to Mohammed Zameer; drmohammedzameer@gmail.com

Academic Editor: Noam Yarom

Molar incisor hypomineralization (MIH) is a qualitative enamel defect of systemic origin affecting 1–4 permanent first molars (PFMs) frequently in association with affected permanent incisors (PIs). The exact etiology of MIH is still unclear but considered to be multifactorial. This present case report to the best of our knowledge is the first case reported which acknowledges MIH in a patient with chronic intestinal pseudoobstruction (CIPO) with underlying neurological disease due to somatic mitochondrial disorder. It also elicits the availability of various contemporary treatment options and their proper selection and early intervention to manage the functional and aesthetic problems caused by enamel defects and to improve the quality of life in the patients.

1. Introduction

Molar incisor hypomineralization (MIH) is a qualitative enamel defect of systemic origin affecting 1–4 permanent first molars (PFMs) frequently in association with affected permanent incisors (PIs). Meanwhile, speculation was raised that the tips of permanent cuspids might present similar defects as they mineralized in the same period as the FPMs and PIs [1]. Further in the literature, MIH-like defects have been reported on second primary molars, permanent canines, premolars, and second permanent molars [2–11]. Although the hypomineralization was initially described as MIH, more recently, it has been noticed that these MIH-like defects can affect any primary or permanent tooth [10–13]. MIH defects can be soft, porous, and vary in their clinical presentation from white to yellow or brownish opacities but always with a distinct demarcation between affected and sound enamel. The porous, brittle enamel can cause loss of tooth structure under the masticatory forces [14]. Thus, the enamel porosities and discolored opacities can result in functional and aesthetic complications in MIH-affected children. Other enamel abnormalities like diffuse opacities, hypoplasia, and amelogenesis imperfecta are clinically similar to MIH defects which can also occur during amelogenesis and are suggested to be designated while evaluation to allow distinction from MIH defects [15].

MIH-affected children have also been shown to have an adverse impact on the Oral Health-Related Quality of Life (OHRQoL) along with considerably increased negative self-perception of oral symptoms [16]. For clinicians, the management of MIH cases can be problematic as the affected

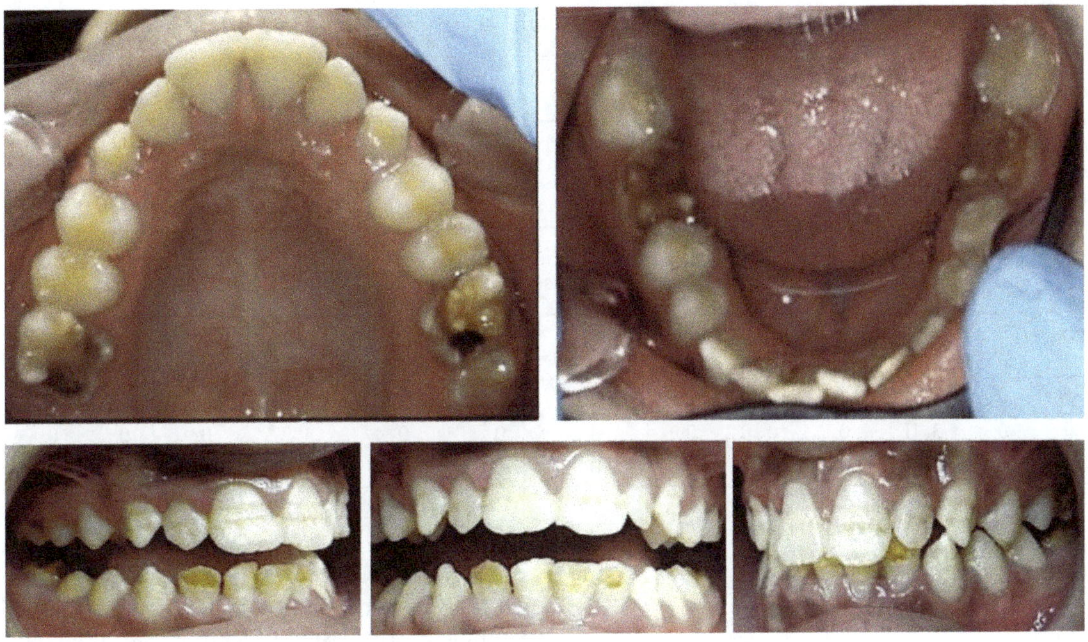

FIGURE 1: Preoperative intraoral photographs.

teeth might be highly sensitive and susceptible to rapid dental caries development. Moreover, limited cooperation of young children, difficulty in achieving anesthesia, and repeated episodes of the marginal breakdown of restorations can complicate their management. Thus, MIH-affected children have shown to spend more time in receiving oral health care in comparison with those without MIH [14, 17, 18].

The exact etiology of MIH is still unclear but is considered to be multifactorial. The causative mechanism of MIH has been associated with both environmental disturbances (prenatal, perinatal, and postnatal disturbances) and genetic factors (genetic variations in TUFT1, TUFT11, AMELX, and ENAM) [19, 20, 21]. To the best of our knowledge, congenital chronic intestinal pseudoobstruction related to underlying neurologic disorder has not been previously described with MIH. The present case report is aimed at narrating the association of congenital chronic intestinal pseudoobstruction (CIPO) with MIH. It also elicits the availability of various contemporary treatment options and their proper selection and early intervention to manage the functional and aesthetic problems caused by enamel defects and to improve the quality of life in the patients.

2. Case Report

A 12-year-old boy with his father presented to the Pediatric Dental Clinic of Armed Forces Hospital (Jazan, KSA) with a chief complaint of discoloration in the lower front teeth since their eruption. Medical history revealed that he was born with preterm delivery by cesarean section due to polyhydramnios at the gestational age of 30 weeks. He was hospitalized for 3 weeks due to prematurity and abdominal distension. He was diagnosed to have a chronic intestinal pseudoobstruction, bacterial overgrowth, chronic diarrhea, and metabolic acidosis. He was managed with sodium bicarbonate, potassium chloride, and pancrelipase/Lipase-Protease-Amylase (Creon™), and the bacterial overgrowth was treated with multiple courses of alternating antibiotics: clindamycin, gentamicin, amoxicillin, and metronidazole. At the age of 9 years, the boy again suffered from acute vomiting, diarrhea, and dehydration. The patient was admitted for rehydration, and further investigations were carried out. The patient was diagnosed with pancreatitis and somatic mitochondrial disorder with pyroglutamic aciduria. He also tested positive for rhinovirus. It was inferred that these findings could be pathognomonic to the enteropathy in the patient's underlying neurological disease.

Intraoral clinical examination was carried out on clean wet teeth. All four FPMs showed extensive enamel breakdown with irregular brown opacities. Mandibular incisors showed demarcated opacities ranging from white-creamy to yellow-brown defects. These opacities in molars and mandibular incisors had clear borders with the adjacent sound enamel. Maxillary incisors and canines showed linear groves with a reduced localized thickness of the enamel and a smooth border with the normal enamel (Figure 1). The patient also reported that the first permanent mandibular molars on both sides often triggered sensitivity especially while eating. The clinical pattern of hypomineralized defects and relevant past medical history led to the diagnosis of MIH. The long data set form formulated by Ghanim et al. was followed to assess the clinical status and extent of MIH and other enamel defects (Tables 1 and 2).

2.1. Management. Three consecutive treatment stages were defined.

TABLE 1: Assessment of the clinical status and extent of MIH along with other enamel defects in maxillary teeth.

Surface	Maxillary right							Maxillary left						
	17	16	15	14	13	12	11	21	22	23	24	25	26	27
Buccal/labial	A	0	0	0	12, I	12, I	12, I	12, I	12, I	12, I	0	0	0	A
Occlusal/incisal	A	3, II	0	0	0	0	0	0	0	0	0	0	3, II	A
Palatal	A	3, II	0	0	0	0	0	0	0	0	0	0	3, II	A

TABLE 2: Assessment of the clinical status and extent of MIH in mandibular teeth.

Surface	Mandibular right							Mandibular left						
	47	46	45	44	43	42	41	31	32	33	34	35	36	37
Buccal/labial	0	3, II	0	0	14, I	22, II	21, I	22, II	22, II	14, I	0	0	3, II	0
Occlusal/incisal	0	3, II	0	0	0	0	0	0	0	0	0	0	3, II	0
Lingual	0	3, II	0	0	0	0	0	0	0	0	0	0	3, II	0

(1) Preventive stage

(i) Appropriate dietary advice to avoid dental erosion and caries

(ii) Professional topical application of arginine-containing desensitizing paste

(iii) At-home oral hygiene practices using arginine-containing desensitizing toothpaste and mouthwash

(2) Aesthetic enhancement stage for anterior teeth

(i) Microabrasion

(ii) Composite veneers

(3) Restorative stage for posterior teeth

(i) Full-coverage restoration using preformed stainless steel crowns (SSCs) for defective molars

The preventive phase started by approaching the child and his parents with appropriate dietary advice. In-office topical application of desensitizing paste containing 8% arginine and calcium carbonate (Elmex sensitive professional desensitizing paste) was carried over for the affected mandibular first molars following the manufacturer's instruction. Simultaneously, the patient was instructed to use arginine-containing desensitizing toothpaste (Elmex sensitive professional toothpaste) and mouthwash (Elmex sensitive professional mouthwash) as a routine at-home oral hygiene practice. Aesthetic enhancement of anterior teeth was accomplished by opting for microabrasion and direct composite restorations for maxillary incisors, lower central incisors, and maxillary and mandibular canines. Complete composite veneering was done for more destructed lower lateral incisors. MIH-affected FPMs were restored with preformed SSCs as a full-coverage restorative approach (Figure 2).

3. Discussion

Amelogenesis is the process of dental enamel formation that can be separated into the initial phase of matrix formation through the secretion of matrix protein and later stages of mineralization and maturation. If any developmental disturbance occurs during the secretory phase, it results in a quantitative defect called hypoplasia. If a disturbance occurs in later stages of mineralization or maturation, it results in a qualitative defect called hypomineralization. MIH is a term that describes a qualitative defect of enamel presenting clinically as variable opacities concomitant with the distinct demarcation between the affected and sound enamel [2, 22].

The literature shows several possible etiological determinants which have been associated with MIH. They are generally identified as systemic factors during the pre-, peri-, and postnatal period, and they include genetic variations [23, 24, 25]. In the period from the final trimester of pregnancy to the third year of the child lies the phase of enamel maturation. Any disturbance to the enamel in this phase can lead to MIH [20, 26]. A considerable association has been found between MIH and premature birth, gastrointestinal system disorders, renal failure, rubella, various drug usage, and chickenpox [26, 27, 28, 29].. In this present case, the patient had a premature birth, was rhinovirus positive, and had CIPO with underlying neurological disease due to somatic mitochondrial disorder.

A minimally interventive conservative approach with microabrasion and the direct composite veneer was opted for all anterior teeth except mandibular lateral incisors similar to the treatment carried out by Pereira [30]. As the conservative approach is not meant to address the depth of destruction in the affected lower lateral incisors and salvage

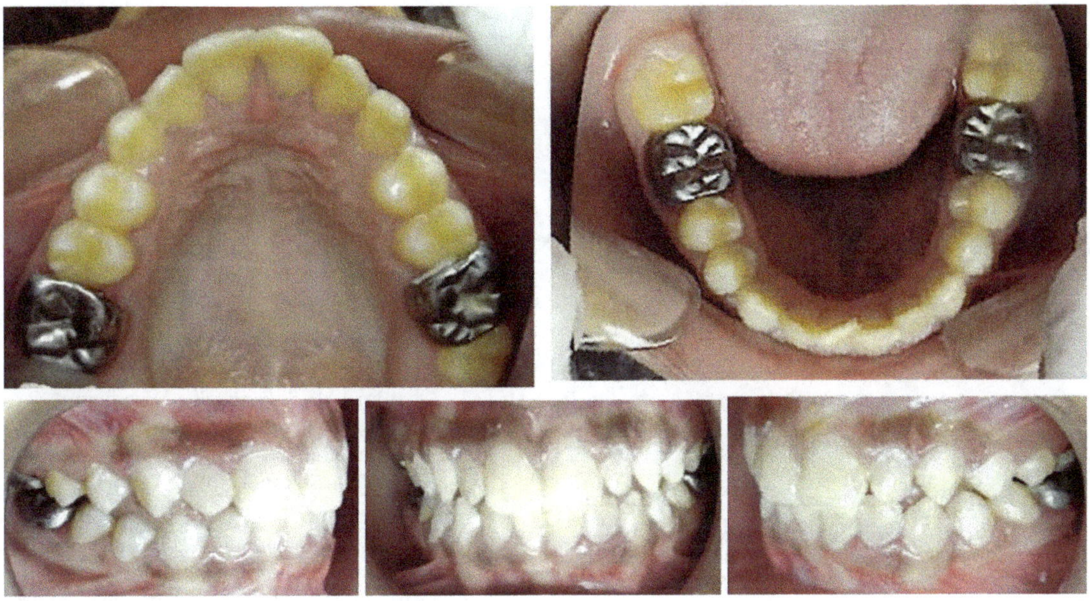

Figure 2: Postoperative intraoral photographs.

them, therefore, direct complete composite veneering was done for the lower lateral incisors.

Arginine paste is used as a dentinal tubule sealant and is recommended as desensitizing toothpaste in MIH-affected teeth. It has also been shown to block hydrodynamic pain mechanisms by reducing the number of exposed sensory afferent nerve endings [21, 31–33]. Hence, we used arginine-based paste in this case to treat MIH-related dentinal hypersensitivity.

In the present case, we have considered all four FPMs for restorative therapy. Based on the severity of damage due to MIH, there was a greater need for full-coverage restoration to restore the form, function, and longevity of the affected teeth. SSCs have been suggested considering their advantages as a treatment modality for severe MIH-affected molars [34]. SSCs can provide full coverage thereby maintaining the structural integrity of mutilated molars, prevents recurrent dental caries, improves oral hygiene, reduces dentinal hypersensitivity, restores crown height and occlusal functionality, and imparts longevity and high success [35–37]. This restorative approach of using SSCs for MIH-affected molars with extensive defects has been adopted in a few previous studies [38, 39]. However, long-term studies are needed to investigate the efficacy of SSCs. This can also be an interim restorative approach for MIH-affected molars in patients with the need of future orthodontic correction and extractions, to manage their malocclusion [38].

Weerheijm and colleagues defined MIH in 2001. They also raised speculation about the manifestation of MIH-like defects in the tips of permanent cuspids along with FPMs and PIs because they are mineralized in the same time frame as the FPMs and PIs. Following which studies were carried out to assess the extent of involvement of teeth other than FPMs and PIs, in a study, 27% of MIH-affected children who were in the permanent dentition stage showed one or more affected canines and premolars [3]. Another study recorded 25.7% MIH-affected individuals of age 14 years which show MIH-like defects in canines [11]. In a study on adolescents, 22.8% MIH-affected individuals of age 16 years reported having MIH-like defects in canine. They also recorded that maxillary canines were 2.3 times more frequently affected than mandibular canines [5]. In the present case, the defects were observed bilaterally in mandibular canines. Other enamel defects like hypoplasia, diffuse opacities, and amelogenesis imperfecta that are clinically similar to MIH defects can also occur due to any disturbances during amelogenesis. These abnormalities should not be misdiagnosed; instead, they are suggested to be assigned as present or absent allowing their distinction from MIH defects [15]. It has been suggested that systemic etiological factors acting for longer periods during enamel mineralization and maturation tend to produce more affected teeth with more severe defects. In the present case, MIH along with hypoplastic defects in maxillary anterior teeth was recorded following the long set data form for use in epidemiological studies on enamel hypomineralization [15].

MIH may lead to posteruptive enamel breakdown leading to dentine exposure, tooth sensitivity with increased caries susceptibility, behavioral management problems due to dental fear and anxiety, aesthetic complications, with a concomitant negative impact on child's self-esteem, personal relationship, and school performance, and an additional financial burden [13, 30, 40, 23]. Hence, early detection and comprehensive treatment of patients with MIH remain a priority.

4. Conclusion

This present case report to the best of our knowledge is the first case reported which acknowledges MIH in a patient with CIPO with underlying neurological disease due to somatic mitochondrial disorder. It also elicits the availability of various contemporary treatment options and their proper selection and early intervention to manage the functional and aesthetic problems caused by enamel defects and to improve the quality of life in the patients.

Consent

Written informed consent was obtained from the parents.

References

[1] K. L. Weerheijm, B. Jälevik, and S. Alaluusua, "Molar–incisor hypomineralisation," *Caries Research*, vol. 35, no. 5, pp. 390-391, 2001.

[2] K. L. Weerheijm, M. Duggal, I. Mejàre et al., "Judgement criteria for molar incisor hypomineralisation (MIH) in epidemiologic studies: a summary of the European meeting on MIH held in Athens, 2003," *European Journal of Paediatric Dentistry*, vol. 4, no. 3, pp. 110–113, 2003.

[3] S. A. Bhaskar and S. Hegde, "Molar-incisor hypomineralization: prevalence, severity and clinical characteristics in 8- to 13-year-old children of Udaipur, India," *Journal of the Indian Society of Pedodontics and Preventive Dentistry*, vol. 32, no. 4, pp. 322–329, 2014.

[4] A. R. Vieira and E. Kup, "On the etiology of molar-incisor hypomineralization," *Caries Research*, vol. 50, no. 2, pp. 166–169, 2016.

[5] A. Schmalfuss, K. R. Stenhagen, A. B. Tveit, C.-G. Crossner, and I. Espelid, "Canines are affected in 16-year-olds with molar-incisor hypomineralisation (MIH): an epidemiological study based on the Tromsø study: "Fit Futures"," *European Archives of Paediatric Dentistry*, vol. 17, no. 2, pp. 107–113, 2016.

[6] G. Dietrich, S. Sperling, and G. Hetzer, "Molar incisor hypomineralisation in a group of children and adolescents living in Dresden (Germany)," *European Journal of Paediatric Dentistry*, vol. 4, no. 3, pp. 133–137, 2003.

[7] M. E. C. Elfrink, A. Ghanim, D. J. Manton, and K. L. Weerheijm, "Standardised studies on molar incisor hypomineralisation (MIH) and hypomineralised second primary molars (HSPM): a need," *European Archives of Paediatric Dentistry*, vol. 16, no. 3, pp. 247–255, 2015.

[8] N. Sidhu, Y. Wang, E. Barrett, and M. Casas, "Prevalence and presentation patterns of enamel hypomineralisation (MIH and HSPM) among paediatric hospital dental patients in Toronto, Canada: a cross-sectional study," *European Archives of Paediatric Dentistry*, vol. 21, no. 2, pp. 263–270, 2020.

[9] C. Serna Muñoz, A. J. Ortiz Ruiz, A. Pérez Silva, L. A. Bravo-González, and A. Vicente, "Second primary molar hypomineralisation and drugs used during pregnancy and infancy. A systematic review," *Clinical Oral Investigations*, vol. 24, no. 3, pp. 1287–1297, 2020.

[10] N. Mittal, "Phenotypes of enamel hypomineralization and molar incisor hypomineralization in permanent dentition: identification, quantification and proposal for classification," *The Journal of Clinical Pediatric Dentistry*, vol. 40, no. 5, pp. 367–374, 2016.

[11] A. Kevrekidou, I. Kosma, I. Kotsanos, K. N. Arapostathis, and N. Kotsanos, "Enamel opacities in all other than molar incisor hypomineralisation index teeth of adolescents," *International Journal of Paediatric Dentistry*, 2020.

[12] R. Steffen, "Therapie der molaren-inzisiven-hypomineralisation in einem schwierigen umfeld," *Praktische Konzepte für den Behandlungsalltag. Quintessenz*, vol. 62, no. 12, pp. 1613–1623, 2011.

[13] Z. Almuallem and A. Busuttil-Naudi, "Molar incisor hypomineralisation (MIH) - an overview," *British Dental Journal*, vol. 225, no. 7, pp. 601–609, 2018.

[14] K. L. Weerheijm, "Molar incisor hypomineralization (MIH): clinical presentation, aetiology and management," *Dental Update*, vol. 31, no. 1, pp. 9–12, 2004.

[15] A. Ghanim, M. Elfrink, K. Weerheijm, R. Mariño, and D. Manton, "A practical method for use in epidemiological studies on enamel hypomineralisation," *European Archives of Paediatric Dentistry*, vol. 16, no. 3, pp. 235–246, 2015.

[16] P. D. Portella, B. L. V. Menoncin, J. F. Souza, J. V. N. B. Menezes, F. C. Fraiz, and L. R. da Silva Assunção, "Impact of molar incisor hypomineralization on quality of life in children with early mixed dentition: a hierarchical approach," *International Journal of Paediatric Dentistry*, vol. 29, no. 4, pp. 496–506, 2019.

[17] M. O. Folayan, T. A. Oyedele, and E. Oziegbe, "Time expended on managing molar incisor hypomineralization in a pediatric dental clinic in Nigeria," *Brazilian Oral Research*, vol. 32, 2018.

[18] F. Al-Othaibi, M. Zameer, S. N. Basheer, and S. A. Peeran, "An interdisciplinary treatment approach to manage molar-incisor hypomineralization (MIH), non-vital immature molar and anterior crowding in a child," *Case Reports in Odontology*, vol. 5, no. 2, pp. 1–5, 2018.

[19] S. Alaluusua, "Aetiology of molar-incisor hypomineralisation: a systematic review," *European Archives of Paediatric Dentistry*, vol. 11, no. 2, pp. 53–58, 2010.

[20] F. Jeremias, M. Koruyucu, E. C. Küchler et al., "Genes expressed in dental enamel development are associated with molar-incisor hypomineralization," *Archives of Oral Biology*, vol. 58, no. 10, pp. 1434–1442, 2013.

[21] A. S. E. da Cunha Coelho, P. C. M. Mata, C. A. Lino et al., "Dental hypomineralization treatment: a systematic review," *Journal of Esthetic and Restorative Dentistry*, vol. 31, no. 1, pp. 26–39, 2019.

[22] F. Crombie, D. Manton, and N. Kilpatrick, "Aetiology of molar-incisor hypomineralization: a critical review," *International Journal of Paediatric Dentistry*, vol. 19, no. 2, pp. 73–83, 2009.

[23] S. M. Allazzam, S. M. Alaki, and O. A. S. El Meligy, "Molar incisor hypomineralization, prevalence, and etiology," *International Journal of Dentistry*, vol. 2014, Article ID 234508, 8 pages, 2014.

[24] D. Fteita, A. Ali, and S. Alaluusua, "Molar-incisor hypomineralization (MIH) in a group of school-aged children in Benghazi, Libya," *European Archives of Paediatric Dentistry*, vol. 7, no. 2, pp. 92–95, 2006.

[25] G. Kılınç, M. Çetin, B. Köse, and H. Ellidokuz, "Prevalence, aetiology, and treatment of molar incisor hypomineralization in children living in Izmir City (Turkey)," *International Journal of Paediatric Dentistry*, vol. 29, no. 6, pp. 775–782, 2019.

[26] M. Koruyucu, S. Özel, and E. B. Tuna, "Prevalence and etiology of molar-incisor hypomineralization (MIH) in the city of Istanbul," *J Dent Sci.*, vol. 13, no. 4, pp. 318–328, 2018.

[27] C. Serna, A. Vicente, C. Finke, and A. J. Ortiz, "Drugs related to the etiology of molar incisor hypomineralization: a systematic review," *Journal of the American Dental Association (1939)*, vol. 147, no. 2, pp. 120–130, 2016.

[28] Y. Sekino, M. Inamori, E. Yamada et al., "Characteristics of intestinal pseudo-obstruction in patients with mitochondrial diseases," *World Journal of Gastroenterology*, vol. 18, no. 33, pp. 4557–4562, 2012.

[29] K. E. Discepolo and S. Baker, "Adjuncts to traditional local anesthesia techniques in instance of hypomineralized teeth," *The New York State Dental Journal*, vol. 77, no. 6, pp. 22–27, 2011.

[30] R. Pereira, "Esthetic approach for treatment of molar incisor hypomineralization: a case report," *Dental Research and Oral Health*, vol. 2, no. 4, pp. 62–72, 2019.

[31] K. Bekes, K. Heinzelmann, S. Lettner, and H.-G. Schaller, "Efficacy of desensitizing products containing 8% arginine and calcium carbonate for hypersensitivity relief in MIH-affected molars: an 8-week clinical study," *Clinical Oral Investigations*, vol. 21, no. 7, pp. 2311–2317, 2017.

[32] Z.-Y. Yang, F. Wang, K. Lu, Y.-H. Li, and Z. Zhou, "Arginine-containing desensitizing toothpaste for the treatment of dentin hypersensitivity: a meta-analysis," *Clinical, Cosmetic and Investigational Dentistry*, vol. 8, pp. 1–14, 2016.

[33] M. O. Sharif, S. Iram, and P. A. Brunton, "Effectiveness of arginine-containing toothpastes in treating dentine hypersensitivity: a systematic review," *Journal of Dentistry*, vol. 41, no. 6, pp. 483–492, 2013.

[34] N. A. Lygidakis, F. Wong, B. Jälevik, A. M. Vierrou, S. Alaluusua, and I. Espelid, "Best clinical practice guidance for clinicians dealing with children presenting with molar-incisor-hypomineralisation (MIH)," *European Archives of Paediatric Dentistry.*, vol. 11, no. 2, pp. 75–81, 2010.

[35] I. Mejàre, E. Bergman, and M. Grindefjord, "Hypomineralized molars and incisors of unknown origin: treatment outcome at age 18 years," *International Journal of Paediatric Dentistry*, vol. 15, no. 1, pp. 20–28, 2005.

[36] S. E. Kopperud, C. G. Pedersen, and I. Espelid, "Treatment decisions on molar-incisor hypomineralization (MIH) by Norwegian dentists - a questionnaire study," *BMC Oral Health*, vol. 17, no. 1, p. 3, 2016.

[37] J. Fütterer, M. Ebel, K. Bekes, C. Klode, and C. Hirsch, "Influence of customized therapy for molar incisor hypomineralization on children's oral hygiene and quality of life," *Clinical and Experimental Dental Research*, vol. 6, no. 1, pp. 33–43, 2019.

[38] G. D. Taylor, K. F. Pearce, and C. R. Vernazza, "Management of compromised first permanent molars in children: cross-sectional analysis of attitudes of UK general dental practitioners and specialists in paediatric dentistry," *International Journal of Paediatric Dentistry*, vol. 29, no. 3, pp. 267–280, 2019.

[39] N. Kotsanos, E. G. Kaklamanos, and K. Arapostathis, "Treatment management of first permanent molars in children with molar-incisor hypomineralisation," *European Journal of Paediatric Dentistry*, vol. 6, no. 4, pp. 179–184, 2005.

[40] A. Ghanim, M. J. Silva, M. E. C. Elfrink et al., "Molar incisor hypomineralisation (MIH) training manual for clinical field surveys and practice," *European Archives of Paediatric Dentistry*, vol. 18, no. 4, pp. 225–242, 2017.

26

Salvaging the Lost Pink Triangle: A Case Series of Papilla Reconstruction

Santhosh Shenoy B,[1] Anahita Punj,[2] Amitha Ramesh,[1] and Avaneendra Talwar[1]

[1]*Department of Periodontics, A.B Shetty Memorial Institute of Dental Sciences, NITTE (Deemed-to-be) University, Deralakatte, Mangalore, Karnataka-575018, India*
[2]*Army College of Dental Sciences, Jai Jawahar Nagar, Chennapur-CRPF Road, Secunderabad, 500087 Telangana, India*

Correspondence should be addressed to Anahita Punj; anahitapunj@gmail.com and Amitha Ramesh; amitharamesh71@yahoo.in

Academic Editor: Giuseppe Alessandro Scardina

Introduction. The interdental papilla may be lost or reduced in height, forming black triangles due to various reasons, which gives an unaesthetic appearance when the patient smiles. Various noninvasive and invasive techniques have been used to augment/reconstruct the interdental papilla, to reclaim the pink triangle. The most satisfactory and natural appearance can be obtained by augmenting or reconstructing the lost papilla as the pink esthetics is as important as the white esthetics. *Cases.* Two female patients and 1 male patient reported to the dental department with the complaint of a small black gap in the gum area between their upper front teeth since 6 months and 1 year, respectively. On examination, the interdental papillae in all three cases were classified as class 1 (Nordland and Tarnow's). The interdental papilla was augmented surgically by using three different approaches in each case. *Result and Conclusion.* Postoperatively and after 1-month follow-up, there was a complete fill of the interdental area by the interdental papilla normal (Nordland and Tarnow's). As a result, the black triangle was successfully converted into a natural pink triangle in all three cases.

1. Introduction

The interdental papilla is a component of the gingiva which is present between the proximal surfaces of the teeth occupying the cervical embrasure space which extends to fill the lingual, buccal, and occlusal pyramidal space of the interdental space [1]. The interdental papilla is triangular when observed two dimensionally and pyramidal when viewed three dimensionally. The shape, position, and presence is dependent upon the presence of underlying alveolar bone proper, the proximal contact point, and the area of the adjacent teeth [1]. This entity is also referred to as the interdental papillary house by Gonzalez et al. [2] where the dimensions of the roof, floor, and lateral walls of the interdental house play important roles in maintaining the interdental papilla.

It is needless to say that in the absence of tooth, alveolar bone proper, and adjacent tooth contact, the interdental papilla will fail to sustain its original form and result in an empty space between teeth, which is commonly referred to as a black triangle. The black triangle can result in unaesthetic appearance while smiling and can result in food impaction and phonetic problems [3]. The etiologies which can result in black triangle include aging, periodontal disease, loss of height of the alveolar bone relative to the interproximal contact, length of embrasure area, root angulations, tooth loss, faulty oral hygiene procedures, interproximal contact position, and triangular-shaped crowns [4, 5].

Once the papilla is lost due to any of the above factors, rebuilding it again and expecting regeneration is cumbersome. Papilla reconstruction or its augmentation is the most esthetically challenging procedure in perioplastic procedure [6]. A number of techniques have been developed by various authors such as Beagle [7], Azzi et al. [8], Han and Takei [9], Carnio [6], and Froum et al. [10] in an attempt to convert the black triangle into an aesthetic pink triangle. The methods include nonsurgical and surgical methods (Table 1). In many cases, surgical methods if performed correctly can give everlasting and natural results. This article attempts to observe and compare the outcome of three different procedures carried out to reconstruct the papilla.

Table 1

S. no.	Year	Author	Technique
1	1956	Kromer [39]	First report of papilla preservation procedure
2	1959	Cohen [40]	Described the interdental papilla
3	1963	Ochsenbein and Bohannon [41]	Palatal approach procedure in which incisions are given from the palatal aspect
4	1967	Frisch et al. [42]	Curtain procedure, which maintains the labial gingiva and lingual and interproximal 2/3rd part is released
5	1973	App [43]	Intact papilla flap: interdental gingiva is retained in the buccal flap
6	1974	Ramfjord and Nissle [44]	Use of submarginal incision to preserve papilla during flap surgery
7	1985	Shapiro [18]	Used periodic curettage of papilla to increase size of papilla
8	1985	Evian et al. [45]	Modified the intact papilla technique
9	1985	Takei et al. [23]	Papilla preservation technique and use of palatal semilunar incision 3 mm apical to gingival margin
10	1988	Checchi and Schonfeld [13]	Modified Evian and Takei's technique and suggested to give buccal incision and coronally advance it to cover graft in the palatal area. Lingual incision was to be given when maximum depth of defect was in labial aspect
11	1992	Beagle [7]	Combines principles of Abrams' roll technique for ridge augmentation with augmentation of Evian's papilla preservation technique. One treatment option for this problem has been to create on acrylic resin mask to mimic the appearance of healthy gingiva
12	1995	Cortellini et al. [24]	Modified papilla preservation technique: here the buccal flap is freed and straight interproximal incisions are given
13	1998	Azzi et al. [8]	Connective tissue from retro molar area is placed in interdental area after raising split thickness flap
14	1999	Cortellini et al. [25]	Simplified papilla preservation technique by giving an oblique incision in the interdental papilla in cases where the interdental distance is less than 2 mm
15	2001	Nemcovsky [26]	Interproximal augmentation of papilla using a new instrument and advancing the papillary flap plus placing connective tissue graft
16	2004	Carnio [6]	Papilla reconstruction using subepithelial connective tissue graft
17	2004 and 2005	Cardaropoli et al. [20, 21]	Use of orthodontics to correct lateral walls of the interdental papilla housing
18	2006	Kotschy and Laky [46]	Bone grafting done in interdental areas to raise the floor of interdental papilla housing
19	2006	Zucchelli and De Sanctis [31]	Papilla amplification flap: giving parabola incisions adjacent to the papilla to be amplified
20	2007	McGuire and Scheyer [47]	Augmentation of papilla by injecting autologous fibroblasts
21	2008	Nordland and Sandhu [15]	Microsurgical technique to augment papilla
22	2009	Akiyama [48]	Papilla reconstruction done using a microscope
23	2016	Froum et al. [10]	New surgical technique for interimplant papilla reconstruction by giving oblique incisions in the vestibular area labially and palatally and creating a tunnel using translingual curette to advance the papillary unit

The table shows the baseline (preoperative) and final (postoperative) changes in classification and gain in soft tissue level in the gingiva.

2. Case Presentation

2.1. Case 1. A 45-year-old adult female patient reported with complaint of deposits in the lower anterior teeth and a black space between the upper front teeth and the gum region since 6 months. On examination, the patient presented with class 1 papilla (Nordland and Tarnow's [11]). The patient was diagnosed with chronic papillary gingivitis [12] with papillary gingival recession type 1 [13] (Figure 1(a)). As the interdental bone was within 5 mm from the contact point, the roll technique [11, 13] was used for reconstruction of the papilla. Scaling and root planning was performed for the patient on the first visit and brushing technique was corrected. After 1 week, surgical procedure was carried using the roll technique. The interdental area was anesthetised by local infiltration using 0.2% lignocaine with 1 : 80000 epinephrine. Next, two

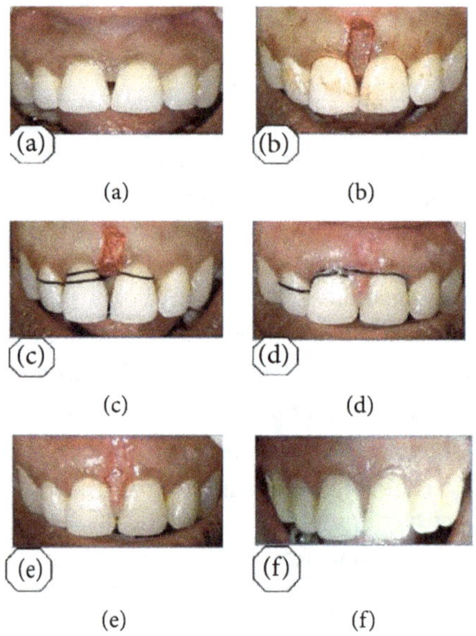

FIGURE 1: (a) Preoperative condition of the papilla between 11 and 21 with square shaped teeth, (b) interproximal and vertical incisions starting at the base of the papilla and connected by horizontal incision, (c) split thickness flap is reflected and rolled partially over to fill the black triangle area and sutured circumferentially around the adjacent teeth, (d) 10 days after operative procedure, (e) 3 weeks after suture removal, and (f) 2 years after procedure.

parallel vertical incisions were placed in the interdental gingiva [12] starting from the coronal end of the papilla near the proximal contact points and was extended apically and joined by a horizontal incision to create a pouch (Figure 1(b)). A partial thickness flap was raised from the apical end and was gently advanced apically towards the contact point. The partial thickness was then rolled and folded on itself and sutured using 3-0 silk suture to keep it in the designated position. While suturing, the suture was circumferentially wound around adjacent teeth to avoid any displacement (Figure 1(c)). Periodontal dressing was given to provide mechanical protection, and the patient was instructed to take analgesics twice a day to avoid postoperative pain. Suture removal was done after 10 days (Figure 1(d)), and there was complete fill of the interdental papilla which was maintained even after 3 weeks (Figure 1(e)) and after 2 years (Figure 1(f)).

2.2. Case 2. A 30-year-old adult female patient reported with complaint of a black space between the upper front teeth and the gum region since 6 months. The patient gave a past history of orthodontic treatment. On examination, the patient presented with class 1 papilla [11]. The patient was diagnosed with chronic papillary gingivitis with papillary gingival recession type 1 [12, 14] (Figure 2(a)). Scaling and root planning was performed for the patient on the first visit. After 1 week, as the interdental bone was slightly more than 5 mm from the contact point (Figure 2(b)), the contact point was moved coronally by building the proximal contours with composite restoration to allow creeping attachment to occur postsurgery (Figure 2(c)). Next, surgical procedure was carried using

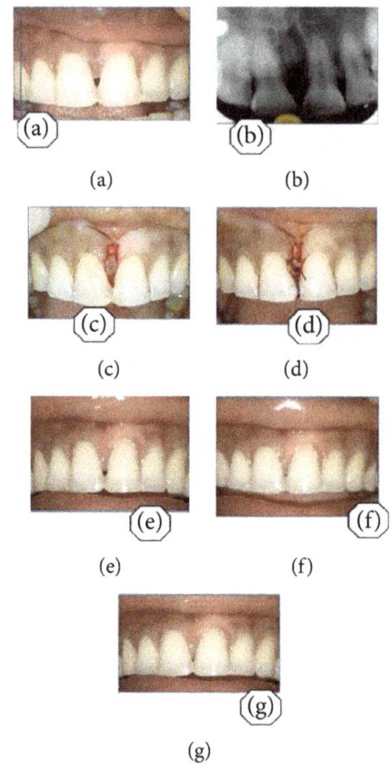

FIGURE 2: (a) Preoperative condition of the papilla between 11 and 21 with triangular-shaped teeth, (b) intraoperative periapical radiograph showing more than 5 mm of vertical distance between the contact point and the bone crest, (c) interproximal and vertical incisions starting at the base of the papilla and connected by horizontal incision, (d) split thickness flap is reflected and rolled partially over to fill the black triangle area and sutured over composite stops, (e) 10 days after operative procedure, (f) 2 months after procedure, and (g) 2.5 years after procedure.

the roll technique in the same manner as in case 1. While suturing, composite stops were used to suspend the suture and avoid any displacement (Figures 2(c) and 2(d)). Periodontal dressing was given to provide mechanical protection, and the patient was instructed to take analgesics twice a day to avoid postoperative pain. Suture removal was done after 10 days (Figure 2(e)), and there was almost complete fill of the interdental papilla, and after 2 months (Figure 2(f)), the interdental papilla completely filled the interdental area. The papilla was maintained in a stable position even after 6 months postprocedure (Figure 2(g)). Unfortunately, the patient was lost to follow-up as she moved to some other city.

2.3. Case 3. A 43-year-old adult male patient reported with complaint of a black space between the upper front teeth and the gum region since 6 months. On examination, the patient presented with class 1 gingival recession and class 1 papilla [11]. The patient was diagnosed as chronic generalised marginal gingivitis with papillary gingival recession type 2 with 11 and 21 (Figure 3(a)) [12, 14]. As the interdental bone was more than 5 mm from the contact point, the pouch and tunnel technique with interposed connective tissue graft using microsurgical instruments was planned. Scaling and root planning was performed for the patient on the first visit.

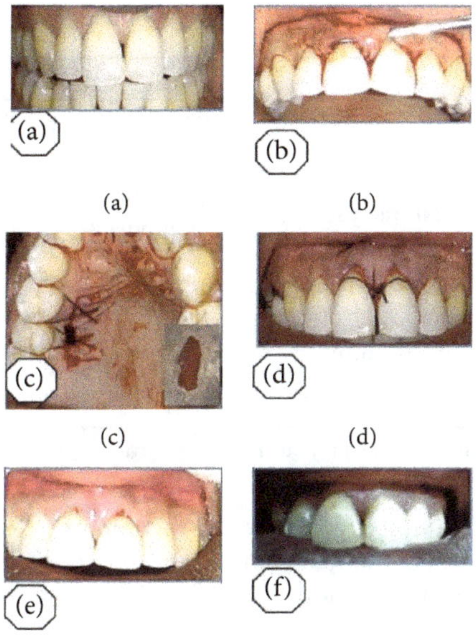

(a) (b) (c) (d) (e) (f)

Figure 3: (a) Preoperative condition of the papilla between 11 and 21 with buccal gingival recession, (b) pouch and tunnel created in the interdental papillary area extending to 11 and 21 distally using microsurgical instruments, (c) connective tissue graft (inset) harvested from the palate and recipient site sutured, (d) connective tissue graft placed inside the tunnel using lasso suturing and positioned using sling sutures, (e) 1 month after operative procedure, and (f) 2 years after the procedure.

After 1 week, surgical procedure was carried by anesthetising the interdental area by local infiltration using 0.2% lignocaine with 1 : 80000 epinephrine. Next, under magnification of 2.5x, a sulcular incision was given around the facial and proximal surfaces; next, using microsurgical tunnelling instruments, a subperiosteal pouch was created by raising a partial thickness flap using sharp dissection (Figure 3(b)). The pouch was extended towards the interdental gingiva, detaching it from the palatal aspect partially. The tunnel was extended beyond the mucogingival junction to allow coronal movement of the interdental gingival unit. Once the interdental gingiva was coronally advanced passively, the amount of connective tissue graft required was estimated by using a tin foil and measuring the amount of space present in the subperiosteal tunnel. The tin foil was used as a guide to harvest the connective tissue graft from the hard palate using the trap door technique. After harvesting the connective tissue graft, the donor site was sutured using 3-0 silk suture with the horizontal mattress suturing technique (Figure 3(c)). The connective tissue graft was then tied at one end with 5-0 resorbable suture as a lasso suture and was inserted into the tunnel created by pulling the suture and tying it to stabilize its position [15]. Similarly, the other end of graft was also stabilized by suturing. Next, 3-0 silk suture was allowed to pass through the labial interdental gingiva, connective tissue graft, and palatal gingiva to bind the graft together and was tied as a sling suture with a composite stop in the middle of the two incisors (Figure 3(d)). Periodontal dressing (Coe-Pak) was given to provide mechanical protection, and the patient was instructed to take analgesics twice a day to avoid postoperative pain. Suture removal was done after 10 days, and there was almost complete fill of the interdental papilla, and after 1 month (Figure 3(e)), the interdental papilla completely filled the interdental area. After approximately 2 years, the interdental papillary fill showed a relapse of about 0.5 mm (Figure 3(f)). In all the three cases, the papilla presence score decreased, quantifying the gain in the papilla as shown in Table 2.

3. Discussion

Treating papillary recession is of utmost importance as the evidence suggests that treated gingival recession defects are unlikely to have an increase in recession depth versus untreated recession defects [16, 17]. Over the years, a number of authors have advocated methods to treat the aesthetically challenging black triangle. Nonsurgical methods such as correction of faulty tooth habits, repeated curettage of papilla every 15 days for 3 months [18], reshaping of contacts and contours using restorations or prosthesis [19], and orthodontic repositioning [20, 21] have been used in mild forms of papillary loss. When the papilla cannot be augmented by nonsurgical methods, surgical techniques become an indispensable part of the treatment plan [22]. The techniques include papilla preservation flap [23], modified papilla preservation [24], and simple papilla preservation flap [25] to prevent inadvertent papillary loss as a result of flap surgery. The other papilla reconstruction techniques include the pedicle flap using the roll technique, semilunar coronally positioned flap, envelope flap which is augmented by use of connective tissue graft [26], hyaluronic acid [27]. Platelet-rich fibrin (PRF) [5], and autogenous graft [28] especially in case the interdental bony crest and contact point are more than 5 mm apart. The use of microsurgical approaches has also been used for papilla reconstruction which cause lesser trauma and better healing outcomes [4]. Similar techniques have been used to create interimplant papilla which include the use of connective tissue graft [6], PRF [29], autogenous bone, metal pins [30], modified instrument design by Froum et al. [10], and papilla amplification flap [31].

In the first case, the patient had chronic localised gingivitis, faulty brushing of teeth, and advanced age which could have resulted in the papilla loss. Since the radiograph showed that the interdental bone crest was within 5 mm from the contact point of 11 and 21, according to Tarnow et al.'s rule [32], it was expected that a simple surgical procedure like Beagle's modified roll technique will result in postoperative papillary fill. The results of this case were similar to those obtained by Kapoor et al. [33]. In the second case, the possible etiologic factors for papillary loss were past orthodontic treatment and triangular shape of the crown. After radiographic examination, as the distance was more than 5 mm, the contact point was moved coronally by building the mesial proximal contacts with composite restoration to allow creeping movement of the gingiva. This result is supported by the fact that decreasing the height of the interdental housing can allow the papilla to maintain its presence [2]. The vertical incisions given in the roll technique used in the two cases in this report are similar to the modification given by Checchi

Table 2

Parameters	Case 1		Case 2		Case 3	
Timeline	Pre-op	Post-op	Pre-op	Post-op	Pre-op	Post-op
Classification [11]	1	0	1	0	1	0
Recession type [14]	Papillary gingival recession type 1	No recession	Papillary gingival recession type 1	No recession	Papillary gingival recession type 2	Buccal gingival recession
Distance from bone crest to contact point	5 mm	5 mm	6 mm	6 mm	6 mm	6 mm
Distance from contact point to gingival margin	3 mm	0 mm	4 mm	0.5 mm	4 mm	0.5 mm
Papilla presence index [49]	2	1	2	1	3r	1r

The table shows the baseline (preoperative) and final (postoperative) changes in classification and gain in soft tissue level in gingiva.

and Schonfeld [13]. In the third case, the possible etiologies included faulty brushing of teeth and past periodontal disease. As in this case, amount of loss was greater and the gingival phenotype was thin; use of connective tissue graft to augment the papilla was used, and to avoid any inadvertent trauma during the surgical procedure, microsurgical instruments were used under 2.5x magnification. The results of this case are in agreement with cases by Carnio [6] and Azzi et al. [8] and a study done by Kaushik et al. [34]. Katsuhiko [35] also carried out papilla reconstruction using connective tissue graft using a microscope. In the third case, there was a relapse of 0.5 mm, which probably occurred due to the physiological process of aging. Montevecchi et al. [22] in their study have mentioned that papilla receded more as the age of the patient advanced. They have also inferred that less than 1 crown width/crown length makes the crown triangular and holds true for cases 1 and 3, while 1 represents square-shaped teeth which is observed in case 1. The cases included in this manuscript are comparing only the central incisor papilla and do not include the lateral incisor papilla to avoid any bias in the results as the critical horizontal and vertical distances for the central and lateral incisors which could support the 90-100% of papillary fill varies [22]. In our present cases, the postoperative discomfort was least in cases 1 and 2 as it did not involve a second surgical site. In case 3, the patient did not complain of any pain 2 days after the procedure owing to his high pain threshold and timely intake of analgesics and adherence to postoperative care. Additionally, there were no complications related to the harvesting of connective tissue graft in the present case which supports the use of grafts if needed. This fact is supported by a study done by Harris et al. [36] where the complication rate such as pain, infection, bleeding, and swelling with the connective tissue grafting procedure was low and was clinically acceptable. Shruthi et al. [37] have compared the Azzi et al. [8] and Han and Takei [9] techniques and found them equally successful. In the present paper, although we have tried to classify the papilla based on different indices to check the postoperative results, an index, called the interdental pressure index, could not be used as it required additional armamentarium and was discovered during the literature review after the procedures were carried out. The index takes into account the inflammatory status of the interdental papilla by evaluating the pressure applied by a modified dynamometer [38]. The number of cases in this report is too small to establish a proper guideline for selection of the best technique for papilla reconstruction.

The present report compares three different techniques for papilla reconstruction which were selected based upon careful diagnosis and treatment planning. An attempt has been made to achieve positive results using simple to moderate techniques for papilla reconstruction which are reproducible and amenable to the patients. On comparing the three cases, Beagle's roll technique with Checchi's modification is simpler and less painful for the patients, but it has its inherent limitations due to which connective tissue graft is used in cases where the bone support and the availability of tissue is limited. The key message is not to promote a particular technique but to diagnose the papillary loss correctly and use the predictable techniques and avoid unnecessary complex procedures if required to suit patients from all walks of life.

References

[1] R. Mutha, P. Mutha, and N. Dani, "Papillary reconstruction: a case report," *Journal of Periodontology & Implant Dentistry*, vol. 7, no. 1, pp. 33-34, 2015.

[2] M. K. Gonzalez, A. L. Almeida, S. L. Greghi, L. F. Pegoraro, J. Mondelli, and T. Moreno, "Interdental papillary house: a new concept and guide for clinicians," *The International Journal of Periodontics & Restorative Dentistry*, vol. 31, no. 6, pp. e87–e93, 2011.

[3] M. Agarwal, M. Mittal, S. Mehrotra, and A. Agarwal, "Black triangle and its reconstruction: A review," *Journal of Dental Sciences & Oral Rehabilitation*, vol. 1, pp. 55-56, 2011.

[4] V. P. Singh, A. S. Uppoor, D. G. Nayak, and D. Shah, "Black triangle dilemma and its management in esthetic dentistry," *Dental Research Journal*, vol. 10, no. 3, pp. 296–301, 2013.

[5] N. Tomar, V. Singal, D. Dureja, and A. Wadhawan, "Reconstruction of interdental papilla with platelet-rich fibrin membrane," *Journal of Current Research in Scientific Medicine*, vol. 2, no. 2, pp. 112–115, 2016.

[6] J. Carnio, "Surgical reconstruction of interdental papilla using an interposed subepithelial connective tissue graft: a case report," *The International Journal of Periodontics & Restorative Dentistry*, vol. 24, no. 1, pp. 31–37, 2004.

[7] J. R. Beagle, "Surgical reconstruction of the interdental papilla: case report," *International Journal of Periodontics & Restorative Dentistry*, vol. 12, pp. 144–151, 1992.

[8] R. Azzi, D. Etienne, and F. Carranza, "Surgical reconstruction of the interdental papilla," *International Journal of Periodontics & Restorative Dentistry*, vol. 18, no. 5, pp. 466–473, 1998.

[9] T. J. Han and H. H. Takei, "Progress in gingival papilla reconstruction," *Periodontology 2000*, vol. 11, no. 1, pp. 65–68, 1996.

[10] S. Froum, M. Lagoudis, G. Rojas, T. Suzuki, and S.-C. Cho, "New surgical protocol to create interimplant papilla: the preliminary results of a case series," *The International Journal of Periodontics & Restorative Dentistry*, vol. 36, no. 2, pp. 161–168, 2016.

[11] W. P. Nordland and D. P. Tarnow, "A classification system for loss of papillary height," *Journal of Periodontology*, vol. 69, no. 10, pp. 1124–1126, 1998.

[12] J. Caton, G. Armitage, T. Berglundh et al., "A new classification scheme for periodontal and peri-implant diseases and conditions - Introduction and key changes from the 1999 classification," *Journal of Clinical Periodontology*, vol. 45, Suppl 20, pp. S1–S8, 2018.

[13] L. Checchi and S. E. Schonfeld, "A technique for esthetic treatment of maxillary anterior infrabony lesions," *Quintessence International*, vol. 19, no. 3, pp. 209–213, 1988.

[14] F. Cairo, M. Nieri, S. Cincinelli, J. Mervelt, and U. Pagliaro, "The interproximal clinical attachment level to classify gingival recessions and predict root coverage outcomes: an explorative and reliability study," *Journal of Clinical Periodontology*, vol. 38, no. 7, pp. 661–666, 2011.

[15] W. P. Nordland and H. S. Sandhu, "Microsurgical technique for augmentation of the interdental papilla: three case reports," *The International Journal of Periodontics & Restorative Dentistry*, vol. 28, no. 6, pp. 543–549, 2008.

[16] L. Chambrone and D. N. Tatakis, "Long-term outcomes of untreated buccal gingival recessions. A systematic review and meta-analysis," *Journal of Periodontology*, vol. 87, no. 7, pp. 796–808, 2016.

[17] G. Agudio, P. Cortellini, J. Buti, and G. P. Pini Prato, "Periodontal conditions of sites treated with gingival augmentation surgery compared with untreated contralateral homologous sites: an 18- to 35-year long-term study," *Journal of Periodontology*, vol. 87, no. 12, pp. 1371–1378, 2016.

[18] A. Shapiro, "Regeneration of interdental papilla using periodic curettage," *The International Journal of Periodontics & Restorative Dentistry*, vol. 5, no. 5, pp. 27–33, 1985.

[19] N. Bichacho, "Papilla regeneration by non-invasive prosthodontics treatment: segmental proximal restorations," *Practical Periodontics and Aesthetic Dentistry*, vol. 10, no. 75, pp. 77-78, 1998.

[20] D. Cardaropoli, S. Re, G. Corrente, and R. Abundo, "Reconstruction of the maxillary midline papilla following a combined orthodontic-periodontic treatment in adult periodontal patients," *Journal of Clinical Periodontology*, vol. 31, no. 2, pp. 79–84, 2004.

[21] D. Cardaropoli and S. Re, "Interdental papilla augmentation procedure following orthodontic treatment in a periodontal patient," *Journal of Periodontology*, vol. 76, no. 4, pp. 655–661, 2005.

[22] M. Montevecchi, V. Checchi, L. Piana, and L. Checchi, "Variables affecting the gingival embrasure space in aesthetically important regions: differences between central and lateral papillae," *The Open Dentistry Journal*, vol. 5, no. 1, pp. 126–135, 2011.

[23] H. H. Takei, T. J. Han, F. A. Carranza Jr., E. B. Kenney, and V. Lekovic, "Flap technique for periodontal bone implants. Papilla preservation technique," *Journal of Periodontology*, vol. 56, no. 4, pp. 204–210, 1985.

[24] P. Cortellini, G. Pini Prato, and M. Tonetti, "The modified papilla preservation technique. A new surgical approach for interproximal regenerative procedures," *Journal of Periodontology*, vol. 66, no. 4, pp. 261–266, 1995.

[25] P. Cortellini, G. Pini Prato, and M. Tonetti, "The simplified papilla preservation flap. A novel surgical approach for the management of soft tissues in regenerative procedures," *Journal of Periodontology*, vol. 19, pp. 589–599, 1999.

[26] C. E. Nemcovsky, "Interproximal papilla augmentation procedure: a novel surgical approach and clinical evaluation of 10 consecutive procedures," *The International Journal of Periodontics & Restorative Dentistry*, vol. 21, no. 6, pp. 553–559, 2001.

[27] S. S. Mansouri, M. Ghasemi, Z. Salmani, and N. Shams, "Clinical application of hyaluronic acid gel for reconstruction of interdental papilla at the esthetic zone," *Journal of Islamic Dental Association of IRAN*, vol. 25, no. 3, pp. 208–214, 2013.

[28] S. Desai, H. Shinde, J. Mudda, and V. Patil, "Simultaneous surgical excision of localized gingival overgrowth and papilla reconstruction with subepithelial connective tissue graft; a case report," *The Internet Journal of Dental Science*, vol. 8, no. 1, pp. 1–8, 2008.

[29] S. Aspalli, G. Nagappa, and A. S. Jain, "Platelet rich fibrin: a panacea for lost interdental papilla," *Journal of Dental Specialities*, vol. 3, no. 2, p. 217, 2015.

[30] M. L. Bhongade, A. Deshpande, A. Jadhav, K. Thakare, and P. Jaiswal, "Interimplant papilla reconstruction by using demineralized freeze dried bone allograft block fixed by titanium screw: a case report," *Case Reports in Dentistry*, vol. 2012, Article ID 809347, 3 pages, 2012.

[31] G. Zucchelli and M. De Sanctis, "The papilla amplification flap for the treatment of a Localized periodontal defect associated with a palatal groove," *Journal of Periodontology*, vol. 77, no. 10, pp. 1788–1796, 2006.

[32] D. P. Tarnow, A. W. Magner, and I. Fletcher, "The effect of the distance from the contact point to the crest of bone on the presence or absence of the interproximal dental papilla," *Journal of Periodontology*, vol. 63, no. 12, pp. 995-996, 1992.

[33] A. Kapoor, P. Biban, S. Goel, S. Kapoor, and A. Kapoor, "Papilla reconstruction: a case report," *IJSS Case Reports & Reviews*, vol. 1, no. 10, pp. 24–26, 2015.

[34] A. Kaushik, P. K. Pal, K. Jhamb et al., "Clinical evaluation of papilla reconstruction using subepithelial connective tissue graft," *Journal of Clinical and Diagnostic Research*, vol. 8, no. 9, pp. ZC77–ZC81, 2014.

[35] A. Katsuhiko, "Papilla reconstruction using dental operating microscope," *The International Journal of Microdentistry*, vol. 1, pp. 25–29, 2009.

[36] R. J. Harris, R. Miller, L. H. Miller, and C. Harris, "Complications with surgical procedures utilizing connective tissue grafts: a follow-up of 500 consecutively treated cases," *The International journal of periodontics & restorative dentistry*, vol. 25, no. 5, pp. 449–459, 2005.

[37] S. Shruthi, S. K. Gujjari, and K. P. Mallya, "Comparison of two

surgical techniques for the reconstruction of interdental papilla," *Journal of Interdisciplinary Dentistry*, vol. 5, no. 1, pp. 17–22, 2015.

[38] L. Checchi, M. Montevecchi, G. Marucci, and V. Checchi, "A proposed new index for clinical evaluation of interproximal soft tissues: the interdental pressure index," *International Journal of Dentistry*, vol. 2014, Article ID 345075, 7 pages, 2014.

[39] H. Kromer, "Behandling av de infraossose iommer," *Den Norske Tannlaegeforenings Tidende*, vol. 86, p. 164, 1956.

[40] B. Cohen, "Morphological factors in the pathogenesis of the periodontal disease," *British Dental Journal*, vol. 7, pp. 31–39, 1959.

[41] C. Ochsenbein and H. M. Bohannon, "The palatal approach to osseous surgery I. Rationale," *Journal of Periodontology*, vol. 34, no. 1, pp. 60–68, 1963.

[42] J. Frisch, R. A. Jones, and S. N. Bhaskar, "Conservation of maxillary anterior Esthetics: a modified surgical approach," *Journal of Periodontology*, vol. 38, no. 1, pp. 11–17, 1967.

[43] G. R. App, "Periodontal treatment for the removable partial prosthesis patient. Another half-century?," *Dental Clinics of North America*, vol. 17, no. 4, pp. 601–610, 1973.

[44] S. P. Ramfjord and R. R. Nissle, "The modified Widman flap," *Journal of Periodontology*, vol. 45, no. 8, pp. 601–607, 1974.

[45] C. I. Evian, H. Corn, and E. S. Rosenberg, "Retained interdental papilla procedure for maintaining anterior esthetics," *The Compendium of Continuing Education in Dentistry*, vol. 6, no. 1, pp. 58–64, 1985.

[46] P. Kotschy and M. Laky, "Reconstruction of supracrestal alveolar bone lost as a result of severe chronic periodontitis. Five-year outcome: case report," *The International Journal of Periodontics & Restorative Dentistry*, vol. 26, no. 5, pp. 425–431, 2006.

[47] M. K. McGuire and E. T. Scheyer, "A randomized double blind, placebo-controlled study to determine the safety and efficacy of cultured and expanded autologous fibroblast injections for the treatment of interdental papillary insufficiency associated with the papilla priming procedure," *Journal of Periodontology*, vol. 78, no. 1, pp. 4–17, 2007.

[48] K. Akiyama, "Papilla reconstruction using dental operating microscope," *The international journal of microdentistry*, vol. 1, pp. 25–29, 2009.

[49] D. Cardaropoli, S. Re, and G. Corrente, "Papilla presence index (PPI) : a new system to assess interproximal papillary levels," *The International Journal of Periodontics & Restorative Dentistry*, vol. 24, pp. 488–492, 2004.

27

Pediatric Pleomorphic Adenoma of the Palate

Jerome A. Lindeboom,[1] Jean-Pierre T. F. Ho,[2] Naomi Donner,[3] and Willem H. Schreuder[4]

[1]*Department of Oral and Maxillofacial Surgery, Amsterdam University Medical Centers and Amstelland Hospital, University of Amsterdam, Netherlands*
[2]*Department of Oral and Maxillofacial Surgery, Amsterdam University Medical Centers and Northwest Clinics, University of Amsterdam, Netherlands*
[3]*Department of Pathology, Amsterdam University Medical Centers, University of Amsterdam, Amsterdam, Netherlands*
[4]*Department of Oral and Maxillofacial Surgery, Amsterdam University Medical Centers, University of Amsterdam, Amsterdam and Department of Head and Neck Surgery, Antoni van Leeuwenhoek Hospital, Amsterdam, Netherlands*

Correspondence should be addressed to Jerome A. Lindeboom; j.a.lindeboom@amsterdamumc.nl

Academic Editor: Giuseppe Colella

Pleomorphic adenoma is the most common salivary gland tumor but is extremely rare in pediatric patients. The parotid gland is the most affected salivary gland, and the minor salivary glands are rarely affected. Here, we report a case of a 12-year-old boy with a pleomorphic adenoma of the palate.

1. Introduction

Salivary tumors are extremely rare in children, with fewer than 5% occurring in children compared to adults. Tumors in the minor salivary glands are uncommon, and pleomorphic adenomas are the most common benign tumors of the palate. Pleomorphic adenoma has a remarkable degree of morphological diversity, with the essential components being the capsule, epithelial and myoepithelial cells, and the mesenchymal or stromal elements [1].

The tumor consists of acini, cords, and thin strands of epithelial cells suspended in stroma, which often has a myxomatous appearance [2]. The tumor is predominately seen in the parotid gland. On the palate, the tumor is mostly located at the transition of the hard and soft palate [3]. Pediatric pleomorphic adenoma of the palate is slightly more common in girls than boys (1.3 : 1), but due to the rarity, it is difficult to provide a reliable estimate [2].

2. Case Report

A healthy 12-year-old boy was referred by an orthodontist with swelling of the palate. The patient did not have any symptoms, and he had no pain or difficulty with speech or swallowing and no history of trauma, fever, fatigue, anorexia, respiratory or gastrointestinal symptoms, or weight changes. The swelling had been present for approximately 5 years, and the dentist observed it during the regular dental control visits, but no further action was taken. The swelling had never bothered the patient. The patient used Ritalin for attention deficit hyperactivity disorder (ADHD). Upon physical examination, a 2 cm nonfluctuating, nontender, immobile, firm nodular swelling was observed with intact overlying mucosa on the left side of the hard palate in the bicuspid-molar region (Figure 1). Clinical and radiographic examination of the dentition did not reveal any pathology. The patient had no palpable cervical lymphadenopathy. MRI showed a well-demarcated mass of the left side of the hard palate without bone invasion (Figures 2(a) and 2(b)). Pathological diagnosis was established by incisional biopsy performed under local anesthesia; histological examination was consistent with a pleomorphic adenoma of the minor salivary glands of the palate. The tumor was excised under general anesthesia with nasotracheal intubation. The mucosa around the tumor was marked and incised with an adequate margin, followed by dissection, with removal of the whole encapsulated mass

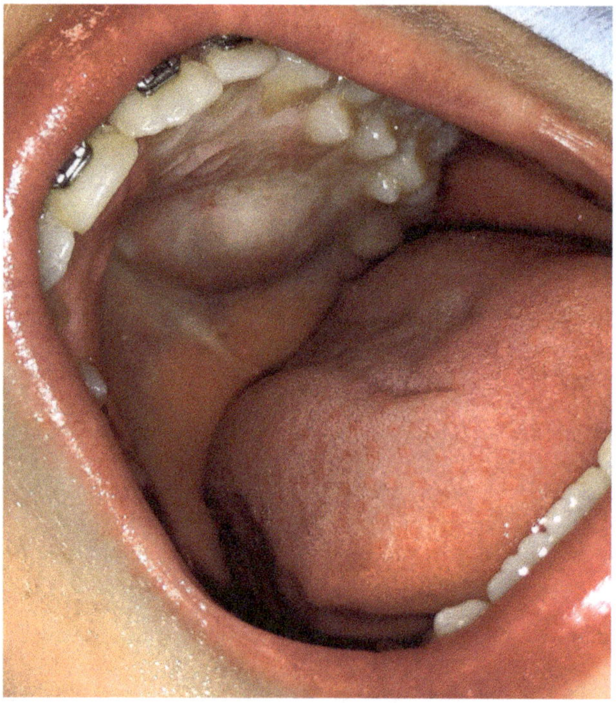

Figure 1: Photograph of the swelling of the left palate with intact overlying mucosa.

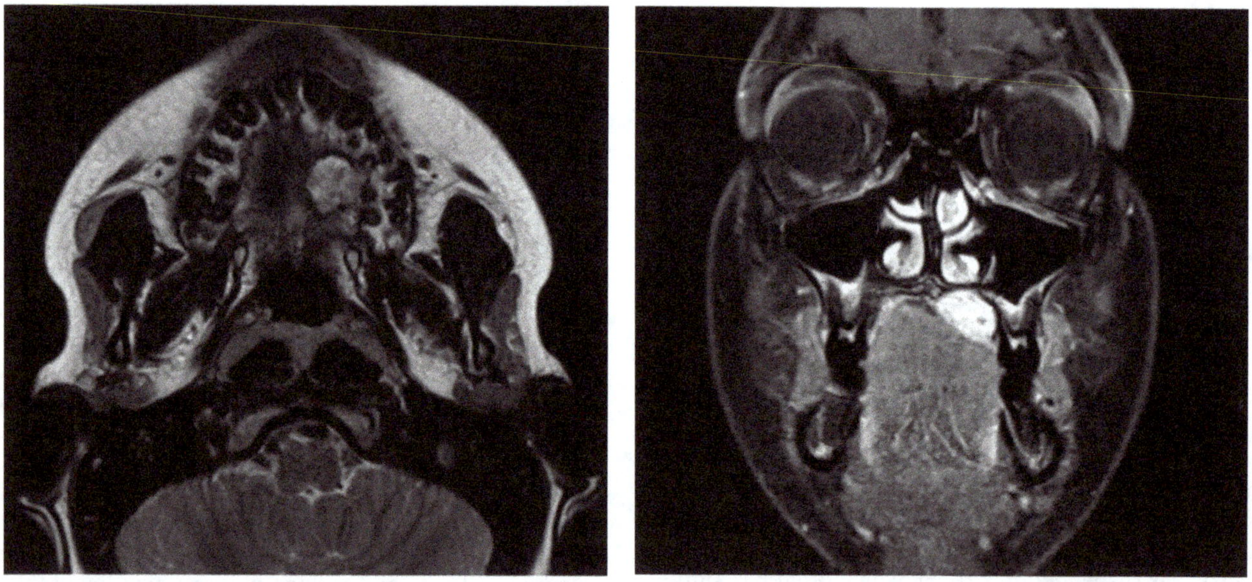

(a) (b)

Figure 2: MRI sections showing a well-defined, homogenous enhancing lesion in the left palate.

and the mucoperiosteum (Figure 3). With a bur under copious sterile saline irrigation, the superficial part of the underlying bone was removed to ensure that no remnants of the lesions could cause recurrence. The defect on the palate was not reconstructed (Figure 4). An iodine tampon dressing was placed, and the wound covered with a fabricated palatal acrylic plate (Figure 5). The postoperative recovery was uneventful and histopathological assessment of the operation specimen confirmed the original diagnosis of pleomorphic adenoma of the palate. Examination showed mucosal tissue with a multinodular lesion consisting of two components in the stroma. There were solid fields of cells with round-oval nuclei and poorly delineated eosinophilic cytoplasm. There was also a spindle cell component located in the myxoid matrix with perivascular condensation. The tumor itself was sharply delineated (Figures 6(a)–6(c)). The wound gradually healed by secondary intention, and complete healing was observed 4 months after surgery (Figure 7). Follow-up 12 months after surgery did not reveal any recurrence. The patient remains under surveillance.

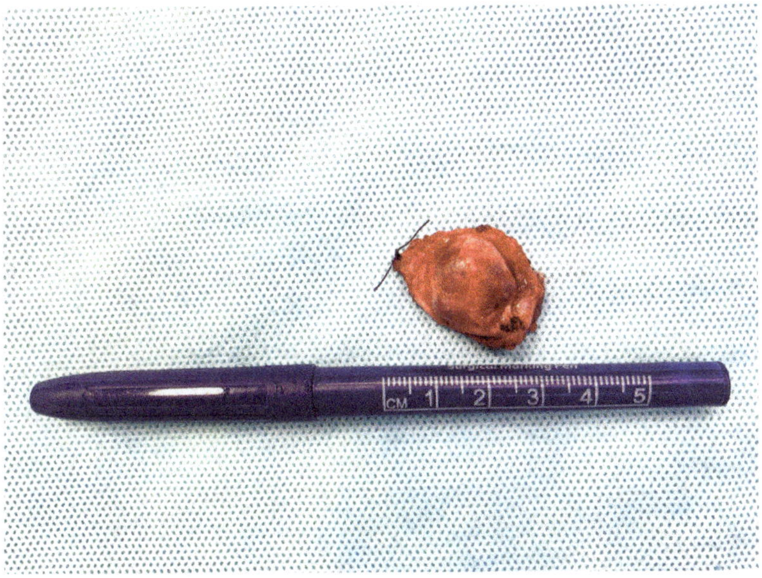

FIGURE 3: Image of the excised palatal tumor, with macroscopically intact capsule.

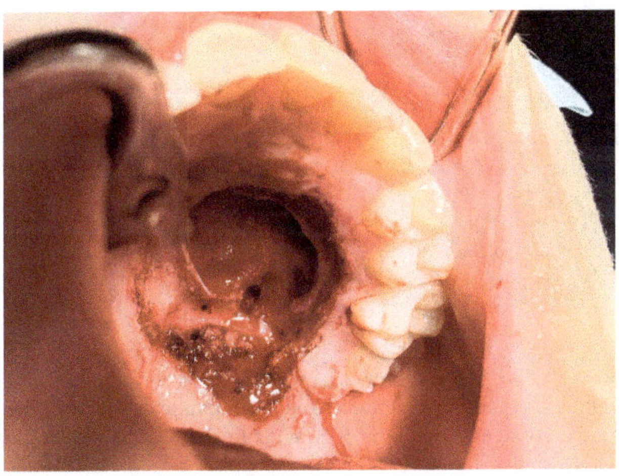

FIGURE 4: Image of the palatal defect after tumor resection.

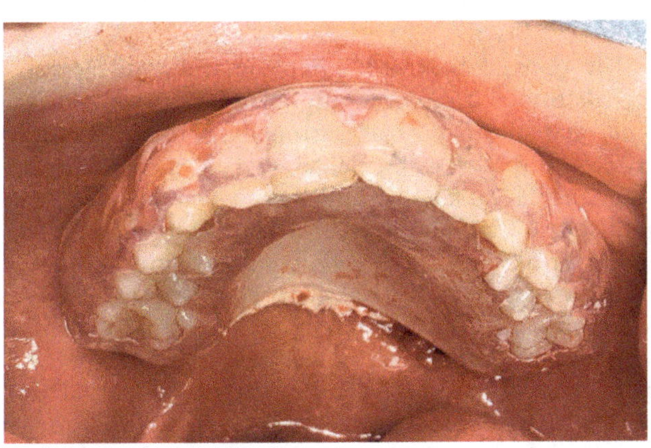

FIGURE 5: The wound was covered with a fabricated palatal acrylic plate.

3. Discussion

Any swelling of the hard palate should be considered a possible minor salivary gland tumor. Pleomorphic adenoma is the most common benign salivary gland tumor but is mainly observed between 30 and 60 years of age [1]. This tumor is rarely observed in children, and involvement of the minor oral salivary gland is even less common. After the minor salivary glands, the palate is the most common intraoral location, followed by the upper lip and buccal mucosa [3, 4]. In a retrospective study of 4341 cases of pleomorphic adenoma, 90 patients younger than 18 years old were identified [1]. Among the 90 pediatric cases, the palatal minor glands were involved in 8 (8.9%).

Pleomorphic adenomas present as a painless, slow-growing firm mass, and patients generally do not exhibit symptoms. In our case, the swelling had been present for years and the patient did not have any symptoms. However, two other pediatric case reports noted that the swelling developed in 4 days and 2 weeks [5, 6].

A biopsy with histopathological assessment is mandatory to establish the diagnosis, especially as there seems to be a predisposition toward malignancy with pediatric salivary gland tumors [7, 8]. Salivary gland lesions are notorious for their extraordinary heterogeneity. However benign and low-grade neoplasms can often be accurately distinguished preoperatively from high-grade malignant tumors to guide clinical management [9]. Additional CT or MRI evaluation is useful in determining the size and extent of palatal lesions, as well as verifying destruction or erosion of the underlying bone [1].

The differential diagnosis of a firm palatal swelling of nonodontogenic origin in children, other than pleomorphic adenoma, is malignant salivary gland tumors, such as mucoepidermoid carcinoma, adenocarcinoma, or acinic cell carcinoma, which emphasizes the importance of histological assessment of swelling of the palate [10]. Other benign and

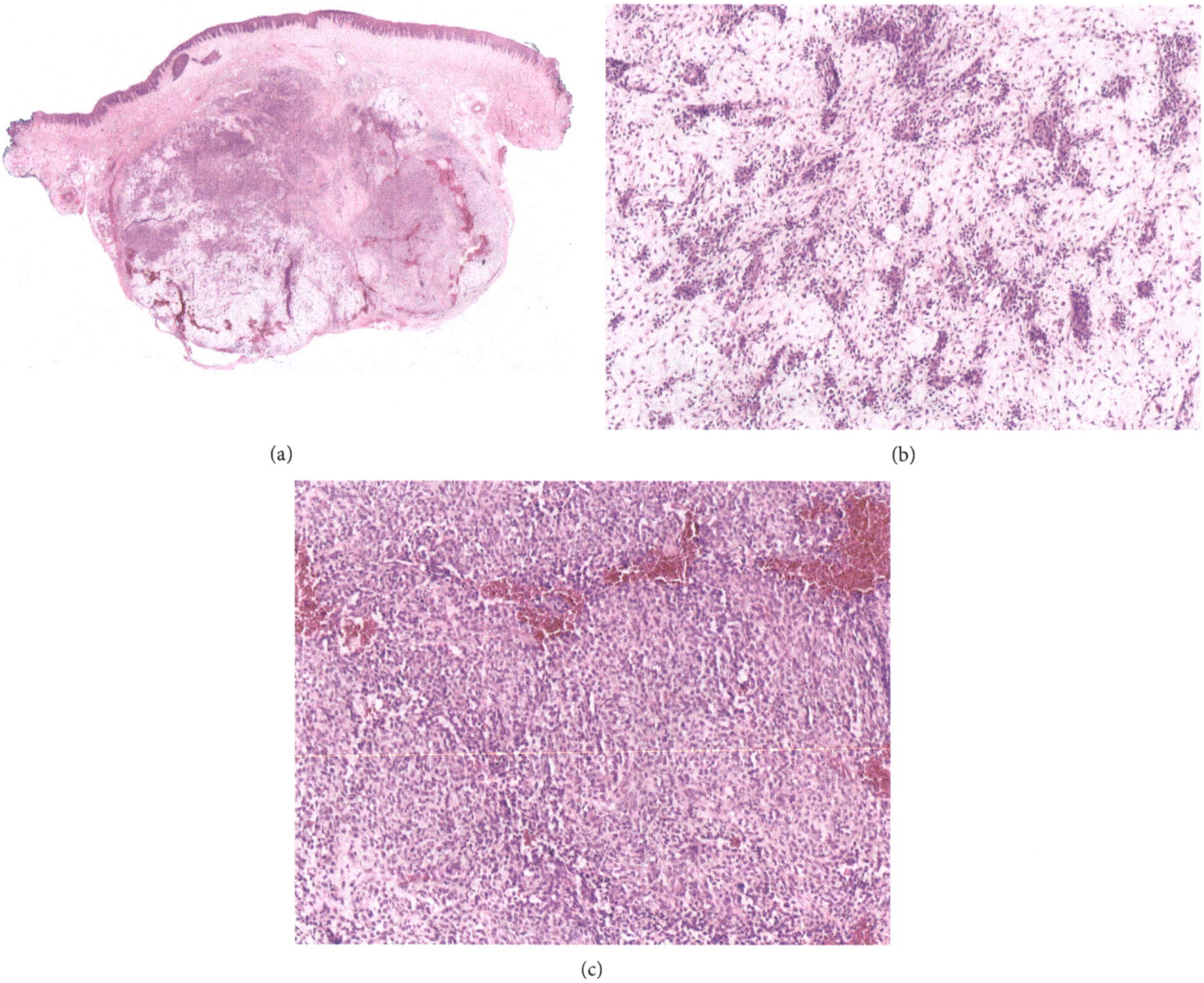

FIGURE 6: (a–c) Histopathological examination of the tissue showed a mucosal excision. In the submucosal stroma, there was a multinodular tumor consisting of 2 components. One component showed solid fields of cells with round to oval nuclei and eosinophilic cytoplasm. There was also a component of spindled cells within a myxoid matrix, with perivascular condensation of the cells. The tumor was clearly demarked from the surrounding stroma.

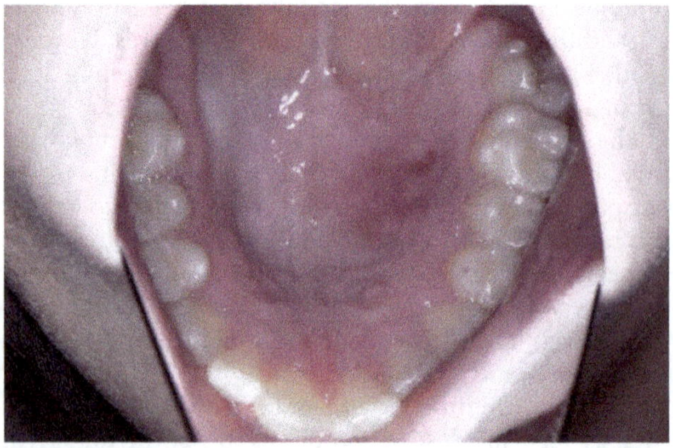

FIGURE 7: Photograph of the postoperative healing 4 months after surgery.

malignant mesenchymal lesions that should be considered are neurofibroma and rhabdomyosarcoma, and lymphomas should be ruled out [11].

The optimal treatment for pleomorphic adenomas of the palate is a wide local surgical excision with an adequate margin of normal surrounding tissue. Complete surgical extirpation is critical to obviate the risk of future malignancy [12]. Simple enucleation should be avoided, as this can lead to local recurrence, particularly if the capsule breaks during surgery [13]. The underlying bone undergoes curettage with a sharp spoon or bur to avoid recurrence, and a local flap is used to reconstruct the palatal mucosal defect [2]. In the present case report, the palatal defect was not reconstructed, but a palatal prosthesis was used to cover the defect to allow it to heal by secondary intention. Recurrence of pleomorphic adenoma of the palate is seldomly seen but is a concern that makes long follow-up of patients necessary [11]. Recurrence on the palate can be considered serious, as they can enter the palatine foramen and reach the base of the skull [10].

4. Conclusion

We described a case of pleomorphic adenoma of the palate in a pediatric patient. The treatment was wide surgical excision of the pleomorphic adenoma with tumor-free margins. Primary reconstruction is not always necessary, as the defect can heal with secondary intention if the bony delimitation between the oral and nasal cavity remains intact.

Consent

Consent to publish the case report was not obtained. The report does not contain any personal information that could lead to identifying the patient.

References

[1] H. Fu, J. Wang, L. Wang, Z. Zhang, and Y. He, "Pleomorphic adenoma of the salivary glands in children and adolescents," *Journal of Pediatric Surgery*, vol. 47, no. 4, pp. 715–719, 2012.

[2] J. S. Daniels, I. Ali, I. M. al Bakri, and B. Sumangala, "Pleomorphic adenoma of the palate in children and adolescents: a report of 2 cases and review of the literature," *Journal of Oral and Maxillofacial Surgery*, vol. 65, no. 3, pp. 541–549, 2007.

[3] C. A. Waldron, S. K. el-Mofty, and D. R. Gnepp, "Tumors of the intraoral minor salivary glands: a demographic and histologic study of 426 cases," *Oral Surgery, Oral Medicine, and Oral Pathology*, vol. 66, no. 3, pp. 323–333, 1988.

[4] D. Wang, Y. Li, H. He, L. Liu, L. Wu, and Z. He, "Intraoral minor salivary gland tumors in a Chinese population: a retrospective study on 737 cases," *Oral Surgery Oral Medicine Oral Pathology Oral Radiology Endodontology*, vol. 104, no. 1, pp. 94–100, 2007.

[5] J. L. López-Cedrún, G. Gonzalez-Landa, and B. Birichinaga, "Pleomorphic adenoma of the palate in children: report of a case," *International Journal of Oral and Maxillofacial Surgery*, vol. 25, no. 3, pp. 206-207, 1996.

[6] H. Shaaban, P. J. Davenport, and J. Bruce, "Recurrent pleomorphic adenoma of the palate in a child," *British Journal of Plastic Surgery*, vol. 54, no. 3, pp. 245–247, 2001.

[7] P. D. Bull, "Salivary gland neoplasia in childhood," *International Journal of Pediatric Otorhinolaryngology*, vol. 49, pp. S235–S238, 1999.

[8] K. Dhanuthai, K. Sappayatosok, and K. Kongin, "Pleomorphic adenoma of the palate in a child: a case report," *Medicina Oral, Patología Oral y Cirugía Bucal*, vol. 14, no. 2, pp. e73–e75, 2009.

[9] M. P. Pusztaszeri and W. C. Faquin, "Update in salivary gland cytopathology: Recent molecular advances and diagnostic applications," *Seminars in Diagnostic Pathology*, vol. 32, no. 4, pp. 264–274, 2015.

[10] M. A. Pogrel, "The management of salivary gland tumors of the palate," *Journal of Oral and Maxillofacial Surgery*, vol. 52, no. 5, pp. 454–459, 1994.

[11] J. Jorge, F. R. Pires, F. A. Alves et al., "Juvenile intraoral pleomorphic adenoma: report of five cases and review of the literature," *International Journal of Oral and Maxillofacial Surgery*, vol. 31, no. 3, pp. 273–275, 2002.

[12] N. D. Dombrowski, N. E. Wolter, A. L. Irace et al., "Pleomorphic adenoma of the head and neck in children: presentation and management," *Laryngoscope*, vol. 129, no. 11, pp. 2603–2609, 2019.

[13] S. Y. Moon, "Surgical Management of the Palatal Pleomorphic Adenoma," *The Journal of Craniofacial Surgery*, vol. 30, no. 6, pp. e580–e582, 2019.

28

Monostotic Fibrous Dysplasia of the Mandible in a 9-Year-Old Male Patient Treated with a Conservative Surgical Treatment: A Case Report and 15-Year Follow-Up

Antoine Berberi[1] **Georges Aoun**[2] **Emile Khalaf**[3] **and Georges Aad**[2]

[1]*Department of Oral and Maxillofacial Surgery, Faculty of Dental Medicine, Lebanese University, Lebanon*
[2]*Department of Oral Medicine and Maxillofacial Radiology, Faculty of Dental Medicine, Lebanese University, Lebanon*
[3]*Beirut Arab University, Lebanon*

Correspondence should be addressed to Antoine Berberi; aberberi@ul.edu.lb

Academic Editor: Pia L. Jornet

Fibrous dysplasia is a developmental disorder of the bone that originates from a genetic defect disturbing the osteogenesis leading to the replacement of normal bone with the excess proliferation of fibrous tissue. It can be associated with hyperpigmentation of the skin and endocrine disorders. Fibrous dysplasia can manifest in a monostotic form affecting one bone or in a polyostotic form involving several bones. Approximately 30% of monostotic forms are observed in the maxilla and the mandible. It frequently appears in the posterior region and is usually unilateral. It is found in teenagers and could become static after adulthood. Patients can present with swelling, facial asymmetry, pain, or numbness on the affected side. Treatment modalities vary between conservative surgical treatment, radical surgical approach, and medical treatment based on bisphosphonates. Here, we present a case of a monostotic form of fibrous dysplasia affecting the posterior left region of the mandible in a 9-year-old male complaining of gradually increased swelling on the left mandibular side of one-year duration. The diagnosis of fibrous dysplasia is established based on clinical, radiographical, and histopathological features. Conservative surgery is implemented with surgical shaving and reencountering of the bone excess to reduce the facial asymmetry. Recurrence is reported 10 years later and is also treated with a localized osteoplasty and remodeling of the bone contours. Five years later, the lesion remains stable. In conclusion, a conservative approach should be adopted as the first line of treatment for young patients suffering from monostotic fibrous dysplasia.

1. Introduction

Fibrous dysplasia (FD) is a benign intraosseous tumor-like process, where the medullary bone is substituted by fibrous connective tissue leading to undeveloped and inadequately calcified bone [1–4]. FD involves an inequity among osteoblastic and osteoclastic activities triggered by a genetic mutation in the stimulatory G protein (GSα) [5].

The increase in the activity of GSα in osteoblast progenitor cells and osteoclasts is stimulated by the amplified production of interleukin-6 stromal cells [5–7].

According to the current World Health Organization classification of bone tumors, FD belongs to tumors with an undefined neoplastic nature [4]. FD can be associated with hormonal dysregulations, most frequently precocious puberty with cutaneous manifestations seen in the McCune-Albright syndrome, MAS, or intramuscular myxomas in Mazabraud's syndrome, MS [1, 2]. FD commonly develops in the first or second decades of life, affects women more than men with a ratio of 2 : 1, and is usually asymptomatic with very low evolution [1, 2]. FD occurs either as a monostotic form affecting a single bone or as a polyostotic form spreading into several bones [1–4]. Monostotic fibrous dysplasia (MFD) is around 10 times more common than polyostotic fibrous dysplasia (PFD) and is frequently unilateral [3, 4]. The lack of stable bone matrix formation can manifest in a multitude of ways, involving facial distortion and asymmetry [5–7]. In the jaws, tooth movement, occlusion problems, pain, paresthesia, and

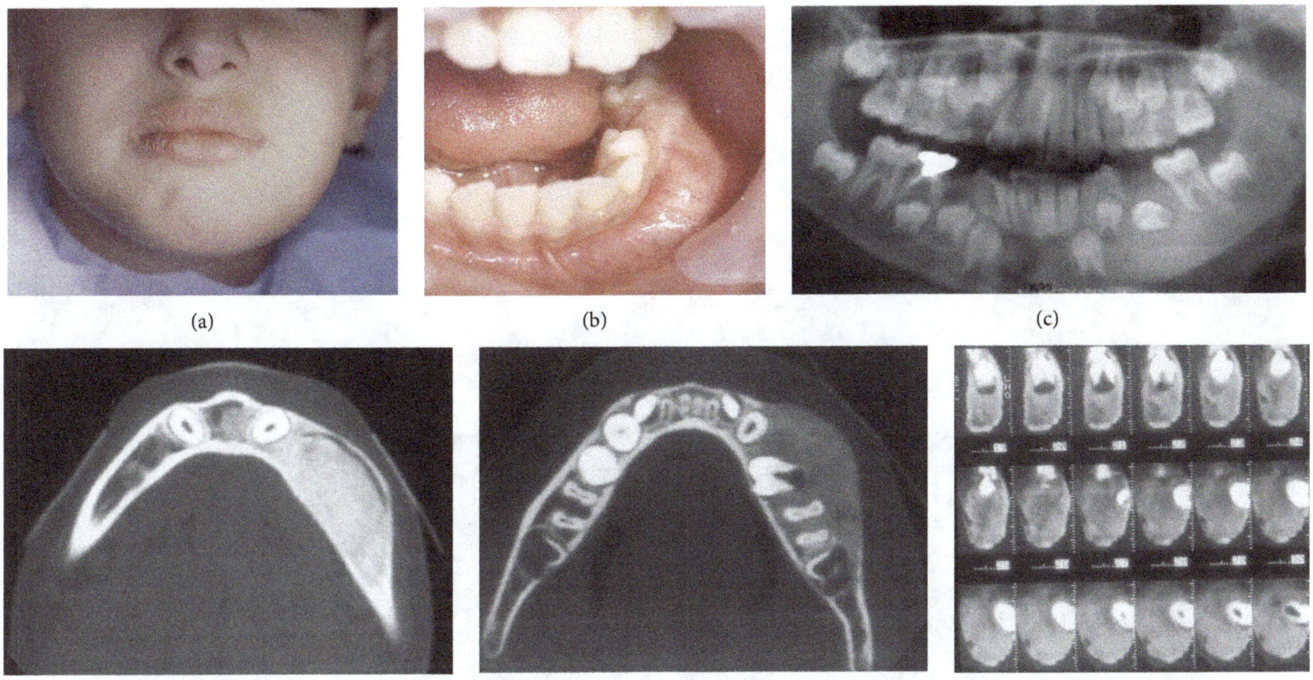

Figure 1: (a) Facial asymmetry on the left side. (b) Swelling in the buccal side of the mandible. (c) Panoramic X-ray showing the radiopaque image englobing the dental germ of the permanent second premolar. (d) The course of the mandibular canal displaced buccally is shown on the axial image of the CBCT. (e) Axial image of the CBCT showing the expansion of the body of the mandible. (f) Para-axial images of the CBCT revealed the ossification of the lesion and the positions of the retained dental germ and the mandibular canal.

interference with dental eruption can be observed [3]. Rapid growth of the bone lesion as well as an increase in the level of alkaline phosphatase could be indicators to possible malignant transformation [2].

In this manuscript, we report a case of MFD in the mandible of a 9-year-old male patient. The diagnosis is established based on different imaging techniques and confirmed with biopsy. Surgery for bone remodeling to correct the patient's facial contour is the treatment adopted.

2. Case Report

A 9-year-old male presented to our clinics with his parents complaining of swelling and asymmetry in the left side of his mandible.

The questionnaires revealed that the expansion of the swelling was slow, gradually increasing during the past year with no pain reported.

Extraoral examination showed a mild facial asymmetry associated with a well-defined swelling on the left side of the mandible measuring 3 to 4 cm (Figure 1(a)). No cutaneous pigmentations on the face, no limitations of mouth opening, and no enlarged submandibular lymph nodes were noticed.

Intraoral examination displayed expansion of the buccal cortical plate, extending from the mandibular left incisal to the first molar, and the first deciduous molar was absent (Figure 1(b)). On palpation, it was hard in constancy, fixed, with no signs of mucosal inflammation observed and no signs of paresthesia.

A panoramic radiograph exposed the loss of trabecular structure and a radiopaque image showing a "ground-glass" feature was observed on the left side of the mandible englobing the dental germ of the permanent second premolar (Figure 1(c)).

The cone-beam computed tomography (CBCT) axial images revealed a radiopacity lesion with an expansion and thinning of the buccal bone cortical with well-defined borders (Figure 1(d)). The dental germ was in the middle of the lesion (Figure 1(e)), and the para-axial images showed the mandibular canal displaced buccally and toward the lower border of the mandible (Figure 1(f)).

Based on the evaluation of the clinical and radiological data, a provisional diagnosis of FD was made, and differential diagnoses of MAS, MS, and hyperparathyroidism were considered.

As the germ needed to be removed, we discussed with the parents the surgical procedure required to extract the germ along with the need for an osteoplasty to remove the excess bone and a biopsy to be taken during the procedure.

Under locoregional analgesia, a conservative surgical excision of the buccal bone was proceeded, with extraction of the dental germ and remodeling of the region disturbed by the asymmetry (Figure 2(a)). Macroscopically, the excised bone was soft with spongy aspects (Figure 2(b)). The histological results were consistent with FD. The hematoxylin-eosin staining revealed irregularly shaped trabeculae of immature bone within proliferating fibroblastic and vascularized stroma (Figure 2(c)).

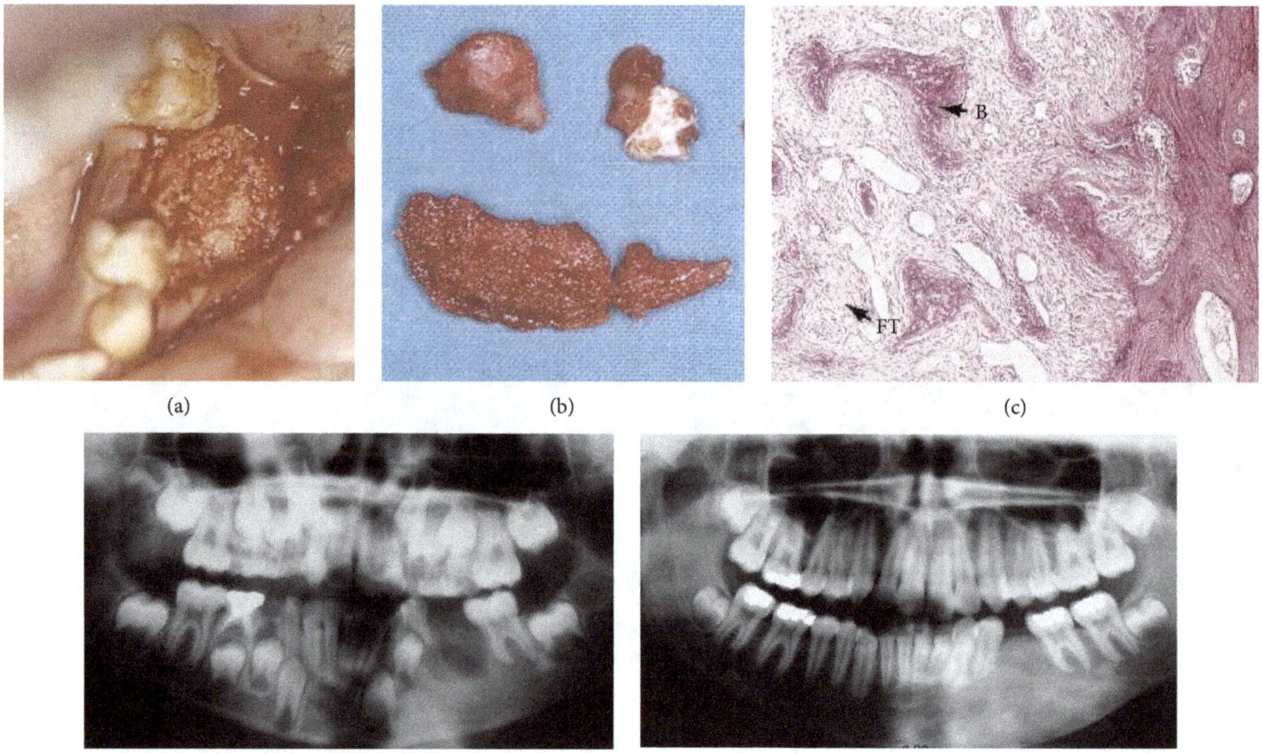

(a) (b) (c) (d) (e)

Figure 2: (a) Clinical view of the excess bone. (b) The excised bone with the dental germ. (c) HE × 10 showing irregularly shaped trabeculae of immature bone within proliferating fibroblastic tissue (B: bone; FT: fibrous tissue). (d) One-week panoramic radiograph. (e) Five-year panoramic radiograph.

The patient was advised to consult his pediatrician for further clinical and radiological investigations. All the laboratory tests and radiological images were in favor of localized FD mandibular lesions.

The patient was followed up yearly, both clinically and radiologically with a panoramic radiograph (Figures 2(d) and 2(e)).

Ten years later, the patient complained of left mandibular asymmetry (Figure 3(a)).

Clinical examination revealed a lingual cortical bone expansion beside the buccal one (Figures 3(b) and 3(c)).

Panoramic X-ray showed the same image of a radiopaque area with the appearance of ground glass aspects in the left hemimandible (Figure 3(d)).

The axial images of the CBCT presented a discontinuity of the buccal cortex, expansion of the lingual one, and expansion of the lesion anteriorly to the middle line of the mandible.

The mandibular canal was still displaced to the lower border of the mandible (Figure 3(e)).

A 3D reconstruction showed an increase in the volume of the left hemimandible, confirming mandibular asymmetry (Figure 3(f)).

After discussing the findings with the patient, a second surgery was decided. Under locoregional analgesia, a wide osteoplasty was performed, and the buccal bone was reshaped until the limit of the mental nerve anteriorly and the position of the mandibular canal apically (Figures 4(a) and 4(b)). The histology results confirmed the previous one.

No complications were recorded in the follow-up period, and the patient was satisfied with the esthetic results (Figure 4(c)).

Five years later the clinical and radiological exams showed a stabilization of the lesion (Figures 4(d)–4(f)).

3. Discussion

FD represents 7% of all benign bone tumors and includes the facial bones in approximately 10%–27% of MFD patients [1–4]. Chen et al. state that MFD affects the maxilla more regularly than the mandible [8]. Kruse et al. reveal that equal distribution between the maxilla and the mandible exists [9]. Lee et al. show that the mandible is touched in 19 cases and the maxilla in 6 [10]. Davidova et al. report that maxilla (23/38) is more involved than the mandible (15/38) [11].

The differential diagnosis of FD comprises simple bone cyst, nonossifying fibroma, osseous-fibrous dysplasia, adamantinoma, low-grade intramedullary osteosarcoma, Paget's disease, MAS, and MS [1, 10, 11].

The CBCT offers complete information about the bone lesions associated with the FD, its border, and the exact relation with the anatomical elements [8].

Treatment modalities of FD such as conservative surgery [9, 10, 12, 13], radical excision [14, 15], and medical treatment with bisphosphonates [16, 17] are suggested. Conservative surgical management implicates surgical excision of the poorly mineralized bone followed by a modeling osteoplasty through an intraoral approach which can potentially help

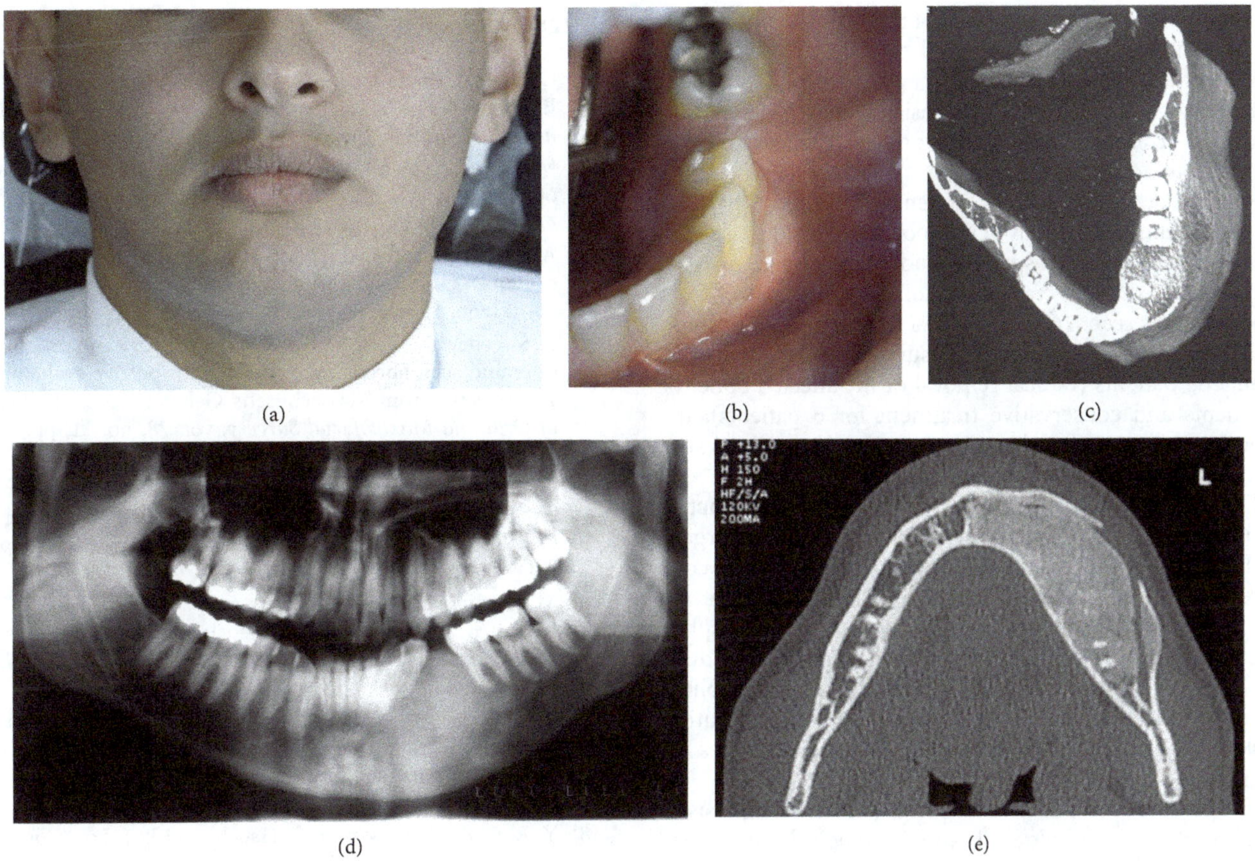

FIGURE 3: (a) Facial asymmetry at 10 years. (b) Clinical view of the intraoral swelling. (c) Panoramic X-ray at 10 years. (d) Axial image of a CBCT showing the expansion of the lesion to the midline and discontinuity of the buccal cortex. (e) 3D reconstruction showed an increase in the volume of the left hemimandible.

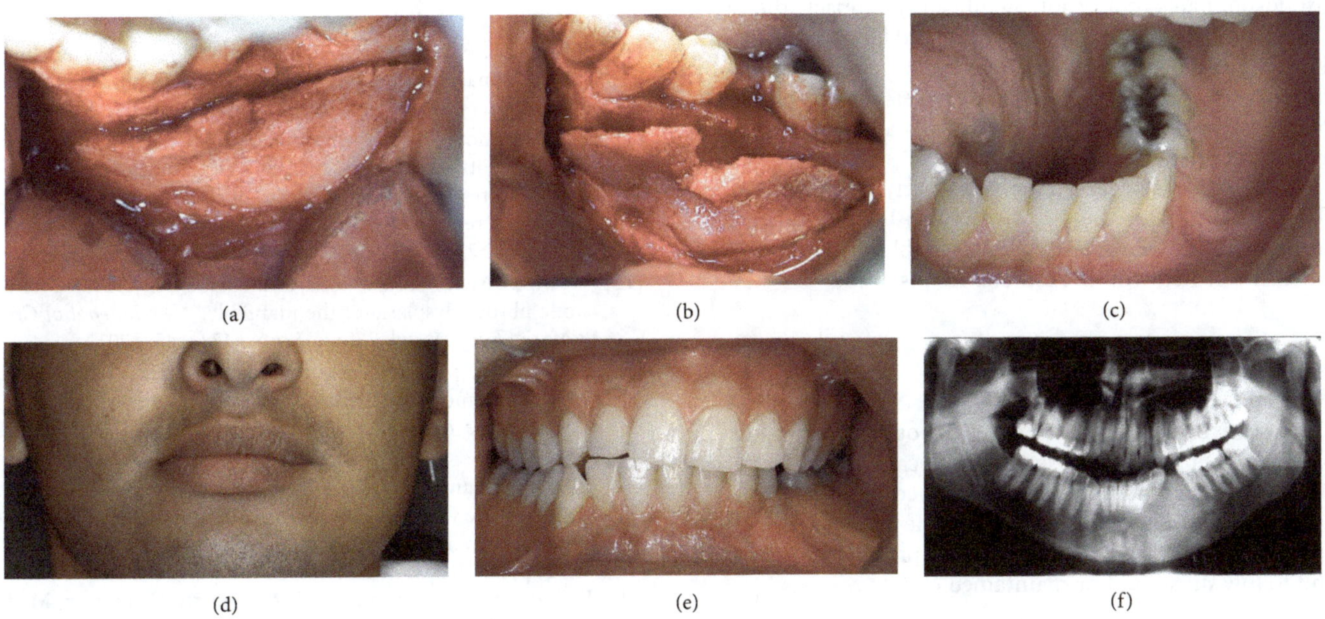

FIGURE 4: (a) Intraoperative view for the surgical approach. (b) The excised bone with respect to the mental foramen. (c) Healing of the soft tissue one month later. (d) Facial stability after 5 years following the second surgery and 15 years after the first surgery. (e) Clinical appearance of the soft healing after 15 years of the first surgery. (f) Panoramic X-ray after 15 years of the first surgery.

with the histological confirmation of the diagnosis [9, 10, 12, 13]. The surgical treatment should take into consideration the age of the patient [4, 9].

The recurrence of fibrous dysplasia is reported in relation to puberty or skeletal maturation; however, its evolution is constant into adulthood [1, 4, 9].

Kruse et al. describe the treatment of MFD in 8 patients with a modeling osteotomy with good results [9]. Valentini et al. state that, in a retrospective study involving 95 patients with FD situated in the craniomaxillofacial area, the following proportions are seen: 76% MFD, 22% PFD, and 2% McCune-Albright syndrome. Of 95 patients, surgical treatment is done for only 68 patients (radical removal of the affected bone for 62 patients and conservative treatment for 6 patients); the remaining patients refused surgery although the authors suggest that radical surgery avoids recurrence [15].

The use of bisphosphonates to decrease osteoclastic activities is considered as a treatment option apart from surgery [16, 17]. Intravenous, not oral, bisphosphonates can be considered in the treatment of persistent, moderate to severe bone pain [18]. Lala et al. state that the use of bisphosphonates improves the clinical situation in children and adults [17]. To note, osteonecrosis of the jaws is a major complication of bisphosphonate treatment [18, 19]. Thus, caution should be considered when prescribing bisphosphonates for a long period in patients suffering from FD [19].

In our case, the patient is young, and the diagnosis is based on clinical, radiological, and histological data. Since the asymmetry is disturbing to the patient, conservative surgical approach is adopted keeping in mind that he is 9 years old, around puberty with a skeletal system that is still in a growth period. At this age, radical excision is very traumatic and can affect the facial growth of the patient. Also, the use of bisphosphonates does not significantly impact the age-dependent decrease in bone turnover, and it does not prevent the progression of FD disease burden in young as stated by Florenzano et al [18]. The CBCT images are very useful to delimitate the lesions, especially when near the mental foramen in the mandibular canal.

Recurrence is observed ten years later, and bone remodeling is adopted for the reasons previously mentioned. Five years later, the clinical situation is stable, and the patient remains satisfied with the esthetic results.

4. Conclusion

Conservative treatment for MFD should be considered, particularly if the patient is young. Localized surgical excision of the demineralized bone followed by an osteoplasty and contour remodeling is one of the most conservative approaches for the treatment of asymmetry. Observation and follow-up should be maintained closely.

Consent

Parents signed the consent form before the first surgery. Patient signed the consent form before the second surgery.

References

[1] C. Ozek, H. Gundogan, U. Bilkay, C. Tokat, T. Gurler, and E. Songur, "Craniomaxillofacial fibrous dysplasia," *The Journal of Craniofacial Surgery*, vol. 13, no. 3, pp. 382–389, 2002.

[2] M. R. DiCaprio and W. F. Enneking, "Fibrous dysplasia, pathophysiology, evaluation, and treatment," *The Journal of Bone and Joint Surgery. American*, vol. 87, no. 8, p. 1848, 2005.

[3] A. B. Burke, M. T. Collins, and A. M. Boyce, "Fibrous dysplasia of bone: craniofacial and dental implications," *Oral Diseases*, vol. 23, no. 6, pp. 697–708, 2017.

[4] K. Sweeney and L. B. Kaban, "Natural history and progression of craniofacial fibrous dysplasia: a retrospective evaluation of 114 patients from Massachusetts General Hospital," *Journal of Oral and Maxillofacial Surgery*, vol. 78, no. 11, pp. 1966–1980, 2020.

[5] G. Ramaswamy, H. Kim, D. Zhang et al., "Gsα controls cortical bone quality by regulating osteoclast differentiation via cAMP/PKA and β-catenin pathways," *Scientific Reports*, vol. 7, no. 1, article 45140, 2017.

[6] M. Riminucci, S. A. Kuznetsov, N. Cherman, A. Corsi, P. Bianco, and P. G. Robey, "Osteoclastogenesis in fibrous dysplasia of bone: in situ and in vitro analysis of IL-6 expression," *Bone*, vol. 33, no. 3, pp. 434–442, 2003.

[7] A. H. G. Cleven, W. H. Schreuder, E. Groen, H. M. Kroon, and D. Baumhoer, "Molecular findings in maxillofacial bone tumours and its diagnostic value," *Virchows Archiv*, vol. 476, no. 1, pp. 159–174, 2020.

[8] Y. R. Chen, F. H. Wong, C. Hsueh, and L. J. Lo, "Computed tomography characteristics of non-syndromic craniofacial fibrous dysplasia," *Chang Gung Medical Journal*, vol. 25, no. 1, pp. 1–8, 2002.

[9] A. Kruse, U. Pieles, M. O. Riener, C. Zunker, M. G. Bredell, and K. W. Grätz, "Craniomaxillofacial fibrous dysplasia: a 10-year database 1996-2006," *The British Journal of Oral & Maxillofacial Surgery*, vol. 47, no. 4, pp. 302–305, 2009.

[10] J. S. Lee, E. FitzGibbon, Y. R. Chen et al., "Clinical guidelines for the management of craniofacial fibrous dysplasia," *Orphanet Journal of Rare Diseases*, vol. 7, Supplement 1, 2012.

[11] L. A. Davidova, I. Bhattacharyya, M. N. Islam, D. M. Cohen, and S. G. Fitzpatrick, "An analysis of clinical and histopathologic features of fibrous dysplasia of the jaws: a series of 40 cases and review of literature," *Head and Neck Pathology*, vol. 14, no. 2, pp. 353–361, 2020.

[12] W. M. De Melo, C. K. Sonoda, and E. Hochuli-Vieira, "Monostotic fibrous dysplasia of the mandible," *The Journal of Craniofacial Surgery*, vol. 23, no. 5, pp. e452–e454, 2012.

[13] N. Alves, R. J. de Oliveira, D. Takehana, and N. F. Deana, "Recurrent monostotic fibrous dysplasia in the mandible," *Case Reports in Dentistry*, vol. 2016, Article ID 3920850, 6 pages, 2016.

[14] M. R. Zenn and J. Zuniga, "Treatment of fibrous dysplasia of the mandible with radical excision and immediate reconstruction: case report," *The Journal of Craniofacial Surgery*, vol. 12, no. 3, pp. 259–263, 2001.

[15] V. Valentini, A. Cassoni, T. M. Marianetti, V. Terenzi, M. T. Fadda, and G. Iannetti, "Craniomaxillofacial fibrous dysplasia: conservative treatment or radical surgery? A retrospective study on 68 patients," *Plastic and Reconstructive Surgery*, vol. 123, no. 2, pp. 653–660, 2009.

[16] A. A. Mäkitie, J. Törnwall, and O. Mäkitie, "Bisphosphonate treatment in craniofacial fibrous dysplasia–a case report and

review of the literature," *Clinical Rheumatology*, vol. 27, no. 6, pp. 809–812, 2008.

[17] R. Lala, P. Matarazzo, S. Bertelloni, F. Buzi, F. Rigon, and C. de Sanctis, "Pamidronate treatment of bone fibrous dysplasia in nine children with McCune-Albright syndrome," *Acta Paediatrica*, vol. 89, no. 2, pp. 188–193, 2000.

[18] P. Florenzano, K. S. Pan, S. M. Brown et al., "Age-related changes and effects of bisphosphonates on bone turnover and disease progression in fibrous dysplasia of bone," *Journal of Bone and Mineral Research*, vol. 34, no. 4, pp. 653–660, 2019.

[19] T. Metwally, A. Burke, J. Y. Tsai, M. T. Collins, and A. M. Boyce, "Fibrous dysplasia and medication-related osteonecrosis of the jaw," *Journal of Oral and Maxillofacial Surgery*, vol. 74, no. 10, pp. 1983–1999, 2016.

29

A Calcifying Odontogenic Cyst Associated with Compound Odontoma Mimicking a Tooth Germ

Eduardo Morato Oliveira[1] **Lucas Alves da Mota Santana**[2] **Erika Rezende Silva**[2] **and Leandro Napier Souza**[1]

[1]*Department of Oral Surgery and Pathology, School of Dentistry, Universidade Federal de Minas Gerais, Belo Horizonte, MG, Brazil*
[2]*Department of Dentistry, Universidade Federal de Sergipe, Aracaju, SE, Brazil*

Correspondence should be addressed to Leandro Napier Souza; leandronapierdesouza@gmail.com

Academic Editor: Konstantinos Michalakis

Calcifying odontogenic cyst (COC) is a rare cyst that affects mainly the anterior region of the jaws. Generally, it appears as a unilocular radiolucent lesion containing peripheral foci of calcification, but with radiographic variations depending on the type of presentation. Here, we report an atypical case of COC associated with odontoma, initially diagnosed as a tooth germ, in the posterior region of the mandible of a 10-year-old male patient. Interestingly, the radiographic aspect appeared as a unilocular radiolucent lesion without peripheral foci of calcification in the edentulous region, having its size increased after traction of the impacted tooth adjacent to that area. Thus, the case presented in this study is aimed at calling dentists' attention to its developmental changes and related pathologies.

1. Introduction

Calcifying odontogenic cyst (COC) is a rare developmental cyst that favorably affects the anterior region of the jaws [1, 2]. It comprises less than 1% of intraosseous cysts arising in the maxillofacial complex, and it was recognized as a distinct pathological entity by Gorlin et al. in 1962 [3, 4]. Asymptomatic swelling, slow growth, and cortical expansion, accompanied or not by root resorption characterize the clinical picture of the cyst [5, 6].

Traditionally, COCs appeared as well-defined unilocular radiolucencies, exhibiting peripheral foci of calcification. Atypical radiographic presentations of COC are uncommon [7]. Here, we report a case of clinical and radiographic evolution of COC associated with odontoma, initially diagnosed as tooth germ in the posterior mandibular region. We also point out that dentists must draw their attention to its developmental changes and related pathologies to diagnose these cases accurately.

2. Case Report

A 10-year-old male patient was referred to orthodontic traction of an impacted right lower first molar (tooth 46). During clinical examination, no alteration was noted except the absence of tooth 46. No abnormalities were detected in previous medical history. A cone-beam computed tomography (CBCT) showed the presence of a radiolucent image measuring <1 cm located between teeth 46 and 48, which was initially interpreted as a dental germ (Figure 1(a)). The patient was submitted to surgery under local anesthesia to achieve tooth crown exposure and bonding of an orthodontic device to traction of its right lower first molar. Six months after the procedure, in a routine panoramic radiograph during orthodontic treatment, a well-defined radiolucent image with radiopaque foci was identified in the region of the suggestive dental germ. Additionally, an increasing volume with cortical expansion and fenestration was observed in a CBCT investigation (Figure 1(b)).

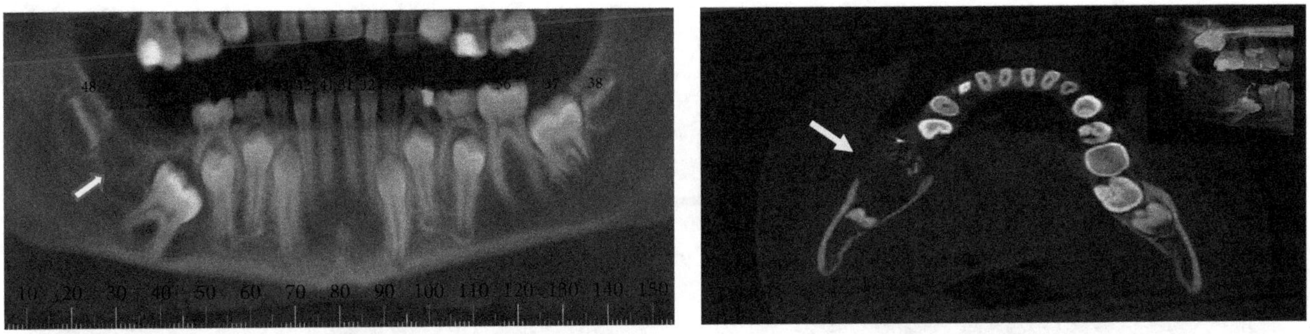

(a) (b)

FIGURE 1: (a) Panoramic reconstruction of an initial CBCT showing a hypodense image (white arrow) in the region of a second molar suggesting the presence of a dental germ. (b) CBCT axial view showing the lesion expansion and cortical fenestration (white arrow). Foci of peripheral calcification in the lesion (in box).

Thereby, a provisional diagnostic hypothesis of odontogenic lesions was made, suggesting adenomatoid odontogenic tumor and COC. The chosen clinical conduct was the surgical enucleation of the lesion. A straight incision was made in the alveolar ridge with flap detachment to facilitate access to the lesion, and an aspiration puncture was performed revealing a liquid content (Figure 2(a)). During surgery, the lesion was completely detached from the mandibular bone, allowing visualization of a capsule with a cystic aspect (Figure 2(b)). The specimen was sent for histopathologic examination, and the microscopic findings revealed a cystic cavity lined by a thin odontogenic epithelium with ameloblastomatous features. Ghost cells and calcification foci were also observed. Furthermore, the formation of dentinoid matrix, immature enamel, and fibrous connective tissue was noticed. Therefore, the diagnosis of COC associated with odontoma was established (Figures 3(a) and 3(b)). One year later, no signs of recurrence were observed and a CBCT revealed new bone formation in the region (Figure 3(c)). Currently, the patient is undergoing clinical and radiographic follow-up with pediatric dentistry specialists and orthodontists for adequate establishment of occlusal dynamics.

3. Discussion

Although COC is a benign lesion and a pathological entity widely known, its occurrence is considered uncommon [1]. Generally, patients are asymptomatic and major clinical signs include alveolar expansion, cortical perforation, and root resorption of adjacent teeth [2]. From all COCs arising in the mandible, about 65% is found in the anterior region in between canines. Approximately, 10-32% of cases are associated with unerupted teeth (especially canine) [1]. Although the age range of COC involvement is wide, Arruda et al.[2] reinforce that one-third of patients are affected in childhood and adolescence. The case reported herein is in accordance with the literature.

Commonly, COC appears as a unilocular radiolucent area with well-defined limits and may exhibit small radiopaque deposits of various aspects [2, 7]. In some cases, the radiographic aspect of COC may be masked, primarily when developing as periapical radiolucent areas. Thus, the differential diagnosis can be established with other lesions of different radiographic aspects, such as ameloblastoma, odontogenic keratocysts, periapical cyst, ameloblastic fibroodontoma, and adenomatoid odontogenic tumor [2, 4, 6, 8].

In the current case, the lesion initially appeared as a well-delimited radiolucent area in the edentulous mandibular bone near an unerupted molar, which did not resemble a COC. During the attempt to traction the impacted tooth, an increasing volume with cortical expansion and fenestration were observed surrounding the radiolucent area, raising the possibility of an odontogenic lesion. Curiously, the lesion resembled a tooth germ in the crypt stage. Due to the exceptionality of the case, a vast literature search was carried out, and to our knowledge, this is the first report of its kind related to COC. On the other hand, the unexpected histological result only increases the notoriety of this report; once, authors described that some cases of delayed eruption may be attributed to physiological disorders impacting interruptions on Nolla's stages [9], thus leading to the most plausible initial diagnosis of a tooth germ, as initially presumed in this report.

Regarding that, the literature argues that the odontogenic tumors can share the same structures of a tooth germ, which is difficult to diagnose with immature structures of dental tissue, especially in children and adolescents [10]. For this reason, the knowledge of histological and radiological aspects of both developing teeth and odontogenic neoplasms is required to the establishment of an accurate clinical conduct.

This comparative analysis is crucial and may avoid diagnostic mistakes to several oral lesions (odontogenic or nonodontogenic origin), especially when malignant lesions are underdiagnosed. In a retrospective study conducted by Bacci et al., [11] the authors reported that upon evaluation of 1,566 samples of biopsy, an erroneous diagnosis between the radiographic examination and the histological analyses was found in 31.5% of the cases. Among such cases, over 80% of these records correspond to malignant or potentially malignant lesions. In another work, Almazrooa et al. [12] reported that the rate of concordance between histopathologic findings and radiographic interpretation of jaw lesions was lower than 50%. Consequently, such diagnostic misunderstandings may influence the treatment of patients as well as prognosis values in cases of malignancy. Therefore, a histologic

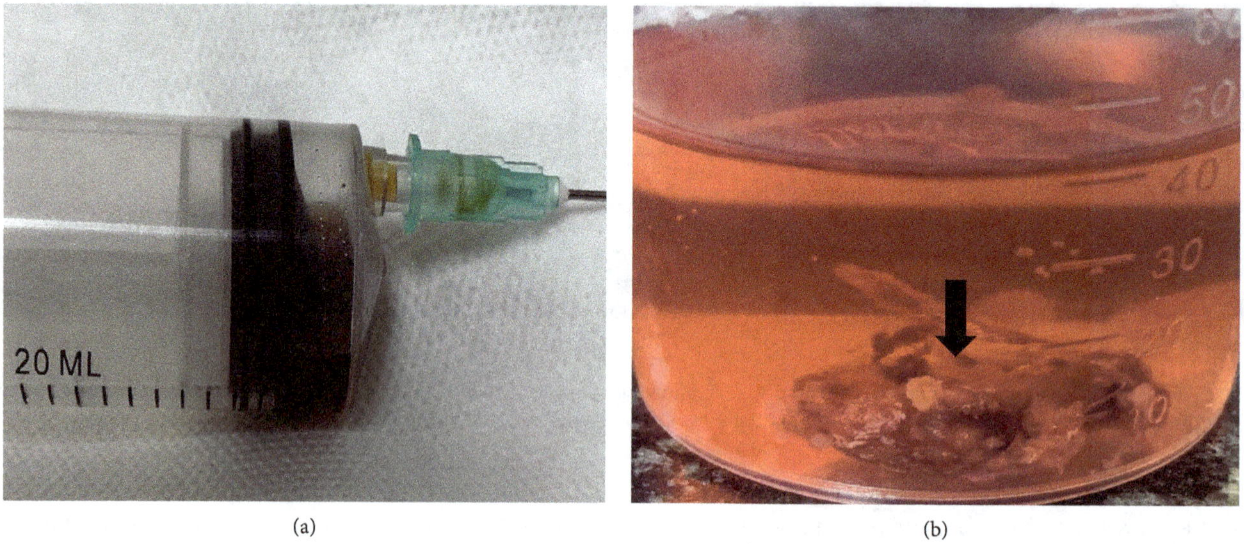

FIGURE 2: (a) Citrus yellow-colored liquid obtained after aspiration puncture of the lesion. Suggestive alteration of odontogenic nature. (b) Anatomopathological specimen obtained after biopsy. Presence of cystic cavity with fibrotic capsule in the lesion (black arrow).

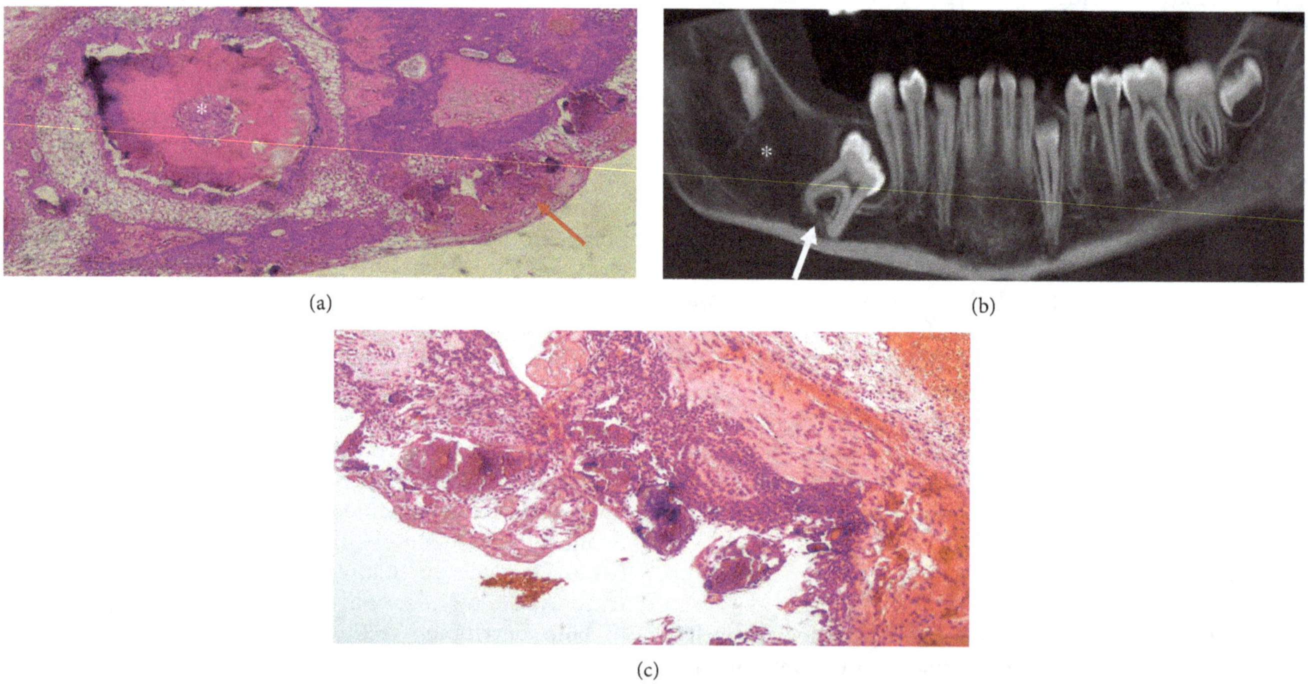

FIGURE 3: (a) Photomicrograph stained by hematoxylin-eosin (200x) revealing features of a calcifying odontogenic cyst with presence of ghost cells (red arrow) associated with odontoma (asterisk). (b) Photomicrography showing a cystic lesion with a fibrous tissue capsule and lining of odontogenic epithelium of ameloblastic type loosely arranged with several amounts of ghost cells (200X). (c) Panoramic reconstruction of a control CBCT evidencing a new bone formation in the area (asterisk). Impacted first molar (white arrow).

examination must be performed in excised tissues and particularly those in which radiographic characteristics may generate confusion.

Also, it is important to highlight that COC may present wide-ranging radiographic patterns, as discussed by different studies. One study by Lida et al.[7] investigated the radiographic profile of 11 cases of COC and only one of them arose from the edentulous mandible. Arruda et al.[2] debated that radiolucent COCs may undergo calcification and progress to a lesion of mixed radiographic appearance, thus causing swelling and cystic expansion. Also, some works suggest that the remaining odontogenic epithelial cords when stimulated may induce the formation of dental tissue in the adjacent connective tissue wall [13].

The most remarkable feature of COC is the presence of ghost cells in an ameloblastoma-like epithelium [4, 14]. In approximately 22% of diagnosed cases, an association with odontoma is seen [15]. Although the origin of the COC is linked to the remnants of the dental lamina [14], recent data suggest that most COC carry a mutation in the CTNNB1 gene responsible for beta-catenin protein synthesis [16]. For most COCs (specifically those with smaller lengths), enucleation is the treatment of choice, with <5% of cases developing a recurrence [17].

As a result, a CBCT evolution of a COC in the mandibular molar area was described, going from a hypodense profile to a mixed appearance, thus calling the attention of dentists that radiographic or tomographic images may lead to misinterpretations between odontogenic lesions and dental apparatus forming structures.

References

[1] S. Kler, S. Palaskar, V. P. Shetty, and A. Bhushan, "Intraosseous calcifying cystic odontogenic tumor," *Journal of Oral and Maxillofacial Pathology*, vol. 13, no. 1, pp. 27–29, 2009.

[2] J. A. A. de Arruda, L. F. Schuch, L. G. Abreu et al., "A multicentre study of 268 cases of calcifying odontogenic cysts and a literature review," *Oral Diseases*, vol. 24, no. 7, pp. 1282–1293, 2018.

[3] R. J. Gorlin, J. J. Pindborg, F. P. Clausen, and R. A. Vickers, "The calcifying odontogenic cyst–a possible analogue of the cutaneous calcifying epithelioma of Malherbe: an analysis of fifteen cases," *Oral Surgery, Oral Medicine, and Oral Pathology*, vol. 15, no. 10, pp. 1235–1243, 1962.

[4] S. Gadipelly, V. B. Reddy, M. Sudheer, N. V. Kumar, and G. Harsha, "Bilateral calcifying odontogenic cyst: a rare entity," *Journal of Maxillofacial and Oral Surgery*, vol. 14, no. 3, pp. 826–831, 2015.

[5] S. Irani and F. Foroughi, "Histologic variants of calcifying odontogenic cyst: a study of 52 cases," *The Journal of Contemporary Dental Practice*, vol. 18, no. 8, pp. 688–694, 2017.

[6] R. Rojo, J. C. Prados-Frutos, I. Gutierrez Lázaro, and J. Á. Herguedas Alonso, "Calcifying odontogenic cysts," *Journal of Stomatology, Oral and Maxillofacial Surgery*, vol. 118, no. 2, pp. 122–124, 2017.

[7] S. Iida, Y. Fukuda, T. Ueda, T. Aikawa, J. E. Arizpe, and M. Okura, "Calcifying odontogenic cyst: radiologic findings in 11 cases," *Oral Surgery, Oral Medicine, Oral Pathology, Oral Radiology, and Endodontics*, vol. 101, no. 3, pp. 356–362, 2006.

[8] A. A. de Carvalhosa, C. R. de Araújo Estrela, A. H. Borges, O. A. Guedes, and C. Estrela, "10-year follow-up of calcifying odontogenic cyst in the periapical region of vital maxillary central incisor," *Journal of Endodontia*, vol. 40, no. 10, pp. 1695–1697, 2014.

[9] O. D. Klein, S. Oberoi, A. Huysseune, M. Hovorakova, M. Peterka, and R. Peterkova, "Developmental disorders of the dentition: an update," *American Journal of Medical Genetics. Part C, Seminars in Medical Genetics*, vol. 163C, no. 4, pp. 318–332, 2013.

[10] P. J. Slootweg, "Update on tooth formation mimicking odontogenic neoplasia," *Head and Neck Pathology*, vol. 1, no. 1, pp. 94–98, 2007.

[11] C. Bacci, L. Donolato, E. Stellini, M. Berengo, and M. Valente, "A comparison between histologic and clinical diagnoses of oral lesions," *Quintessence International*, vol. 45, no. 9, pp. 789–794, 2014.

[12] S. Almazrooa, N. O. Binmadi, H. M. Khalifa, F. M. Jadu, A. M. Jan, and D. E. Meisha, "The agreement rate between radiographic interpretation and histopathologic diagnosis of jaw lesions," *Radiology research and practice*, vol. 2019, 2019.

[13] A. M. Neelima, *Textbook of Oral and Maxillofacial Surgery*, Jaypee Brothers Medical Publishers, New Delhi, 2012.

[14] A. K. El-Naggar, J. K. C. Chan, T. Takata, J. R. Grandis, and P. J. Slootweg, "The fourth edition of the head and neck World Health Organization blue book: editors' perspectives," *Human Pathology*, vol. 66, pp. 10–12, 2017.

[15] C. Ledesma-Montes, R. J. Gorlin, M. Shear et al., "International collaborative study on ghost cell odontogenic tumours: calcifying cystic odontogenic tumour, dentinogenic ghost cell tumour and ghost cell odontogenic carcinoma," *Journal of Oral Pathology & Medicine*, vol. 37, no. 5, pp. 302–308, 2008.

[16] A. Yukimori, Y. Oikawa, K. I. Morita et al., "Genetic basis of calcifying cystic odontogenic tumors," *PLoS One*, vol. 12, no. 6, article e0180224, 2017.

[17] A. Buchner, "The central (intraosseous) calcifying odontogenic cyst: an analysis of 215 cases," *Journal of Oral and Maxillofacial Surgery*, vol. 49, no. 4, pp. 330–339, 1991.

Permissions

All chapters in this book were first published by Hindawi Publishing Corporation; hereby published with permission under the Creative Commons Attribution License or equivalent. Every chapter published in this book has been scrutinized by our experts. Their significance has been extensively debated. The topics covered herein carry significant findings which will fuel the growth of the discipline. They may even be implemented as practical applications or may be referred to as a beginning point for another development.

The contributors of this book come from diverse backgrounds, making this book a truly international effort. This book will bring forth new frontiers with its revolutionizing research information and detailed analysis of the nascent developments around the world.

We would like to thank all the contributing authors for lending their expertise to make the book truly unique. They have played a crucial role in the development of this book. Without their invaluable contributions this book wouldn't have been possible. They have made vital efforts to compile up to date information on the varied aspects of this subject to make this book a valuable addition to the collection of many professionals and students.

This book was conceptualized with the vision of imparting up-to-date information and advanced data in this field. To ensure the same, a matchless editorial board was set up. Every individual on the board went through rigorous rounds of assessment to prove their worth. After which they invested a large part of their time researching and compiling the most relevant data for our readers.

The editorial board has been involved in producing this book since its inception. They have spent rigorous hours researching and exploring the diverse topics which have resulted in the successful publishing of this book. They have passed on their knowledge of decades through this book. To expedite this challenging task, the publisher supported the team at every step. A small team of assistant editors was also appointed to further simplify the editing procedure and attain best results for the readers.

Apart from the editorial board, the designing team has also invested a significant amount of their time in understanding the subject and creating the most relevant covers. They scrutinized every image to scout for the most suitable representation of the subject and create an appropriate cover for the book.

The publishing team has been an ardent support to the editorial, designing and production team. Their endless efforts to recruit the best for this project, has resulted in the accomplishment of this book. They are a veteran in the field of academics and their pool of knowledge is as vast as their experience in printing. Their expertise and guidance has proved useful at every step. Their uncompromising quality standards have made this book an exceptional effort. Their encouragement from time to time has been an inspiration for everyone.

The publisher and the editorial board hope that this book will prove to be a valuable piece of knowledge for researchers, students, practitioners and scholars across the globe.

List of Contributors

Vincenzo Grassia, Ludovica Nucci, Paola Martina Marra and Letizia Perillo
Multidisciplinary Department of Medical-Surgical and Dental Specialties, University of Campania Luigi Vanvitelli, Naples, Italy

Gaetano Isola
Department of General Surgery and Surgical-Medical Specialties, School of Dentistry, University of Catania, Italy

Angelo Itro
Complex Operative Unit of Stomatological Surgery in Developmental Age, University of Campania Luigi Vanvitelli, Naples, Italy

M. V. Ashith and Dhruv Ahuja
Department of Orthodontics and Dentofacial Orthopedics, Manipal College of Dental Sciences Mangalore(Manipal Academy of Higher Education Manipal), Mangalore, Karnataka, India

NS Suma
Department of Orthodontics, SVS Institute of Dental Sciences, Mahabubnagar, India

K. Mithun
Department of Orthodontics, AJ Institute of Dental Sciences, Mangalore, Karnataka, India

Mohammed Alhussain
Ministry of Health, Riyadh, Saudi Arabia

Naif Almosa
Department of Pediatric Dentistry and Orthodontics, College of Dentistry, King Saud University, Riyadh, Saudi Arabia

Hourya Alnofaie
Division of Oral and Maxillofacial Surgery, Basic Dental Sciences Department, College of Dentistry, Princess Nourah Bint Abdulrahman University, Riyadh, Saudi Arabia

C. Moreno-Soriano
Department of Odontostomatology, Faculty of Medicine and Health Sciences (Dentistry), University of Barcelona, L'Hospitalet de Llobregat, Barcelona, Spain

A. Estrugo-Devesa, P. Castañeda-Vegaan and E. Jané-Salas
Department of Odontostomatology, Faculty of Medicine and Health Sciences (Dentistry), University of Barcelona, L'Hospitalet de Llobregat, Barcelona, Spain
Oral Health and Masticatory System Group, Institut d'Investigació Biomédica de Bellvitge (IDIBELL, Bellvitge Institute of Biomedical Research), L'Hospitalet de Llobregat, Barcelona, Spain

J. López-López
Department of Odontostomatology, Faculty of Medicine and Health Sciences (Dentistry), University of Barcelona, L'Hospitalet de Llobregat, Barcelona, Spain
Oral Health and Masticatory System Group, Institut d'Investigació Biomédica de Bellvitge (IDIBELL, Bellvitge Institute of Biomedical Research), L'Hospitalet de Llobregat, Barcelona, Spain
Medical-Surgical Area of Dentistry Hospital University of Barcelona-University of Barcelona, L'Hospitalet de Llobregat, Barcelona, Spain

Nazanin Samiei
Periodontics Department, School of Dentistry, Tehran University of Medical Sciences, Tehran, Iran

Hadi Kaseb Ghane
Department of Prosthodontics, Dental Branch, Islamic Azad University of Medical Sciences, Tehran, Iran

Reza Fekrazad
Radiation Sciences Research Center, Laser Research Center in Medical Sciences, AJA University of Medical Sciences, Tehran, Iran
International Network for Photo Medicine and Photo Dynamic Therapy (INPMPDT), Universal Scientific Education and Research Network (USERN), Tehran, Iran

Seyed Mohsen Sadeghi
School of Dentistry, Department of Endodontics, Qom University of Medical Sciences, Qom, Iran

Samaneh Moradi
School of Dentistry, Department of Endodontics, Isfahan University of Medical Sciences, Isfahan, Iran

Samaneh Soltani
School of Dentistry, Department of Periodontology, Qom University of Medical Sciences, Qom, Iran

Shogo Hasegawa, Hitoshi Miyachi and Toru Nagao
Department of Maxillofacial Surgery, School of Dentistry, Aichi-Gakuin University, 2-11 Suemori-Dori, Chikusa, Nagoya, Aichi 464-8651, Japan

Jun Sasaki
Department of Maxillofacial Surgery, School of Dentistry, Aichi-Gakuin University, 2-11 Suemori-Dori, Chikusa, Nagoya, Aichi 464-8651, Japan
Department of Maxillofacial Surgery, Okazaki City Hospital, 3-1 Goshoai, Koryujicho, Okazaki, Aichi 444-8553, Japan

Makiko Okubo-Sato, Kenji Yamagata, Satoshi Fukuzawa, Kazuhiro Terada, Fumihiko Uchida, Naomi Ishibashi-Kanno and Hiroki Bukawa
Department of Oral and Maxillofacial Surgery, Institute of Clinical Medicine, Faculty of Medicine, University of Tsukuba, 1-1-1 Tennodai, Tsukuba, Ibaraki 305-8575, Japan

Régis Augusto Aleixo Alves, André Luiz Gomide Morais, Thábata Frederico Izelli, Cyntia R. A. Estrela and Carlos Estrela
Department of Stomatology Sciences, Federal University of Goiás, Goiânia, Brazil

Damian Chybicki, Małgorzata Lipczyńska-Lewandowska, Gaja Torbicka and Anna Janas-Naze
Department of Oral Surgery, Central Clinical Hospital, Medical University of Lodz, Poland

Erika Antonia dos Anjos Ramos, Luciana Munhoz, Stephanie Kenig Viveiros and Emiko Saito Arita
Department of Stomatology, School of Dentistry, University of São Paulo, 2227 Lineu Prestes Avenue, 05508-000 São Paulo, SP, Brazil

Basílio Almeida Milani
Department of Maxillofacial Surgery, Hospital Municipal do Campo Limpo, 1661 Estrada da Itapecerica, 05835-005 São Paulo, Brazil

Tomás Zecchini Barrese
Department of Pathological Sciences, School of Medicine, Santa Casa de Sao Paulo School of Medical Sciences, 61 Dr. Cesário Motta Junior Street, 01221-020 São Paulo, SP, Brazil

Celine Moukarzel, Naim El Haddad and Anthony Rizk
Postgraduate Department, MOI, Faculty of Dentistry, Goethe University, Frankfurt, Germany

Daniel Saad
Postgraduate Department, MOI, Faculty of Dentistry, Goethe University, Frankfurt, Germany Private Practice, Beirut, Lebanon

Nivedhitha Malli Sureshbabu, Mahalakshmi Nandakumar and Deepak Selvam
Department of Conservative Dentistry and Endodontics, Saveetha Dental College, Saveetha Institute of Medical and Technical Sciences, Saveetha University, 162, Poonamallee High Road, Chennai, 600077 Tamil Nadu, India

Kathiravan Selvarasu
Department of Oral and Maxillofacial Surgery, Saveetha Dental College, Saveetha Institute of Medical and Technical Sciences, Saveetha University, 162, Poonamallee High Road, Chennai, 600077 Tamil Nadu, India

Jayanth Kumar V
Department of Oral Medicine and Radiology, Saveetha Dental College, Saveetha Institute of Medical and Technical Sciences, Saveetha University, 162, Poonamallee High Road, Chennai, 600077 Tamil Nadu, India

Tatiana Miranda Deliberador, Suyany Gabriely Weiss, Alexandre Teixeira Domingues Neto, Isabela Zago Zetola, Maria Eduarda Santana Prix, Darlan Rigo Júnior, Heloysa Hoffman Martins and Carmen Lucia Mueller Storrer
School of Health Sciences, Positivo University, 5300 Professor Pedro Viriato Parigot de Souza Street, Campo Comprido, Curitiba, PR, Brazil 81280-330

Satomi Arimoto and Masaya Akashi
Division of Oral and Maxillofacial Surgery, Department of Surgery Related, Kobe University Graduate School of Medicine, Kobe, Japan

Manabu Shigeoka
Division of Pathology, Department of Pathology, Kobe University Graduate School of Medicine, Kobe, Japan

Alice Alberti, Beatrice Zotti and Luca Francetti
Department of Biomedical, Surgical and Dental Sciences, Università degli Studi di Milano, Milan, Italy
IRCCS Istituto Ortopedico Galeazzi, Milan, Italy

Stefano Corbella
Department of Biomedical, Surgical and Dental Sciences, Università degli Studi di Milano, Milan, Italy
IRCCS Istituto Ortopedico Galeazzi, Milan, Italy
Institute of Dentistry, I.M. Sechenov First Moscow State Medical University, Moscow, Russia

W. Chinadet and P. Chompu-inwai
Division of Pediatric Dentistry, Department of Orthodontics and Pediatric Dentistry, School of Dentistry, Chiang Mai University, Thailand

T. Sutharaphan
Phrae Hospital, Phrae, Thailand

Kamel Alraei
Department of Oral and Maxillofacial Surgery, Al-Noor Specialist Hospital, Makkah, Saudi Arabia

Jameel Sharqawi
Department of Oral and Maxillofacial Surgery, Royal Commission Hospital, Jubail, Saudi Arabia

Somaya Harcher
General Dentist, Saudi Arabia

Ibrahim Ghita
Department of Hematology, Al-Noor Specialist Hospital, Makkah, Saudi Arabia

Yoshiaki Ihara, Yuka Nakamichi, Yuichi Tashimo, Shinji Nozue, Kota Hayashi, Mitsunori Ishiguro and Koji Takahashi
Division of Oral Rehabilitation Medicine, Department of Special Needs Dentistry, School of Dentistry, Showa University, Tokyo, Japan

Shiv Prasad Sharma
Specialist Oral and Maxillofacial Surgeon, Zulfi General Hospital, Ministry of Health, King Abdulla Street, 11932, Saudi Arabia

Silviu Brad
Department of Radiology "Victor Babes", University of Medicine and Pharmacy, Timisoara 300041, Romania

Laura Andreea Schiller
Department of Radiology "Victor Babes", University of Medicine and Pharmacy, Timisoara 300041, Romania
Department of Oral Surgery, Stomdas Clinic (Private Practice), Bacau 600125, Romania

Albert Cristian Schiller
Department of Prosthetic Dentistry "Victor Babes", University of Medicine and Pharmacy, Timisoara 300041, Romania
Department of Endodontics, Stomdas Clinic (Private Practice), Bacau 600125, Romania

Adalbert Schiller
Department of Nephrology "Victor Babes", University of Medicine and Pharmacy, Timisoara 300041, Romania

Aida Gabriela Dascalu
Department of Orthodontics "Victor Babes", University of Medicine and Pharmacy, Timisoara 300041, Romania

Jean Carlos Barbosa Ferreira, Rodrigo Tavares de Sá and Giovanni Gasperini
Department of Oral and Maxillofacial Surgery, Clinical Hospital, Federal University of Goiás, Goiânia, Brazil

Eneida Franco Vêncio
Department of Oral Medicine (Oral Pathology), Dental School, Federal University of Goiás, Goiânia, Brazil

Alberto Murri Dello Diago, Luigi Generali, Roberto Apponi, Vittorio Colombini and Vittorio Checchi
Department of Surgery, Medicine, Dentistry and Morphological Sciences-Unit of Dentistry and Oral-Maxillo-Facial Surgery, University of Modena and Reggio Emilia, Modena, Italy

Alessio Danilo Inchingolo, Sabino Ceci, Luisa Limongelli, Daniela Azzollini, Pietro Paolo Mezzapesa, Grazia Marinelli, Giuseppina Malcangi, Giovanni Coloccia, Gianfranco Favia and Francesco Inchingolo
Department of Interdisciplinary Medicine, Section of Dental Medicine, University of Bari "Aldo Moro", 70124 Bari, Italy

Alberto Corriero, Nicola Brienza and Mario Ribezzi
Unit of Anesthesia and Resuscitation, Department of Emergencies and Organ Transplantations, Aldo Moro University, Bari, Italy

Luigi Curatoli and Nicola Quaranta
Department Neurosciences & Sensory Organs & Musculoskeletal System, University of Bari "Aldo Moro", 70124 Bari, Italy

Maria Massaro
Azienda Ospedaliero-Universitaria Consorziale Policlinico di Bari, Bari, Italy

Ioana Roxana Bordea
Department of Oral Rehabilitation, Faculty of Dentistry, Iuliu Haţieganu University of Medicine and Pharmacy, 400012 Cluj-Napoca, Romania

Antonio Scarano and Felice Lorusso
Department of Innovative Technologies in Medicine and Dentistry, University of Chieti-Pescara, 66100 Chieti, Italy

Mohammed Zameer, Syed Ali Peeran and Faisal Mohammad Alzahrani
Armed Forces Hospital, Jazan, Saudi Arabia

Syed Nahid Basheer
Department of Restorative Dentistry, College of Dentistry, Jazan, Saudi Arabia

Syed Wali Peeran
Department of Periodontology & Oral Implantology, Faculty of Dentistry, University of Sebha, Sebha, Libya

Sameen Badiujjama Birajdar
Sanjeevani Dental Clinic, Raichur, India

Ali Mohammed A. Alkhayrat
College of Dentistry, Jazan, Saudi Arabia

Santhosh Shenoy B, Amitha Ramesh and Avaneendra Talwar
Department of Periodontics, A.B Shetty Memorial Institute of Dental Sciences, NITTE (Deemed-to-be) University, Deralakatte, Mangalore, Karnataka-575018, India

Anahita Punj
Army College of Dental Sciences, Jai Jawahar Nagar, Chennapur-CRPF Road, Secunderabad, 500087 Telangana, India

Jerome A. Lindeboom
Department of Oral and Maxillofacial Surgery, Amsterdam University Medical Centers and Amstelland Hospital, University of Amsterdam, Netherlands

Jean-Pierre T. F. Ho
Department of Oral and Maxillofacial Surgery, Amsterdam University Medical Centers and Northwest Clinics, University of Amsterdam, Netherlands

Naomi Donner
Department of Pathology, Amsterdam University Medical Centers, University of Amsterdam, Amsterdam, Netherlands

Willem H. Schreuder
Department of Oral and Maxillofacial Surgery, Amsterdam University Medical Centers, University of Amsterdam, Amsterdam and Department of Head and Neck Surgery, Antoni van Leeuwenhoek Hospital, Amsterdam, Netherlands

Antoine Berberi
Department of Oral and Maxillofacial Surgery, Faculty of Dental Medicine, Lebanese University, Lebanon

Georges Aoun and Georges Aad
Department of Oral Medicine and Maxillofacial Radiology, Faculty of Dental Medicine, Lebanese University, Lebanon

Emile Khalaf
Beirut Arab University, Lebanon

Eduardo Morato Oliveira and Leandro Napier Souza
Department of Oral Surgery and Pathology, School of Dentistry, Universidade Federal de Minas Gerais, Belo Horizonte, MG, Brazil

Lucas Alves da Mota Santana and Erika Rezende Silva
Department of Dentistry, Universidade Federal de Sergipe, Aracaju, SE, Brazil

Index

www.ingramcontent.com/pod-product-compliance
Lightning Source LLC
LaVergne TN
LVHW082232200926
848484LV00008B/2340